BLUEPRINTS IN
CARDIOLOGY

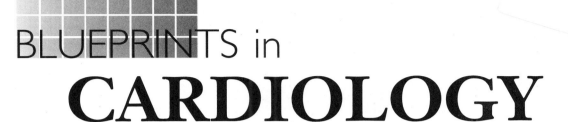

BLUEPRINTS in
CARDIOLOGY

Editor

Eric H. Awtry, MD, FACC
Assistant Professor of Medicine
Boston University School of Medicine
Director of Education, Section of Cardiology
Boston Medical Center
Boston, Massachusetts

Authors

Arjun V. Gururaj, MD
Teaching Fellow in Internal Medicine
Boston University School of Medicine
Fellow in Electrophysiology
Division of Cardiology
Boston Medical Center
Boston, Massachusetts

Melanie Maytin, MD
Teaching Fellow in Medicine
Boston University School of Medicine
Fellow, Section of Cardiology
Boston Medical Center
Boston, Massachusetts

Michael W. Tsang, MD
Teaching Fellow in Medicine
Boston University School of Medicine
Fellow, Section of Cardiology
Boston Medical Center
Boston, Massachusetts

Benoy J. Zachariah, MD, MRCP
Teaching Fellow in Medicine
Boston University School of Medicine
Clinical Fellow in Interventional Cardiology
Boston Medical Center
Boston, Massachusetts

Faculty advisor

Joseph Loscalzo, MD, PhD
Wade Professor of Medicine
Boston University School of Medicine
Chairman, Department of Medicine
Boston Medical Center
Boston, Massachusetts

Blackwell
Publishing

Blackwell Science
l Publishing company

well Publishing, Inc., 350 Main Street, Malden, Massachusetts 02148-5018, USA
kwell Science Ltd, Osney Mead, Oxford OX2 0EL, UK
ackwell Science Asia Pty Ltd, 550 Swanston Street, Carlton, Victoria 3053, Australia
Blackwell Verlag GmbH, Kurfürstendamm 57, 10707 Berlin, Germany

02 03 04 05 5 4 3 2 1

ISBN: 0-632-04628-7

Library of Congress Cataloging-in-Publication Data

Blueprints in cardiology / editor, Eric H. Awtry ; authors, Melanie
Maytin . . . [et al.].
    p. ; cm.—(Blueprints series)
  ISBN 0-632-04628-7 (pbk.)
  1. Heart—Diseases—Outlines, syllabi, etc. 2. Cardiology—Outlines, syllabi, etc.
  [DNLM: 1. Heart Diseases—Outlines. 2. Cardiology—Outlines. WG 18.2 B658 2002] I. Awtry, Eric.
II. Maytin, Melanie. III. Blueprints.
  RC682 .B558 2002
  616.1′2–dc21

                                                                                    2002005758

A catalogue record for this title is available from the British Library

Acquisitions: Nancy Duffy
Development: Angela Gagliano
Production: Debra Lally
Cover design: Hannus Design
Typesetter: SNP Best-set Typesetter Ltd., Hong Kong
Printed and bound by Capital City Press in Vermont, USA

For further information on Blackwell Publishing, visit our website:
www.blackwellscience.com

Notice: The indications and dosages of all drugs in this book have been recommended in the medical literature and conform to the practices of the general community. The medications described and treatment prescriptions suggested do not necessarily have specific approval by the Food and Drug Administration for use in the diseases and dosages for which they are recommended. The package insert for each drug should be consulted for use and dosage as approved by the FDA. Because standards for usage change, it is advisable to keep abreast of revised recommendations, particularly those concerning new drugs.

Contents

Preface

Today's medical trainees are faced with the seemingly insurmountable task of mastering an ever-expanding body of knowledge. Not only is the student expected to understand the pathophysiological basis of disease, but also to recognize the disease in the clinical setting, determine the appropriate tests with which to fully evaluate the disease, interpret the results of these tests, and apply all of this information to the development of an appropriate treatment plan. These skills are then tested both at the bedside and in a series of USMLE examinations.

While no student can be expected to know every aspect of medicine, certain fundamental principles must be identified and learned. This can be difficult given the current state of information overload. In no specialty is this truer than in the field of cardiology. The past several decades have witnessed the introduction of a vast array of increasingly more complex diagnostic modalities and the development of innumerable pharmacological and non-pharmacological therapies. In addition, a veritable tidal wave of clinical trials has been performed, aimed at determining the appropriate use of these diagnostic and therapeutic options.

In this new addition to the *Blueprints* series, we have attempted to cover the core competencies in cardiology. We have discussed those skills that are essential to success in clinical rotations (including key cardiac symptoms and physical findings, as well as the interpretation of cardiac tests), and have covered a broad array of cardiac disorders that consistently appear on the board examinations. Although memorization of specific facts is an essential component of the learning process, we strongly feel that a true understanding of disease requires knowledge of disease process. Throughout the text, we briefly review the pathophysiology of cardiac diseases and use this review as a guide to understanding the clinical presentation and treatment of these diseases.

We hope that you find *Blueprints in Cardiology* informative and useful. We welcome feedback and suggestions you may have about this book or any in the *Blueprints* series. Send to *blue@blacksci.com*.

Eric H. Awtry
Arjun V. Gururaj
Melanie Maytin
Michael W. Tsang
Benoy J. Zachariah
Joseph Loscalzo

Acknowledgments

To my wife, Sandhya Wahi-Gururaj, MD, MPH., and my parents for all their support.

—A.G.

To my wife Nina and daughter Roshini for their support and patience while I was working on this book.

—B.Z.

To E.H.A. for keeping me on track and for understanding when I wasn't. To J.L. for affording me the opportunity. To D.L.B. and M.T.S. for being consummate mentors and wonderful friends, and for always pushing me to "raise the bar."

—M.M.

I would like to thank the students and residents of Boston Medical Center, whose enthusiasm for learning make teaching so enjoyable and projects such as this so rewarding. To my co-authors and editor: thank you for your insight, expertise, and commitment to this project. Finally, I would like to thank my wife Kyle and children Jake, Nicholas, and Zachary for their endless support, patience, and encouragement.

—E.H.A.

Reviewers

Brian L. Dunfee
Temple University
Class of 2002
Philadelphia, Pennsylvania

Deborah Lam
Northwestern University
Class of 2002
Evanston, Illinois

Saeed Sadeghi, MD
PGY3 resident
Department of Internal Medicine
Keck School of Medicine at University of Southern California
University of Southern California Medical Center
Los Angeles, California

Pradnya Mitroo MD
Internal Medicine PGY1
Thomas Jefferson University Hospital
Philadelphia, Pennsylvania

Abbreviations

A_2:	aortic component of the second heart sound
ABE:	acute bacterial endocarditis
ABI:	ankle-brachial index
ACS:	acute coronary syndrome
ACE:	angiotensin-converting enzyme
AF:	atrial fibrillation
AI:	aortic insufficiency
AMI:	acute myocardial infarction
Ao:	aorta
AP:	action potential
AS:	aortic stenosis
ASD:	atrial septal defect
ASH:	asymmetric septal hypertrophy
AV:	aortic valve
AV node:	atrioventricular node
AVNRT:	atrioventricular nodal reentrant tachycardia
AVRT:	atrioventricular reentrant tachycardia
BID:	twice daily
BP:	blood pressure
BPM:	beats per minute
CAD:	coronary artery disease
CABG:	coronary artery bypass graft
CEA:	carotid endarterectomy
CHB:	complete heart block

CHD:	congenital heart disease
CHF:	congestive heart failure
CI:	cardiac index
CK:	creatinine kinase
CMP:	cardiomyopathy
CNS:	central nervous system
CO:	cardiac output
CPR:	cardiopulmonary resuscitation
CSM:	carotid sinus massage
CT:	computed tomography
CVD:	cerebrovascular disease
CVA:	cerebrovascular accident
DCM:	dilated cardiomyopathy
DM:	diabetes mellitus
DVT:	deep venous thrombosis
ECG:	electrocardiogram
EEG:	electroencephalogram
EF:	ejection fraction
EPS:	electrophysiological study
ETT:	exercise tolerance test
HB:	heart block
HCM:	hypertrophic cardiomyopathy
HDL:	high-density lipoprotein
HF:	heart failure
HIV:	human immunodeficiency virus
HOCM:	hypertrophic obstructive cardiomyopathy
HR:	heart rate
HTN:	hypertension
IABP:	intra-aortic balloon pump
ICD:	implantable cardioverter-defibrillator
IDL:	intermediate density lipoprotein
IE:	infectious endocarditis
IHSS:	idiopathic hypertrophic subaortic stenosis
INR:	international normalized ratio
IVC:	inferior vena cava
JVP:	jugular venous pressure
LA:	left atrium
LBBB:	left bundle branch block
LDL:	low-density lipoprotein

LMWH:	low molecular weight heparin
Lp(a):	lipoprotein (a)
LV:	left ventricle
LVEDP:	left ventricular end diastolic pressure
LVOT:	left ventricular outflow tract
MAT:	multifocal atrial tachycardia
MI:	myocardial infarction
MR:	mitral regurgitation
MRA:	magnetic resonance angiography
MRI:	magnetic resonance imaging
MS:	mitral stenosis
MV:	mitral valve
MVP:	mitral valve prolapse
NSTE:	non-ST elevation (MI)
NSVT:	nonsustained ventricular tachycardia
NVE:	native valve endocarditis
P_2:	pulmonic component of the second heart sound
PA:	pulmonary artery
PAC:	premature atrial complex
PAD:	peripheral arterial disease
PCN:	penicillin
PCW(P):	pulmonary capillary wedge (pressure)
PDA:	patent ductus arteriosus
PE:	pulmonary embolism
PMI:	point of maximal impulse
PPH:	primary pulmonary hypertension
PS:	pulmonic stenosis
PTA:	percutaneous transluminal angioplasty
PTCA:	percutaneous transluminal coronary angioplasty
PV:	pulmonary valve
PVC:	premature ventricular complex
PVE:	prosthetic valve endocarditis
PVR:	pulmonary vascular resistance
RBBB:	right bundle branch block
RA:	right atrium
RCM:	restrictive cardiomyopathy
RF:	rheumatic fever, or radio frequency (ablation)
RHD:	rheumatic heart disease
RIND:	reversible ischemic neurological deficit

RV:	right ventricle
RVH:	right ventricular hypertrophy
RVI:	right ventricular infarction
S_1:	first heart sound
S_2:	second heart sound
S_3:	third heart sound
S_4:	forth heart sound
SA:	sinoatrial
SBE:	subacute bacterial endocarditis
SBP:	systolic blood pressure
SCD:	sudden cardiac death
SIDS:	sudden infant death syndrome
SLE:	systemic lupus erythematosus
SND:	sinus node dysfunction
SPH:	secondary pulmonary hypertension
SSS:	sick sinus syndrome
STE:	ST elevation (MI)
SV:	stroke volume
SVR:	systemic vascular resistance
SVT:	supraventricular tachycardia
TAO:	thromboangiitis obliterans
TdP:	torsade de pointes
TEE:	transesophageal echocardiography
TG:	triglyceride
TIA:	transient ischemic attack
TID:	three times daily
TOF:	tetralogy of Fallot
TPA:	tissue plasminogen activator
TR:	tricuspid regurgitation
TV:	tricuspid valve
UA:	unstable angina
VF:	ventricular fibrillation
VLDL:	very low density lipoprotein
VPC:	ventricular premature complex
VSD:	ventricular septal defect
VT:	ventricular tachycardia
VTE:	venous thromboembolic
WPW:	Wolff-Parkinson-White

Signs and Symptoms

Chest Pain
- Angina
- Myocardial infarction
- Aortic dissection
- Pericarditis
- Pulmonary embolism
- Pneumonia
- Pleurisy
- Pneumothorax
- Pulmonary hypertension
- Gastroesophageal reflux disease
- Esophageal spasm
- Costochondritis
- Rib fracture
- Anxiety

Dyspnea
- Congestive heart failure
- Myocardial ischemia
- Myocardial infarction
- Restrictive heart disease
- Pericardial tamponade
- Pulmonary embolism
- Pneumonia
- Chronic obstructive pulmonary disease
- Asthma
- Bronchitis
- Pleural effusion
- Pneumothorax
- Pulmonary hypertension
- Interstitial lung disease
- Upper airway obstruction
- Anemia
- Obesity

Syncope
- Tachyarrhythmias
- Bradyarrhythmias
- Aortic stenosis
- Mitral stenosis
- Hypertrophic cardiomyopathy
- Vasovagal syncope
- Carotid sinus sensitivity
- Orthostasis
- Atrial myxoma
- Pulmonary embolism
- Pulmonary hypertension
- Cerebrovascular accident
- Seizure
- Hypoglycemia
- Anxiety

Palpitations
- Atrial premature beats
- Ventricular premature beats
- Tachyarrhythmias
- Bradyarrhythmias
- Hyperthyroidism
- Anxiety
- Anemia

Edema
- Heart failure
- Nephrotic syndrome
- Cirrhosis
- Venous insufficiency
- Deep venous thrombosis
- Hypothyroidism
- Lymphedema

Left-Sided Heart Failure
- Myocardial ischemia
- Myocardial infarction
- Ischemic cardiomyopathy
- Dilated cardiomyopathy
- Valvular heart disease (MS, MR, AS, AI)
- Myocarditis
- Infiltrative heart disease
- Hypertension
- Restrictive cardiomyopathy
- Tachyarrhythmias
- Thyrotoxicosis
- Arteriovenous fistula
- Anemia

Right-Sided Heart Failure
- Left-sided heart failure
- Right ventricular infarction
- Pulmonary embolism
- Primary pulmonary hypertension
- Secondary pulmonary hypertension (e.g., COPD, chronic embolic disease)
- Constrictive pericarditis
- Pericardial tamponade
- Tricuspid regurgitation

Important Cardiovascular Formulas

Alveolar-arterial gradient = $[(P_{atm} - P_{H20})(FIO_2) - (PCO_2/0.8)] - PaO2$

Blood pressure = $CO \times SVR$

$CO = SV \times HR$ (units: l/min)

$CI = CO/BSA$ (units: $l/min/m^2$) (where BSA is the body surface area in m^2)

LDL cholesterol = total cholesterol − (HDL + TG/5) (providing TG are <400 mg/dl)

Maximum predicted heart rate = 220 − age

Mean pulmonary artery pressure = 1/3 PA systolic pressure + 2/3 PA diastolic pressure

Mean systemic arterial pressure = 1/3 systemic systolic pressure + 2/3 systemic diastolic pressure

Pulmonary vascular resistance = $[(mean\ PAP - PCWP)/CO] \times 80$ (units: dynes-sec-cm^{-5})

Pulse pressure = systolic BP − diastolic BP

Stroke volume = LV end diastolic volume − LV end systolic volume

Systemic vascular resistance = $[(MAP - CVP)/CO] \times 80$ (units: dynes-sec-cm^{-5})

BP: blood pressure
CI: cardiac index
CO: cardiac output
CVP: central venous pressure
FIO_2: percent inspired oxygen (21% on room air)
HR: heart rate
MAP: mean arterial pressure
P_{ATM}: atmospheric pressure (760 mmHg at sea level)

P_{H20}: partial pressure of water (47 mmHg)
P_aCO_2: arterial CO_2 concentration
PA: pulmonary artery
PAP: pulmonary arterial pressure
PCWP: pulmonary capillary wedge pressure
SV: stroke volume
SVR: systemic vascular resistance
TG: triglycerides

Part I
History and Physical Examination

Chest Pain

Despite major innovations in diagnostic technology and advances in medical therapy, a well-performed history and physical examination remain the cornerstone of good patient care. In addition to providing important clues about a patient's illness, a thorough evaluation helps to direct further diagnostic testing and therapy. It also provides the physician an opportunity to establish rapport with the patient; strong physician-patient relationships establish trust and help to ensure compliance with treatment regimens. Conversely, an inadequate or poorly obtained history may trigger inappropriate or incomplete testing and contribute to additional morbidity and mortality.

The cardinal symptoms of heart disease include chest pain, dyspnea, and palpitations. These symptoms will be discussed in this and the following chapters. A thorough history of each symptom includes information regarding symptom duration, frequency, quality, severity, aggravating or alleviating factors, and associated symptoms. With regard to chest pain, location and radiation are also important features.

CLINICAL MANIFESTATIONS

History

Angina is the cardinal symptom of coronary artery disease (CAD) and results from inadequate oxygen delivery to the myocardium. It is usually an uncomfortable sensation rather than a pain, and may be described as:

- an ache
- heartburn
- indigestion
- a choking sensation
- constriction
- pressure

The symptom is generally substernal in location, but may radiate or localize to the precordium, neck, jaw, shoulders, arms, or epigastrium. Patients with angina often use a clenched fist to indicate the site of discomfort (Levine's sign). Anginal pain is generally triggered by exertion, relieved by rest, and resolves more rapidly (within 1 to 5 minutes) with sublingual nitroglycerin. Other precipitating factors include cold weather, walking on inclines, emotional upset, fright, and the postprandial state. Occasionally, it may occur spontaneously in the early morning hours.

Anginal chest pain may occur in several patterns:

- **Stable angina** is angina that occurs in a well-defined, reproducible pattern—usually on exertion.
- **Unstable angina** refers to angina that is new, occurs at rest, or occurs more frequently than the person's usual angina.
- The pain of a **myocardial infarction** is usually more intense and longer lasting than angina, radiates more widely, and is often accompanied by dyspnea, diaphoresis, palpitations, nausea, and vomiting.

Importantly, many patients, especially diabetics, do not have typical anginal chest pain during an ischemic episode or a myocardial infarction. Rather, they may present with atypical chest pain, restlessness, dyspnea, or diaphoresis.

Physical Examination

Physical findings can be quite helpful in the evaluation of chest pain and may occasionally implicate specific etiologies. A pericardial friction rub is pathognomonic for pericarditis. A late-peaking systolic murmur at the upper sternal border indicates aortic stenosis. Unequal pulses or blood pressure in the arms and the presence of an aortic insufficiency murmur strongly suggest aortic dissection.

Angina may be associated with a normal physical examination; however, an S_3, S_4, or murmur of mitral regurgitation is often heard during the ischemic episode.

DIFFERENTIAL DIAGNOSIS OF CHEST PAIN

The key to differentiating innocuous causes of chest pain from those that are potentially life threatening lies in the history (see Table 1–1). The chest pain of aortic stenosis, hypertrophic cardiomyopathy, and pulmonary hypertension may be indistinguishable from angina. **Aortic dissection** classically presents with severe substernal chest pain that is tearing in quality, comes on abruptly, and radiates to the interscapular or lumbar region. The sudden onset of chest pain that is associated with dyspnea may herald a **pulmonary embolism**; this pain is usually worse upon inspiration (pleuritic) and may be substernal or more lateral in location. A similar pain can occur with **pneumonia** or a **spontaneous pneumothorax**. **Pericarditis** causes chest pain that is substernal or precordial, radiates to the shoulder, is often pleuritic, sharp, worse when swallowing or lying supine, and improved by leaning forward.

Several gastrointestinal disorders (e.g., peptic ulcer disease, gastroesophageal reflux disease, pancreatitis, gall bladder disease) can present with chest pain, but frequently have an abdominal component to the discomfort or are temporally associated with eating, and may be relieved with antacids. **Esophageal spasm** may mimic angina but it is not related to exertion and is frequently provoked by food. Pain resulting from diseases of the muscles, ligaments, or bones of the chest tends to be localized and is exacerbated by movement or certain postures. Sharp, stabbing chest pains localized to the precordium and lasting only a few seconds are rarely cardiac in etiology and are usually associated with anxiety.

Several other historical factors are important to note when evaluating a patient with chest pain. These include:

- risk factors for CAD (see Chapter 9) (suggests angina)
- cocaine use (suggests coronary spasm)
- recent viral illness (suggests pericarditis or pneumonia)
- recent prolonged immobility (suggests pulmonary embolism)
- history of bullous lung disease (suggests pneumothorax)
- recent injury (suggests musculoskeletal pain)
- history of Marfan's syndrome (suggests aortic dissection)

DIAGNOSTIC EVALUATION

The initial tests for patients with chest pain should include an electrocardiogram (ECG) and a chest x-ray. The ECG may demonstrate regional ST segment depression/elevation indicating myocardial ischemia/infarction, or may reveal the diffuse ST segment elevation of pericarditis. A chest x-ray may reveal rib fractures, focal infiltrates of pneumonia, wedge-shaped peripheral infiltrates of pulmonary emboli, or the radiolucency of a pneumothorax. It may also suggest aortic dissection (widened mediastinum), or hiatal hernia (stomach in the thoracic cavity).

If an acute coronary syndrome is suspected, medical therapy (see Chapters 14 and 15) should be immediately started and serial ECGs and cardiac enzymes (creatine kinase and troponin) checked to confirm or exclude a myocardial infarction. For patients in whom the diagnosis remains uncertain but CAD is suspected, a stress test can be performed for clarification. Chest pain associated with ST segment depression during a stress test is diagnostic of angina. Cardiac catheterization remains the gold standard for the diagnosis of coronary artery disease and may be necessary to rule out significant CAD in a subset of patients for whom other tests are unable to confirm or exclude the diagnosis.

TABLE 1–1

Differential Diagnosis of Chest Pain

Diagnosis	Characteristic Features	Physical Findings	Diagnostic Tests (Finding)
Angina	Substernal, exertional, relieved with rest or nitroglycerin; lasts 5–15 minutes	S_3, S_4, or MR murmur during pain; vascular bruits	ECG, Exercise stress test (ST depression)
Myocardial infarction	Similar to angina, only more severe and prolonged	S_3, S_4, congestive heart failure, tachycardia	ECG (ST depression or elevation); increased cardiac enzymes
Aortic stenosis	Similar to angina	Murmur of aortic stenosis	Echocardiogram (stenotic aortic valve)
Aortic dissection	Sudden, severe, tearing pain, radiating to the back	Unequal arm pulses and BP; hypertension; AI murmur	TEE, MRI, or CT scan (dissection flap)
Pericarditis	Sharp, pleuritic pain that is worse with swallowing and worse when lying down; may radiate to shoulder	Pericardial friction rub	ECG (diffuse ST elevation)
Pulmonary hypertension	Similar to angina	Loud P2, signs of right heart failure	Echocardiogram, Swan-Ganz catheter (increased PA pressure)
Pulmonary embolism	Sudden onset of pleuritic chest pain associated with shortness of breath	Tachypnea, hypoxia, tachycardia, signs of acute right heart failure	VQ scan, spiral CT scan, PA angiogram (perfusion or filling defect)
Pneumonia	Sharp, pleuritic pain associated with cough, shortness of breath	Rhonchi over affected lung area	CXR (pulmonary infiltrate)
Spontaneous pneumothorax	Sudden sharp chest pain	Decreased breath sounds and hyper-resonance over affected lung	CXR (air in pleural space; lung collapse)
Esophageal rupture	Follows vomiting or esophageal instrumentation, constant	Mediastinal crunch	CXR (pneumothorax, left pleural effusion), Barium swallow
Gastroesophageal reflux	Burning substernal pain aggravated by eating or lying down	None	Upper GI series, endoscopy (reflux of gastric contents)
Esophageal spasm	Sudden severe pain that can mimic angina	None	Esophageal manometry (increased esophageal pressure)
Musculoskeletal pain	Sharp or achy pain, worse with movement, tender to touch	Tenderness over involved area	None
Herpes zoster	Sharp, burning pain in dermatomal distribution	Vesicular rash over affected area	Tzanck prep of vesicular fluid (giant cells)
Anxiety	Variable quality and location of pain; stressful situations	Chest wall tenderness	Diagnosis of exclusion

MR: mitral regurgitation; ECG: electrocardiogram; BP: blood pressure; AI: aortic insufficiency; TEE: transesophageal echocardiogram; MRI: magnetic resonance imaging; PA: pulmonary artery; VQ: ventilation/perfusion; CT: computed tomography; CXR: chest x-ray; GI: gastrointestinal.

In patients with pulmonary emboli, arterial blood gases usually reveal hypoxia and/or widened A-a gradient, and ventilation/perfusion (V/Q) scanning or spiral CT scanning may confirm the diagnosis. Patients suspected of having an aortic dissection should undergo urgent transesophageal echocardiography, CT scanning with intravenous contrast, or magnetic resonance imaging (MRI). Patients suspected of having a gastroesophageal cause of their chest pain may need a barium swallow (esophageal reflux or rupture), endoscopy (esophagitis, gastritis, peptic ulcer disease), hepatobiliary hydroxyiminodiacetic acid (HIDA) scan or abdominal ultrasound (gall bladder disease), esophageal manometry (esophageal spasm), or continuous esophageal pH measurement (reflux) to confirm the diagnosis.

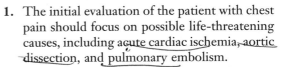

◆ **KEY POINTS** ◆

1. The initial evaluation of the patient with chest pain should focus on possible life-threatening causes, including acute cardiac ischemia, aortic dissection, and pulmonary embolism.

2. Angina classically causes chest pain that is substernal, precipitated by exertion, and relieved with rest or after sublingual nitroglycerin.

3. A variety of pulmonary, musculoskeletal, and gastrointestinal disorders can present with chest pain and may be difficult to distinguish from true angina.

2 Dyspnea

Dyspnea is an uncomfortable awareness of breathing. It is a common symptom of cardiac and pulmonary diseases, and may also result from neurological conditions, chest wall problems, and anxiety states.

DIFFERENTIAL DIAGNOSIS OF DYSPNEA (see Table 2–1)

Cardiac causes of dyspnea predominantly relate to increased pressure in the left ventricle and/or atrium. This pressure is transmitted back to the lungs where it results in transudation of fluid into the interstitial and alveolar spaces, and interferes with alveolar gas exchange. This can occur as a result of:

- valvular heart disease (mitral or aortic regurgitation or stenosis)
- left ventricular systolic dysfunction (ischemic or non-ischemic cardiomyopathies)
- left ventricular diastolic dysfunction (e.g., left ventricular hypertrophy, acute myocardial ischemia, infiltrative cardiomyopathy)
- pericardial diseases (pericardial constriction or tamponade)

Pulmonary causes of dyspnea may result from abnormalities of the tracheobronchial tree, alveolae, pulmonary vasculature, or pleura. These include:

- pneumonia
- chronic obstructive pulmonary disease (COPD)
- asthma
- pulmonary embolism (PE)
- pneumothorax
- pulmonary fibrosis
- pulmonary hypertension
- pleural effusion
- airway obstruction
- diaphragmatic paralysis

Dyspnea may also be a feature of anemia, hyperthyroidism, obesity, neurological disorders that effect the respiratory muscles, physical deconditioning, and anxiety.

CLINICAL MANIFESTATIONS

History

Several historical features may help differentiate between causes of dyspnea. The sudden onset of dyspnea may occur with angina, pulmonary edema, pneumothorax, or PE. Slowly progressive dyspnea may result from COPD, pleural effusions, anemia, or chronic congestive heart failure (CHF). Other historical features that implicate specific causes of dyspnea include:

TABLE 2–1

Differential Diagnosis of Dyspnea

Categorical Cause of Dyspnea	Specific Cause of Dyspnea	Diagnostic Test(s) of Choice
Cardiac	Congestive heart failure/pulmonary edema	CXR, echocardiogram, metabolic stress test; BNP
	Ischemia	ECG, Exercise stress test
	Valvular disease (AS, AI, MS, MR)	Echocardiogram
	Pericardial (tamponade, constriction)	Echocardiogram
	Restrictive heart disease (infiltrative or hypertrophic heart diseases)	Echocardiogram
Pulmonary	COPD	CXR, PFTs
	Asthma	PFTs, methacholine challenge
	Pneumonia	CXR
	Pleural effusion	CXR
	Pulmonary embolism	V/Q scan, spiral CT scan, PA angiogram
	Pneumothorax	CXR
	Pulmonary fibrosis	CXR, high resolution CT scan
	Pulmonary hypertension	Echocardiogram, PA catheter
	Airway obstruction	CXR, PFTs, bronchoscopy
Other	Anemia	Hematocrit
	Hyperthyroidism	TSH
	Diaphragmatic paralysis	PFTs, CXR

CXR: chest x-ray; BNP: brain natriuretic peptide; ECG: electrocardiogram; AS/I: aortic stenosis/insufficiency; MS/R: mitral stenosis/regurgitation; COPD: chronic obstructive pulmonary disease; PFTs: pulmonary function tests; V/Q: ventilation-perfusion; CT: computed tomography; TSH: thyroid stimulating hormone.

- chest pain (angina, myocardial infarction (MI), pneumonia, PE, pneumothorax)
- cough (pneumonia, bronchitis, asthma)
- fever (pneumonia, bronchitis)
- hemoptysis (PE, bronchitis)
- history of smoking (COPD)
- cardiac risk factors (angina, MI)
- chest wall trauma (pneumothorax)

It is also important to note the pattern of dyspnea. Dyspnea is frequently precipitated by exertion irrespective of its cause. Dyspnea that occurs at rest usually indicates severe cardiac or pulmonary disease. Paroxysmal nocturnal dyspnea suggests left heart failure; this usually occurs 2 to 4 hours into sleep and requires that the patient sit up or get out of bed to obtain relief. Orthopnea is often a symptom of heart failure, but can also occur as a result of pulmonary disorders.

Physical Examination

The physical examination of the person with dyspnea usually demonstrates tachypnea. Patients may also be cyanotic, reflecting poor oxygenation or low cardiac output. In patients with cardiac diseases causing dyspnea, examination may reveal evidence of valvular heart disease (e.g., murmurs, opening snap of mitral stenosis (MS), widened pulse pressure of aortic regurgitation) or evidence of CHF (S_3, pulmonary rales, elevated jugular venous pressure). Patients with pneumonia may have fever and focal lung findings, whereas patients with COPD may have diffusely reduced air entry and wheezes. Decreased breath sounds may indicate pleural effusion or pneumothorax, whereas a pleural rub indicates pleuritis associated with PE or pneumonia. Wheezes may be heard with heart failure or bronchospasm, while stridor indicates upper airway obstruction.

DIAGNOSTIC EVALUATION

The approach to patients with dyspnea depends in part on the acuity of the problem. Patients with acute dyspnea require a rapid evaluation to exclude life-threatening causes, whereas patients with chronic dyspnea require less urgent evaluation.

The initial test of choice for most patients with dyspnea is the chest x-ray. This can be diagnostic in a variety of settings including:

- pneumonia (focal infiltrate)
- CHF (Kerley B lines, vascular cephalization, cardiomegaly, pulmonary edema)
- pleural effusion (blunted costophrenic angle)
- pneumothorax (mediastinal shift, loss of lung markings)

The chest x-ray may also suggest the diagnosis in the setting of:

- PE (peripheral infiltrate, loss of vascular markings)
- COPD (hyperinflation, bullous changes)
- cardiac tamponade (large, "water bottle"–shaped cardiac silhouette

If dyspnea is associated with chest pain, or the patient has known or suspected coronary artery disease (CAD), an ECG should be obtained to exclude acute ischemia as the cause. Suspected cardiac causes of dyspnea should be evaluated with an echocardiogram to evaluate ventricular systolic and diastolic function, and to exclude valvular heart disease.

A complete blood count should be obtained to evaluate for anemia. Arterial blood gas analysis rarely clarifies the underlying diagnosis, but it can be helpful in assessing physiological significance and severity of the disease. An elevated serum brain natriuretic peptide (BNP) level during an acute episode of dyspnea suggests CHF as the cause.

The extent to which dyspnea is attributable to lung disease can be assessed with pulmonary function tests (PFTs). With PFTs, flow-volume loops, lung volumes, and diffusion capacity can be measured to assess for restrictive or obstructive lung diseases. CT scanning is appropriate to evaluate patients suspected of having interstitial lung disease or pulmonary emboli, the latter of which may also be diagnosed with a ventilation-perfusion lung scan.

Often it is not clear if a patient's dyspnea is the result of cardiac or pulmonary disease. In this setting, metabolic exercise testing (see Chapter 6) or invasive assessment of intracardiac and pulmonary vascular pressures with a pulmonary artery catheter (Swan-Ganz catheter) may help distinguish between the two possibilities.

◆ KEY POINTS ◆

1. Dyspnea is the uncomfortable awareness of breathing.
2. Dyspnea most commonly results from cardiac or pulmonary disease.
3. Life-threatening causes of dyspnea include pulmonary embolism, pneumothorax, pneumonia, and myocardial ischemia/infarction.

3 Palpitations

Palpitations are the subjective awareness of the heart beating and are usually the result of a change in heart rate, heart rhythm, or the force of cardiac contraction.

ETIOLOGIES

A wide variety of disorders can produce palpitations (Table 3–1). The most common causes are arrhythmias, medications, and psychiatric disorders.

CLINICAL MANIFESTATIONS

History

Patients may describe palpitations as a fluttering, skipping, or pounding sensation in their chests and may have associated lightheadedness, dizziness, or dyspnea. Arrhythmias are the predominant cause and include supraventricular (SVT) and ventricular (VT) tachycardias, and premature atrial (PAC) and ventricular (PVC) contractions. The pattern of palpitations may suggest the underlying cause. Patients can often reproduce the rhythm by tapping their fingers on a table—a rapid regular rhythm suggests sinus tachycardia, SVT, or VT, whereas a rapid, irregular rhythm suggests atrial fibrillation (AF), or frequent premature beats.

Abrupt onset and termination suggests SVT or VT. Associated syncope is more likely with VT than SVT. Single "missed beats" or "flip-flops" are usually from atrial or ventricular premature contractions. Rapid regular palpitations associated with a pounding sensation in the neck suggests a specific type of SVT called AV nodal re-entrant tachycardia (AVNRT) (see Chapter 23). A very slow rate suggests sinus bradycardia or heart block. Palpitations triggered by mild exertion suggest underlying heart failure, valvular disease, anemia, thyrotoxicosis, or poor physical fitness. Occasionally, VT that arises from the right ventricle (RV) outflow tract may present as exercise-induced palpitations. Although anxiety can cause palpitations (typically owing to sinus tachycardia), other more worrisome diagnoses should be excluded. Many young women with SVT are wrongly labeled with anxiety or panic disorder as the cause of their palpitations.

A history of excessive caffeine intake or of cocaine use suggests SVT or PACs as the cause. A thorough review of the patient's medications should be performed to exclude pro-arrhythmic medications (e.g., antiarrhythmic agents, antipsychotic agents) or stimulants (e.g., beta-agonists, theophylline).

Physical Examination

The examination of the person with palpitations is frequently unrevealing; however, clues to the underlying disease may be found and include:

- murmurs (valvular heart disease)
- elevated jugular venous pressure (JVP), rales (heart failure)
- enlarged thyroid gland (thyrotoxicosis)

TABLE 3–1

Common Causes of Palpitations

Cardiac	Tachyarrhythmias (see Chapter 23) Bradyarrhythmias (see Chapter 24) Valvular heart disease (e.g., mitral valve prolapse) Implanted pacemaker Cardiomyopathy (dilated or hypertrophic)	Medications/ Drugs	Sympathomimetic agents (e.g., theophylline, albuterol) Vasodilators Cocaine Amphetamines Caffeine Nicotine
Metabolic disorders	Thyrotoxicosis Hypoglycemia Pheochromocytoma Electrolyte abnormalities (hyper- or hypokalemia, hypomagnesemia)	Psychiatric	Panic attacks Anxiety disorder Depression Emotional stress
		Other	Pregnancy Anemia Fever

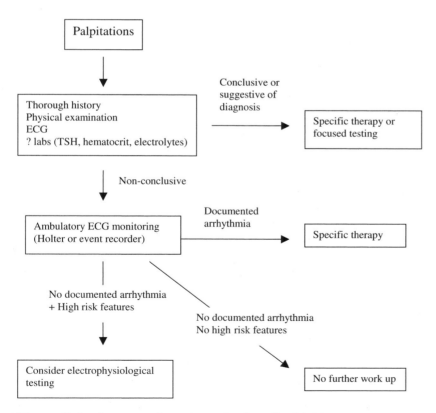

Figure 3–1 An approach to the evaluation of palpitations.

DIAGNOSTIC EVALUATION
(see Figure 3–1)

The most helpful diagnostic study in the evaluation of palpitations is a 12-lead ECG performed during the patient's symptoms. Unfortunately, a routine ECG performed in the absence of symptoms is rarely diagnostic. The routine ECG may, however, provide clues to the presence of cardiac conditions such as pre-excitation syndrome (short PR, delta wave), cardiomyopathy (Q waves, ventricular hypertrophy), or valvular heart disease (ventricular hypertrophy, atrial enlargement).

Prolonged monitoring with a 24-hour ambulatory ECG, ambulatory event monitor, or an implantable loop recorder is usually necessary to determine the cause of infrequent palpitations. An echocardiogram should be performed if underlying heart disease is suspected. A serum TSH level should be routinely obtained to exclude hyperthyroidism as a cause of PACs or SVT. A very aggressive diagnostic strategy should be pursued in those patients with a high likelihood of VT—this includes those with significant valvular disease, myocardial disease, or prior myocardial infarction, and those with a family history of syncope or sudden death. Rarely, electrophysiological studies may be necessary to determine the cause of palpitations.

 KEY POINTS ◆

1. Although they are often the result of benign conditions, palpitations may indicate the presence of life-threatening disorders.

2. The history is crucial to identifying possible etiologies of palpitations.

3. An ECG (12 lead or rhythm strip) during symptoms is essential to confirm the diagnosis.

4. Prolonged ECG monitoring may be required before the diagnosis is established.

Physical Examination of the Cardiovascular System

A thorough physical examination can provide clues to the presence and severity of cardiovascular disease, and alert one to the presence of life-threatening conditions even before the results of any diagnostic workup are available.

GENERAL APPEARANCE

Dyspnea, tachypnea, use of accessory respiratory muscles, discomfort from pain, diaphoresis, and cyanosis may all indicate underlying cardiac disease.

PULSE

The pulse should be examined for rate, regularity, volume, and character. Some abnormalities in the character of the pulse may be diagnostic for certain cardiovascular conditions:

- **Irregularly irregular**: Atrial fibrillation, multifocal atrial tachycardia.
- **Collapsing**: Aortic insufficiency
- **Bisferiens** (double impulse): Combined aortic stenosis (AS) and insufficiency
- **Pulsus parvus** (weak) **et tardus** (delayed): Severe aortic stenosis
- **Pulsus alternans** (alternating strong and weak pulse): Severe LV dysfunction

- **Pulsus paradoxus** (marked inspiratory decrease in strength of pulse): Cardiac tamponade, pericardial constriction, severe obstructive airway disease.

JUGULAR VENOUS PRESSURE (JVP)

The jugular venous pulsation is best visualized with the patient lying with the head tilted up 30–45°. The central venous pressure can be estimated by adding 5 cm (the vertical distance between the center of the right atrium (RA) and the sternal angle) to the maximum vertical height of the pulsations above the sternal angle. The JVP is elevated in heart failure and not identifiable in volume depletion. When heart failure is present, firm pressure over the abdominal right upper quadrant will cause persistent elevation of the JVP (hepatojugular reflux). Characteristic abnormalities of the jugular venous waveforms occur in a variety of cardiac disorders (Figure 4–1).

INSPECTION AND PALPATION OF THE CHEST

The point of maximal impulse (PMI) of the LV apex should be located and palpated. It is usually in the 5th intercostal space at the mid-clavicular line; it is displaced laterally with right ventricle (RV) dilation and infero-laterally with LV dilation. It is diffuse with dilated cardiomyopathy or LV aneurysm, and may demonstrate

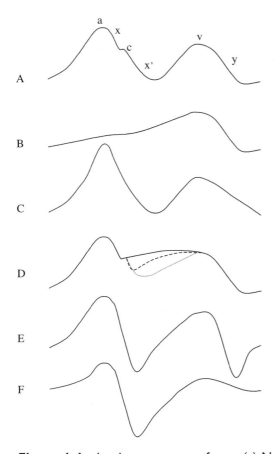

Figure 4–1 Jugular venous waveforms. (a) Normal. (b) Absent a wave in atrial fibrillation. (c) Prominent a wave and shallow y descent in tricuspid stenosis. (d) CV wave in varying degrees of tricuspid regurgitation. (e) Rapid x and y descents in constrictive pericarditis. (f) Rapid x descent and absent y descent in pericardial tamponade.

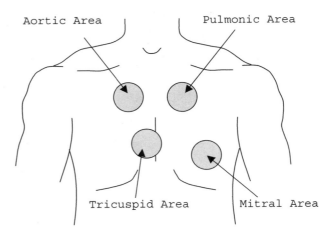

Figure 4–2. Locations of maximal intensity of murmurs depending on the valve of origin.

a double impulse with hypertrophic cardiomyopathy, AS, or hypertension. A left parasternal heave may be evident with RVH.

AUSCULTATION OF THE CHEST

Heart Sounds

The entire precordium should be systematically examined for normal heart sounds (S_1 and S_2), gallops (S_3 or S_4), and other additional sounds (e.g., clicks, snaps). These auscultatory findings are strongly correlated with specific cardiac disorders (see Table 4–1).

The second heart sound comprises the aortic valve (A2) and pulmonic valve (P2) closure sounds, and is abnormal in a variety of disease states. Normally, P2 follows A2, and the split widens with inspiration. A widely split S2 that still varies normally with respiration may result from right bundle branch block (RBBB), severe RV failure, or severe pulmonary hypertension. Wide splitting that does not vary with respiration (**fixed splitting**) is characteristic of an atrial septal defect (ASD). Paradoxical splitting (splitting that narrows with inspiration) is a feature of LBBB, patent ductus arteriosus (PDA), and severe AS.

Murmurs

Murmurs usually arise from blood flow across an abnormal valve, but can also be the result of increased blood flow across a normal valve. The origin of a murmur can often be inferred from its auditory character, its timing within the cardiac cycle (see Table 4–2), and its area of maximal intensity (see Figure 4–2). Various maneuvers may be performed at the bedside to clarify the nature of a particular murmur (see Table 4–3).

Murmur intensity can be graded on a scale of one to six. A grade 1 murmur is barely audible, a grade 2

TABLE 4–1

Abnormal Heart Sounds and Their Significance

Heart Sound	Associated Disease State
Loud S_1	Mitral stenosis
Variable intensity S_1	Atrial fibrillation, AV dissociation
Loud A_2	Hypertension
Soft A_2	Aortic stenosis
Loud P_2	Pulmonary hypertension
Fixed split S_2	Atrial septal defect
Paradoxically split S_2	LBBB, severe AS, PDA
Widely split S_2 with normal variation	RBBB
S_3	Left ventricular dysfunction
S_4	Hypertension, AS, HCM
Early systolic ejection click	Bicuspid aortic valve, pulmonary stenosis, Pulmonary hypertension
Mid-systolic click	Mitral valve prolapse
Opening snap	Mitral stenosis
Pericardial knock	Constrictive pericarditis

Electrocardiogram

Timing of Heart Sounds

AS: aortic stenosis; PDA: patent ductus arteriosus; LBBB: left bundle branch block; RBBB: right bundle branch block; EC: ejection click; MSC: mid-systolic click; OS: opening snap; HCM: hypertrophic cardiomyopathy.

murmur is easily audible, a grade 3 murmur is loud, and grade 4 to grade 6 murmurs are all associated with palpable precordial thrills. Grade 4 murmur can be heard only with the stethoscope firmly on the chest, grade 5 murmurs can be heard with just the edge of the stethoscope on the chest, and grade 6 murmurs can be heard without the stethoscope.

Several general principles worth remembering during cardiac auscultation are:

- Aortic events are best heard with the patient leaning forward and at end expiration.
- Mitral events are best heard in the left lateral position, during expiration.

TABLE 4–2

Classification of Murmurs

Category	Graphic Representation	Examples
Early-peaking systolic ejection murmur		Benign flow murmur, aortic sclerosis
Late-peaking systolic ejection murmur		Aortic stenosis, pulmonic stenosis, hypertrophic cardiomyopathy
Holosystolic murmur		Mitral regurgitation, tricuspid regurgitation, ventricular septal defect
Mid-systolic murmur		Mitral valve prolapse with mitral regurgitation
Decrescendo diastolic murmur		Aortic insufficiency, pulmonic insufficiency
Diastolic rumble (with pre-systolic accentuation)		Mitral stenosis
Continuous murmur ("machinery" murmur)		Patent ductus arteriosus, arterio-venous fistulas
Pericardial friction rub		Pericarditis

MSC: mid-systolic click; OS: opening snap.

- With the exception of the pulmonary ejection click, all right-sided events are louder with inspiration.
- Left-sided events are usually louder with expiration.

Pericardial friction rubs may be mistaken for systolic and diastolic murmurs. They tend to have a scratchy quality and vary significantly with respirations. Classically there are three components of a pericardial rub:

- an atrial systolic component
- a ventricular systolic component
- a ventricular diastolic component

TABLE 4–3

Differential Diagnosis of Systolic Murmurs

	Location	Character	Radiation	Accentuating Maneuvers	Attenuating Maneuvers	Other Findings
AS	Right upper SB	Ejection systolic	Neck, carotids	Leg raising, post-Valsalva, post-PVC	Hand grip	Paradoxically split S_2; soft A_2; S_4
HOCM	3rd–4th left ICS	Ejection systolic	Upper left SB	Sudden standing, Valsalva	Squatting, post-Valsalva	Mitral regurgitation
MR	Apex	Holosystolic	Axilla	Hand grip	Inspiration, Valsalva	S_3
MVP with MR	Apex	Late systolic	Varies	Sudden standing, Valsalva	Supine posture, post-Valsalva	Mid-systolic click
VSD	3rd–4th left ICS	Holosystolic	None	Hand grip	Valsalva	S_3
PS	Left upper SB	Ejection systolic	None	Inspiration, passive leg raising	Expiration, sudden standing	Ejection click
TR	Left lower SB	Holosystolic	None	Inspiration, passive leg raising	Expiration	Pulsatile liver

AS: aortic stenosis; HOCM: hypertrophic obstructive cardiomyopathy; MR: mitral regurgitation; MVP: mitral valve prolapse; VSD: ventricular septal defect; PS: pulmonary stenosis; TR: tricuspid regurgitation; SB: sternal border; ICS: Intercostal space.

Frequently, however, only one or two components are heard.

THE LUNGS

It is essential to examine the lungs in every cardiac patient, paying special attention to the following features:

- inspiratory crackles (rales)—indicate left heart failure
- bronchospasm (wheezing)—may indicate peribronchial edema ("cardiac asthma")
- diminished breath sounds and dullness to percussion at the lung bases—may represent pleural effusions

Several other physical findings are worth noting:

- Hepatomegaly, ascites, and peripheral edema may reflect RV failure.
- A pulsatile liver is seen with tricuspid regurgitation.
- Central cyanosis is commonly associated with congenital heart disease, whereas peripheral cyanosis is associated with diminished cardiac output.
- Digital clubbing may be seen with congenital cyanotic heart disease and endocarditis.

Part II
Diagnostic
Modalities

5

The Electrocardiogram

The electrocardiogram (ECG) is a visual representation of the electrical impulses generated by the heart with each beat. Ever since Willem Einthoven developed the ECG in the early 1900s, it has become an invaluable tool in the diagnosis of a variety of cardiac conditions. This section will present the fundamental electrophysiology of the cardiac cycle and the components and appearance of the normal ECG, and will briefly outline criteria for some abnormal findings.

BASIC CARDIAC ELECTROPHYSIOLOGY

The mechanical process of ventricular contraction begins with an electrical impulse generated in a region of the superior right atrium known as the sinoatrial (SA) node (Figure 5–1). The sinus impulse quickly spreads through the atria resulting in atrial contraction, and then continues through the atrioventricular (AV) node, the His bundle, and the right and left bundle branches, eventually reaching the ventricular myocardium where it results in synchronized biventricular contraction. If ventricular contraction results from impulses that originate in the SA node, then normal sinus rhythm is said to be present. Abnormalities of this process result in various arrhythmias (dysrhythmias).

THE LEAD SYSTEM

The electrical impulses in the heart can be recorded by means of electrodes strategically placed on the surface of the body. The standard ECG has 12 leads: 6 limb leads and 6 precordial or chest leads. The limb leads (I, II, III, aVR, aVL, aVF) record cardiac electrical impulses in a vertical or frontal plane (Figure 5–2). The precordial leads (V1–6) are placed over the left chest and record electrical impulses in a horizontal plane.

The ECG is generated by simultaneously recording the electrical activity of the heart at each electrode or pair of electrodes. Any net electrical impulse directed toward the positive aspect of a lead is represented by an upward deflection of the ECG tracing in that lead. The magnitude of the deflection reflects the strength of the electrical signal, which depends, in part, on the mass of myocardium that is being depolarized, and, in part, on the electrical impedance of interposed tissue.

THE NORMAL ECG (Figure 5–3)

Every cardiac cycle's electrical impulse is inscribed on the ECG as a waveform with the following components: P wave, QRS complex and T wave (Figure 5–4).

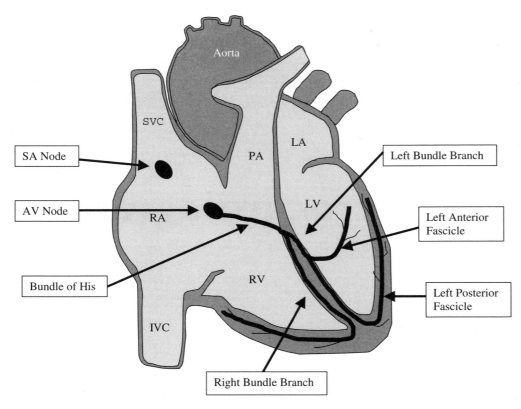

Figure 5–1   The anatomy of the cardiac conduction system.

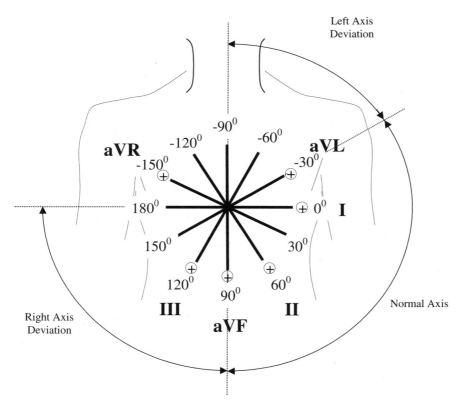

Figure 5–2   Orientation of limb leads and axis. Positive pole of lead denoted by +.

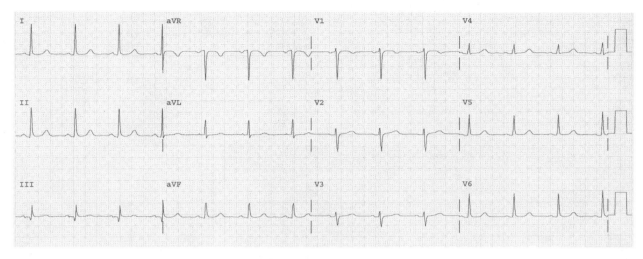

Figure 5–3   Normal 12-lead ECG. (See text for details.)

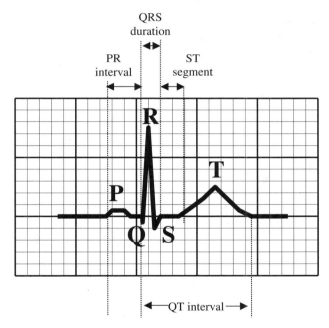

Figure 5–4   Normal electrocardiographic waveforms and intervals.

The P Wave

The onset of the P wave heralds the onset of atrial depolarization. The normal electrical impulse travels from the SA node and depolarizes the atria in a superior-to-

inferior direction, resulting in a P wave on the ECG that is upright (positive) in lead II and downward (negative) in lead aVR. An impulse arising from a site other than the SA node will depolarize the atria in a different direction and results in a different P wave morphology. The normal P wave is ≤1 mV in amplitude in lead V1, ≤2.5 mV in amplitude in lead II, and ≤0.12 seconds in duration in lead II. Increases in these parameters occur with atrial enlargement.

The PR Interval

The PR interval is measured from the onset of the P wave to the onset of the QRS complex and is a measure of the time it takes for the sinus impulse to traverse the atria, AV node, and His-Purkinje system before depolarizing the ventricles. The normal PR interval can vary between 0.12–0.20 seconds; this variability is mainly the result of autonomic tone. A prolonged PR segment reflects slowing of the impulse through the conduction system. An abnormally short PR segment may represent accelerated conduction through the AV node or a "short circuit" between the atria and the ventricles (a **bypass tract**).

The QRS Complex

The QRS complex is measured from the onset of the Q or R wave to the end of the S wave. The initial 0.04 seconds of this complex represents depolarization of the septum, which occurs from left to right. This results in a small initial negative deflection ("septal q wave") in leads I and V6 because the impulse is directed away from the positive poles of these leads. The remainder of the QRS complex reflects depolarization of the right and left ventricles. Because of its greater mass, the electrical forces from the left ventricle predominate, resulting in a QRS complex that is mainly positive in leads I and V6

and negative in aVR and V1. Thus, the appearance of the QRS complex in normal sinus rhythm is characterized by:

- initial "septal Q waves" in leads I and V6
- predominantly positive QRS complex in leads I and V6

TABLE 5–1

Diagnostic Criteria for Common ECG Abnormalities

Abnormality	Diagnostic Criteria
Left atrial enlargement	P wave duration in lead II $\geq$0.12 sec **OR** P wave in V_1 $\geq$1 mV deep and $\geq$0.04 sec long
Right atrial enlargement	P wave in V1 >1.5 mV in amplitude **OR** P wave in II >2.5 mV in amplitude
Left ventricular hypertrophy	S wave in V_1 + the R wave in V_5 or V_6 >35 mV **OR** S wave in V_2 + the R wave in V_5 or V_6 >45 mV **OR** R wave in V_5 >26 mV **OR** R wave in lead aVL >11 mV **OR** R wave in lead I >14 mV
Right ventricular hypertrophy	R/S ratio in V_1 >1 **OR** R wave in V_1 + the S wave in V_5 or V_6 $\geq$11 mV **OR** R wave in V_1 >7 mV **OR** R/S ratio in V_5 or V_6 $\leq$ 1
Left axis deviation	Axis −30° to −105°
Right axis deviation	Axis >+100
Pathologic Q wave	Duration $\geq$0.04 sec **AND** Amplitude >1/3 the height of the R wave
Peaked T wave	T wave amplitude >6 mV in limb leads **OR** T wave amplitude >10 mV in precordial leads
Left bundle branch block	QRS duration $\geq$0.12 sec **AND** Broad monophasic R wave in leads I, V_5, V_6
Right bundle branch block	QRS duration $\geq$0.12 sec **AND** rsR pattern in V_1 **AND** Wide S wave in V_5, V_6, and lead I
Left anterior fascicular block	QRS axis −45° to −90° **AND** qR complex in leads I, aVL **AND** rS complex in leads III, aVF **AND** QRS duration $\leq$0.10 sec
Left posterior fascicular block	QRS axis +100° to +180° **AND** Deep S wave in lead I, Q wave in lead III **AND** QRS duration $\leq$ 0.10 sec

- predominantly negative QRS complex in leads aVR and V1
- incremental increase in the amplitude of R waves from V2 to V5

The normal QRS duration (the total time for ventricular depolarization) is less than 100 milliseconds. Longer QRS durations suggest conduction block or delay.

The ST Segment

The ST segment corresponds to the time during which the ventricles have completely depolarized but not yet begun to repolarize. During this time there is no net electrical activity in the heart and the ECG records a flat segment at the electrical baseline. This segment becomes abnormal during myocardial ischemia (ST segment depression) and infarction (ST segment elevation).

The T Wave

The onset of the T wave denotes the onset of ventricular repolarization. The T wave in most circumstances follows the same direction (polarity) as the predominant portion of the QRS complex, and, thus, is normally upright in leads I and V6 and inverted in lead aVR. However, the normal T wave can be either upright or inverted in leads V1, aVL, and III. Changes in T wave morphology may reflect myocardial ischemia or infarction, and can also occur as a result of metabolic abnormalities.

QT Interval

The QT interval is measured from the onset of the QRS complex to the end of the T wave. The normal duration of the QT interval depends on many factors, including a person's age, gender, and heart rate. Nonetheless, a QT interval greater than 0.46 seconds or greater than 50% of the associated R wave to R wave interval is abnormally long. A prolonged QT interval may reflect a primary congenital abnormality of myocardial repolarization or be secondary to medications or metabolic abnormalities, and predisposes to malignant ventricular arrhythmias.

QRS Axis (Figure 5–2)

The electrical axis is the overall direction of the electrical depolarization of the heart. If this direction is horizontal and to the right, the axis is assigned a value of zero. Axes directed more clockwise are assigned positive values, whereas axes directed more counterclockwise are assigned negative values. The axis can be estimated by identifying the limb lead in which the QRS complex is most isoelectric (positive and negative deflections are of equal size); the axis is perpendicular to this lead. Because the ventricles depolarize predominantly from superior to inferior and from right to left, the QRS axis normally falls between −30° and +90°.

ABNORMAL ECG PATTERNS

A variety of cardiac disorders are associated with specific patterns on ECG. Although it is beyond the scope of this text to provide a comprehensive discussion of this topic, the reader should be familiar with the ECG patterns associated with some common abnormalities, as outlined in Table 5–1.

◆ KEY POINTS ◆

1. The electrocardiogram is a visual representation of the electrical activity of the heart.
2. The normal electrocardiographic waveform consists of a P wave, QRS complex, and T wave representing atrial depolarization, ventricular depolarization, and ventricular repolarization, respectively.
3. The P wave in sinus rhythm has a characteristic appearance and is upright in lead II and downward in lead aVR.
4. The QRS is normally a predominantly negative complex in lead V1 and transitions to a predominantly positive complex by V4.
5. The normal electrical axis of the heart is −30° to +90°.
6. Certain cardiac abnormalities are associated with specific patterns on ECG.

6

Stress Testing

Stress testing is one of the most widely used tools in cardiology. It provides diagnostic and prognostic information in patients with suspected or known coronary heart disease, and is a useful tool for assessing the adequacy of therapy. Stress testing can also objectively assess the functional capacity of a patient, and help determine the nature of a patient's functional limitations.

INDICATIONS

The most common (and, perhaps, most useful) indication for stress testing is to determine whether a patient's symptoms relate to underlying coronary artery disease. For patients in whom the diagnosis of CAD is already certain, stress testing may be useful to:

- assess risk and determine long-term prognosis
- assess exercise capacity
- evaluate the efficacy of therapy
- assist in therapeutic decision making (i.e., determine who may benefit from cardiac catheterization and revascularization)
- detect exercise-related arrhythmias
- localize a region of ischemia in order to target percutaneous revascularization

CONTRAINDICATIONS

There are small but real risks associated with stress testing, including myocardial infarction (MI), serious arrhythmias, and death (approximate rate of 1 in 2,500 tests). Most of these complications occur in patients with certain high-risk markers; therefore, patients should be carefully screened before undergoing exercise testing to ensure that no contraindications exist (see Table 6–1).

TESTING MODALITIES

Stress testing can be performed in several ways (Table 6–2). The stress can be induced by exercise (either walking on a treadmill or riding a bicycle) or by pharmacological means with dobutamine or coronary vasodilators. Treadmill exercise is the best-standardized modality and allows for more flexible protocols, as speed and incline can be varied independently. The Bruce protocol is the most commonly used and consists of incremental increases in the speed and slope of the treadmill every three minutes. Bicycle testing may, however, be better tolerated in patients who have orthopedic or balance problems. The aim of the exercise is to increase myocardial oxygen demand (MVO_2). In patients with coronary artery disease (CAD), the increased MVO_2 may exceed the ability of the coronary arteries to supply oxygenated blood, resulting in ischemia.

TABLE 6–1

Absolute and Relative Contraindications to Exercise Stress Testing

Absolute:
- Acute myocardial infarction (within 2 days)
- Unstable angina (until medically stabilized)
- Acute myocarditis, pericarditis, or endocarditis
- Uncontrolled hypertension (resting SBP >200 mmHg or DBP >120 mmHg)
- Uncontrolled tachy- or bradyarrhythmias
- Decompensated, symptomatic congestive heart failure
- Severe or symptomatic aortic stenosis
- Acute/recent deep venous thrombosis or pulmonary embolism
- Acute aortic dissection
- Recent cerebrovascular accident

Relative:
- Moderate valvular stenoses (unless symptomatic)
- Hypertrophic obstructive cardiomyopathy
- Suspected left main coronary artery disease
- High grade AV block
- Acute illness, such as active infection, thyrotoxicosis, severe anemia
- Inability to exercise adequately

TABLE 6–2

Stress Testing Modalities

Exercise ECG
Exercise echocardiography
Exercise with nuclear imaging
Dobutamine echocardiography
Dipyridamole with nuclear imaging
Adenosine with nuclear imaging

Dobutamine produces an increase in heart rate, contractility, and blood pressure, thereby mimicking exercise and increasing MVO_2. Dipyridamole or adenosine cause coronary vasodilation preferentially in normal coronary arteries. This results in a flow mismatch with blood flow in normal coronary arteries increased relative to diseased coronary arteries. Pharmacological stress testing with these agents yields sensitivities and specificities comparable to exercise stress testing. Pharmacological stress is not without risk; dobutamine can induce ventricular arrhythmias and precipitate myocardial ischemia, while dipyridamole can cause bronchospasm.

MONITORING MODALITIES

All patients who undergo stress testing are assessed for symptoms and have continuous ECG monitoring to identify ischemic changes (ST depression or elevation) or arrhythmias. The sensitivity and specificity of stress testing can be improved with the use of echocardiographic or nuclear imaging to identify objectively areas of myocardial ischemia.

The isotopes used in myocardial perfusion imaging are thallium-201 (^{201}Tl) and technetium-99m (^{99m}Tc) sestamibi. Sestamibi is a newer agent that has superior image quality, and allows for the assessment of left ventricular function as well as ischemia. After intravenous injection, these isotopes are taken up by viable myocardial cells in quantities proportional to their regional blood flow. Regions of the myocardium that are well perfused appear brighter on nuclear imaging than regions that are poorly perfused (because of CAD) (Figure 6–1). When used during stress testing, nuclear or echocardiographic imaging is performed at both rest and at peak exercise.

CHOICE OF TESTING MODALITIES (PHYSIOLOGICAL VS. PHARMACOLOGICAL)

In general, if a patient can exercise, an exercise test is preferred over a pharmacological stress test (see Figure 6–2) because it is a more physiological study. Pharmacological stress testing is employed when the patient is unable to exercise adequately. With exercise or dobutamine stress testing, the patient must attain at least 85%

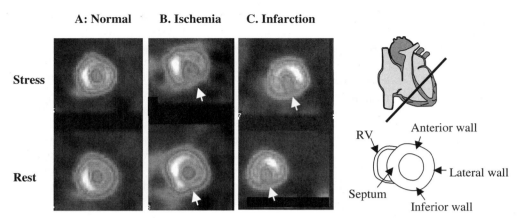

Figure 6–1 Nuclear imaging during stress testing. (a) Normal scan. Both rest and stress images demonstrate homogeneous perfusion of the myocardium. (b) Ischemia. The stress image demonstrates a large inferior wall perfusion defect that "fills in" in the rest images. (c) Infarction. Both rest and stress images demonstrate a large inferior wall perfusion defect.

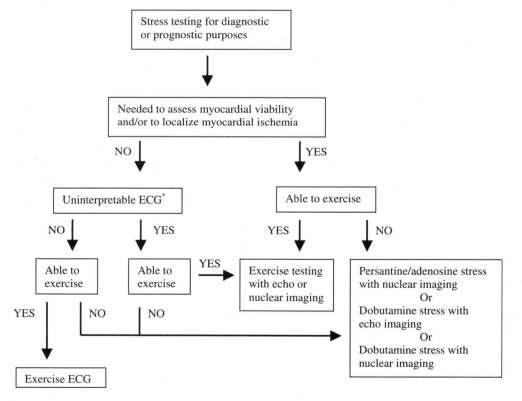

Figure 6–2 Selection of stress test modality. *Uninterpretable ECG includes left ventricular hypertrophy, left bundle branch block, intraventricular conduction delays, paced ventricular rhythms, digitalis effect, resting ST-T wave abnormalities.

of his/her maximum predicted heart rate (maximum predicted heart rate = 220 − age) in order to achieve a sufficient level of myocardial stress to precipitate ischemia. When dipyridamole or adenosine is used as the stress modality, it is presumed that maximum coronary vasodilation occurs with the standard dose, and a heart rate response is not required.

The level of physiological stress achieved can be compared between different exercise protocols and related to routine daily activities by reporting the level of stress in terms of metabolic equivalents (METs) (see Table 6–3). One MET equals the body's oxygen requirement at rest ($\sim$3.5 mL O_2/min/kg body weight).

CHOICE OF MONITORING MODALITIES (ECG ALONE VS. IMAGING)

If a patient can exercise and has no significant ST segment abnormalities on his/her resting ECG, then ECG monitoring alone is usually adequate. In patients with abnormal resting ECGs (left bundle branch block [LBBB], left ventricular hypertrophy, digoxin effect, paced rhythms, persistent ST segment depression), the ECG is not adequate to identify ischemia, and an additional imaging modality is necessary. When pharmacological stress testing is used, an imaging modality is always necessary because of the low sensitivity of drug-induced ST segment changes. The use of echocardiographic or nuclear imaging improves the sensitivity and specificity of the test in these settings. The decision as to which imaging modality should be employed depends on the expertise of the institution. The reported sensitivities among the various modalities are similar (see Table 6–4).

INTERPRETATION OF EXERCISE ECG TESTING

ST segment depression is the most common electrocardiographic manifestation of ischemia. Other stress-induced ECG findings suggestive of ischemia include ST segment elevation, ventricular ectopy or arrhythmias, QRS widening, and increased R wave amplitude. Several different types of ST segment changes may be

TABLE 6–3

Activities of Daily Living (ADLs) and Their Corresponding Metabolic Equivalent (MET*) Level

METS	Equivalent Workload
1	ADLs, e.g., eat, dress, use the toilet
3–4	Walk at 2.5 mph pace, bowl, light household chores
4–5	Push power lawn mower, play golf (walk, carry clubs), mop floors, strip and make bed, walk down a flight of stairs without stopping
5–6	Carry anything up a flight of stairs without stopping, have sexual intercourse, garden, rake, weed, walk at 4 mph pace on level ground
7–10	Carry at least 24 lbs up a flight of stairs, shovel snow, carry objects that are at least 80 lbs, jog/walk at a 5 mph pace
>10	Strenuous sports, e.g., swimming, basketball, skiing, singles tennis
18	Elite endurance athlete
20	World class athlete

*One MET = 3.5 mL O_2/min/kg.

seen, although horizontal or down-sloping ST depressions are the most specific (see Figure 6–3). Although chest pain occurs only in approximately 1/3 of stress tests, its presence increases the likelihood of underlying coronary heart disease.

When echocardiography or nuclear imaging are performed, ischemia is defined as a region of myocardium that appears normal at rest but abnormal with exercise. Infarction is a region that appears abnormal at both rest and exercise. Either of these findings is strong evidence of CAD.

Certain findings during stress testing are markers for adverse prognosis. These include:

- ST segment depression of ≥2 mm or in ≥5 leads
- ST segment elevation
- angina pectoris
- ventricular tachycardia

TABLE 6–4

Comparison of the Diagnostic Value of Various Types of Stress Tests

Type of Stress Test	Sensitivity	Specificity	PPV	NPV
Exercise ECG	65–70%	80–84%	91%	41%
Dobutamine echo	78–85%	70–88%	92%	69%
Nuclear imaging	80–90%	70–80%	85%	72%

*The reported values for exercise nuclear imaging include the average of both sestamibi and thallium studies. PPV: positive predictive value; NPV: negative predictive value.

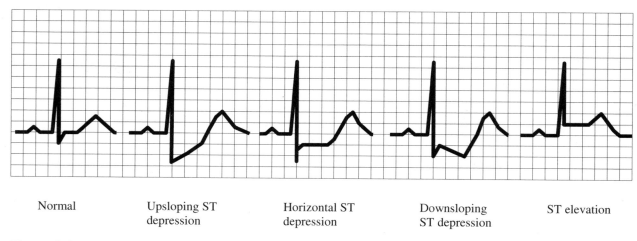

Normal   Upsloping ST depression   Horizontal ST depression   Downsloping ST depression   ST elevation

Figure 6–3   Patterns of ST segment changes during stress testing. Most physicians use the criteria of 1 mm ST segment depression if the pattern is horizontal or downsloping, and 1.5 mm if upsloping. ST segment elevation greater than 1 mm is a significant finding.

- exercise-induced hypotension (>20 mmHg drop in systolic blood pressure [SBP])
- low exercise capacity (≤5 MET level)

The theory of conditional probability, or Bayes' theorem, is an integral component of the interpretation of stress testing when it is used for diagnosing ischemic heart disease. This theorem states that the post-test probability of a particular disease depends upon the incidence of the disease in the population being studied. That is, an abnormal stress test in a person with a very low likelihood of having CAD is probably a false positive test, and a negative test in a person with a very high probability of having CAD is likely a false negative test.

Therefore, stress testing for the diagnosis of CAD is most helpful in patients who have an intermediate probability of CAD.

STRESS TESTING IN WOMEN

Women under the age of 55 to 60 years often have "false-positive ST depression," i.e., ST segment depression in relation to exertion that is not due to epicardial coronary artery disease. Consequently, other exercise variables, such as exercise time and hypotension, must be considered when diagnosing coronary heart disease in women. Given the lower prevalence of ischemic heart disease in women as compared with men, all modalities of stress testing are less accurate in this population.

CARDIOPULMONARY STRESS TESTING

Cardiopulmonary exercise testing (CPET) measures respiratory gas exchange during treadmill or bicycle exercise protocols. It uses these data to provide information regarding peak oxygen uptake, anaerobic threshold, and minute ventilation. Indications for CPET include:

- objective assessment of functional capacity
- determination of the appropriateness and timing of cardiac transplantation
- determination whether a patient's dyspnea or low exercise capacity is the result of cardiac disease, pulmonary disease, deconditioning, or poor motivation

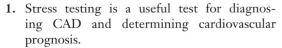

◆ KEY POINTS ◆

1. Stress testing is a useful test for diagnosing CAD and determining cardiovascular prognosis.

2. Stress testing can be accomplished with exercise protocols or pharmacological agents. If a patient can exercise, an exercise protocol is preferred.

3. During stress testing, ischemia can be identified by monitoring the patient's symptoms and ECG, or by echocardiographic or nuclear imaging.

4. If a patient's ECG is abnormal at rest, then an imaging modality is necessary to identify ischemia during stress.

5. The post-test probability of CAD depends, in part, on the pre-test probability of CAD in the population being studied.

7 Echocardiography

Echocardiography refers to a group of tests that utilize reflected ultrasonic waves (echoes) to generate images of the heart and other related structures. Since its discovery and application to medicine over 30 years ago, it has become widely used and is an indispensable tool for the assessment of cardiac structure and function.

PRINCIPLES AND TECHNIQUES

Two-dimensional (2-D) echocardiography is the most common technique used clinically and produces 2-D images of the heart in multiple planes (see Figure 7–1). The images can be obtained by either transthoracic or transesophageal techniques. In transthoracic echocardiography, the ultrasonic **transducer** is placed on various locations (or "windows") on the surface of the chest to obtain different views or planes of the heart. The probe emits an ultrasound beam that moves across a sector so that a pie-shaped slice of the heart is interrogated and images obtained. This technique allows visualization of cardiac structures and measurement of wall thickness and chamber sizes.

During the study, the heart is imaged continuously throughout the cardiac cycle. By comparing images in systole and diastole, the motion of various regions of the heart can be assessed and overall systolic function (ejection fraction) can be estimated. Regions of the left ventricle that do not contract well during systole provide evidence of prior myocardial infarction or non-ischemic

injury. Transthoracic echocardiography is also an effective method by which to visualize the pericardium and identify and assess the significance of pericardial effusions.

Doppler echocardiography is often used in addition to 2-D echocardiography to record blood flow within the cardiovascular system. It utilizes the principle of the Doppler effect to determine the direction and velocity of blood flow relative to the transducer. This information can also be recorded in a spatially correct format superimposed on a 2-D echocardiogram. **Color Doppler echocardiography** takes such information and uses various shades of red to depict blood moving toward the transducer, and various shades of blue for blood moving away from the transducer. Doppler techniques are used to assess the presence and severity of valvular stenosis or regurgitation, and to identify intracardiac shunts. A summary of the uses and limitations of transthoracic echocardiography can be found in Table 7–1.

Transesophageal echocardiography (TEE) utilizes standard echocardiography principles; however, the transducer is placed at the end of a probe and inserted into the patient's esophagus. The distance from the transducer to the heart is thereby minimized, allowing for improved image resolution compared to transthoracic echocardiography (see Figures 31–1, 46–1). TEE is especially well suited for assessing valvular anatomy and function, identifying valvular vegetations in patients with endocarditis, visualizing aortic

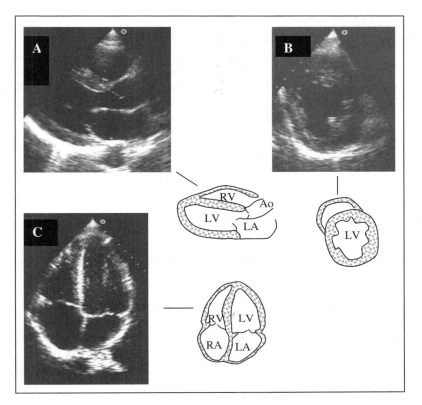

Figure 7–1 Two-dimensional images of the heart from various transducer positions. (a) Parasternal long axis view. (b) Parasternal short axis view. (a) Apical 4-chamber view. RV: Right ventricle; LV: left ventricle; RA: right atrium; LA: left atrium; Ao: aorta.

TABLE 7–1

Uses and Limitations of Echocardiography

Uses	- Assessment of: - LV systolic and diastolic function - LV segmental wall motion (e.g., post-MI) - RV systolic function - Wall thickness (e.g., LV hypertrophy) - Valvular disease (acquired or congenital) - Infective endocarditis - Congenital heart disease - Cardiac shunts (ASD, VSD, PDA)	- Cardiomyopathies (hypertrophic, dilated or infiltrative) - Pericardial disease (effusion, tamponade) - Cardiac tumors and thrombi - Aortic aneurysm - Aortic dissection
Limitations		- Poor transmission of ultrasound waves through bone or air (lung) - Study quality is operator-dependent

LV: left ventricle; MI: myocardial infarction; ASD: atrial septal defect; VSD: ventricular septal defect; PDA: patent ductus arteriosus.

TABLE 7-2

**Advantages and Disadvantages of
Transesophageal Echocardiography (TEE)**

Advantages	- Image quality superior to transthoracic echo
	- Better visualization of valves and atria
	- Particularly useful in assessing prosthetic valves, vegetations, aortic disease, and intracardiac masses
	- Can be used during cardiac surgery
Disadvantages	- Invasive
	- Requires conscious sedation
	- Risk of aspiration
	- Risk of trauma to teeth, pharynx, and esophagus

atherosclerosis and aortic dissections, and identifying potential cardiac sources of emboli in patients with embolic neurological events. The advantages and disadvantages of TEE are listed in Table 7–2.

Other techniques and applications of echocardiography include:

- **Intravascular ultrasound** (IVUS): A miniaturized ultrasound transducer is placed on the tip of a vascular catheter allowing for imaging of atherosclerotic plaques from within an artery.

- **Contrast echocardiography**: Agitated saline or microbubbles are injected intravenously. The bubbles are highly refractory under ultrasound and, thus, opacify the cardiac chambers, allowing better definition of left and right ventricular wall motion, identification of intracardiac shunts, and assessment of myocardial perfusion.

- **Three-dimensional (3-D) echocardiography**: Allows visualization of cardiac structures in a 3-D format. Current utility limited to congenital heart disease, valvular abnormalities, and research.

◆ KEY POINTS ◆

1. Echocardiography utilizes ultrasonic waves and their reflected signals to generate images of the heart.

2. Echocardiography permits the assessment of cardiac structure, valvular function, ventricular systolic and diastolic function, and estimation of left ventricular ejection fraction. Serial images can be obtained over time, allowing for the assessment of disease progression.

3. Transesophageal echocardiography provides higher image resolution than transthoracic echocardiography. TEE is well-suited for imaging valvular structures and thoracic aortic pathology, and for the identification of potential intracardiac sources of emboli.

8

Cardiac Catheterization

Cardiac catheterization involves the percutaneous placement of catheters into the vasculature and cardiac chambers. This allows for the measurement of intracardiac pressures, assessment of ventricular function, and visualization of the coronary anatomy. This information is an essential part of the assessment of a variety of cardiac disorders.

TECHNIQUES

Access to the vasculature is most often obtained via the femoral artery and vein, although the brachial or radial arteries and the subclavian or internal jugular veins may be used as well. A sheath with a one-way valve is placed in the vessel, through which various catheters may be advanced and positioned into the desired cardiac chamber or vessel (see Figure 8–1). A full diagnostic cardiac catheterization encompasses several techniques, including right heart catheterization, left heart catheterization, assessment of oxygen saturation, measurement of cardiac output, coronary angiography, and contrast ventriculography. The specific techniques performed during a particular procedure depend upon the information required.

RIGHT HEART CATHETERIZATION (RHC)

Hemodynamics

During RHC a balloon-tipped catheter is advanced through the right-sided cardiac structures, allowing for the direct measurement of pressure in the right atrium, right ventricle, and pulmonary artery (see Figure 8–1b and Figure 8–2). The catheter can then be advanced as far as possible in the pulmonary artery (the pulmonary capillary wedge position); pressure measured in this position is an indirect measurement of the left atrial pressure.

Oximetry

Blood samples can be drawn sequentially from the various right-sided cardiac chambers and vessels (venae cavae to pulmonary artery). If a sudden increase in saturation is noted, it identifies the location where oxygenated blood from the left side of the heart is entering the right heart circulation (i.e., intracardiac shunting through an atrial or ventricular septal defect or patent ductus arteriosus). The magnitude of the oxygen "step up" can be used to quantify the size of the shunt.

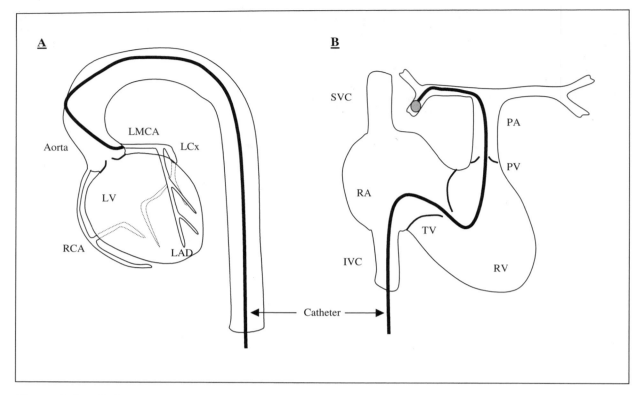

Figure 8–1   (a) Coronary angiography. An intravascular catheter is advanced from the femoral artery, through the aorta, and placed into the ostium of the left main coronary artery. Catheters can also be placed into the ostium of the right coronary artery and across the aortic valve into the left ventricular chamber (LV). (b) Right heart catheterization. A balloon-tipped catheter is advanced through the inferior vena cava (IVC), into the right atrium (RA), across the tricuspid valve (TV), into the right ventricle (RV), across the pulmonary valve (PV), and is "wedged" into a branch of the pulmonary artery (PA). LAD: left anterior descending coronary artery; LCx: left circumflex coronary artery; LMCA: left main coronary artery; RCA: right coronary artery; SVC: superior vena cava.

Cardiac output (CO)

Cardiac output can be measured by injecting a known volume of saline, at a known temperature, into the right atrium and monitoring the temperature changes distally in the pulmonary artery (thermodilution technique). CO can also be assessed by measuring oxygen consumption with a metabolic rate meter (Fick technique) or by making assumptions about a person's oxygen consumption (assumed Fick). Using these techniques, the following formula applies:

$$\text{cardiac output} = O_2 \text{ consumption} \div AV\ O_2 \text{ difference}$$

The AV O_2 difference equals the oxygen carrying capac-ity of blood (13.6 mL of O_2/g of hemoglobin/liter of blood) × (serum hemoglobin concentration) × (arteri-ovenous difference in percent O_2 saturation).

Systemic vascular resistance (SVR) can be calculated from the cardiac output and arterial blood pressure using the following formula:

$$SVR = [(\text{mean arterial BP} - \text{RA pressure}) \div CO] \times 80$$

SVR is expressed in units of dynes-sec-cm^{-5}. Measure-ment of the CO, SVR, and chamber pressures can be very useful in delineating the cause of a patient's hemo-dynamic abnormalities and determining the appropriate treatment (see Table 8–1).

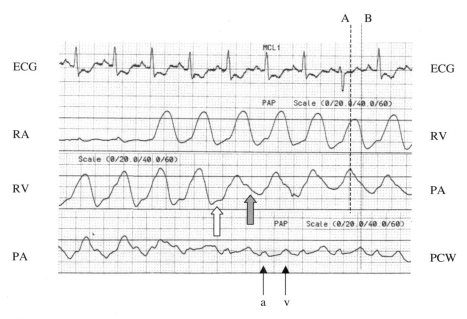

Figure 8–2 Continuous pressure recording during right-heart catheterization.
Line 1: An electrocardiogram (ECG) rhythm strip (similar to lead V_1).
Line 2: Demonstrates the rise in pressure from the right atrium (RA) to the right ventricle (RV) (distinct RA wave forms not well seen).
Line 3: Demonstrates the change in pressure as the catheter is advanced from the RV to the pulmonary artery (PA). Note the similar systolic pressure and the rise in diastolic pressure. Also note that the pressure rises during diastole in the RV (white arrow) but falls during diastole in the PA (gray arrow).
Line 4: As the catheter is advanced from the PA to the pulmonary capillary wedge (PCW) position, the systolic pressure falls and distinct a and v waves are seen. Note that the peak of the PA wave form occurs during the ST segment on the ECG (line A); whereas the peak of the v wave in the PCW tracing occurs after the peak of the T wave on the ECG (line B). This feature may help to distinguish the two pressure wave forms in patients with large V waves on the PCW pressure tracing.

INDICATIONS FOR RIGHT HEART CATHETERIZATION

Right heart catheterization may be performed alone or as part of a complete diagnostic cardiac catheterization. The major indications for right heart catheterization include:

- assessment of filling pressures and cardiac output in patients in heart failure, especially when complicated by hypotension or renal failure
- assessment of volume status and vascular resistance in patients with sepsis
- evaluation of intracardiac shunts
- evaluation of pericardial disease (tamponade, constriction, etc.)
- perioperative monitoring of patients with a high risk of periprocedural heart failure

LEFT HEART CATHETERIZATION (LHC)

Hemodynamics

During LHC, a catheter is passed through the femoral artery and advanced retrograde through the aorta, across the aortic valve, and into the left ventricle (LV). Left ventricular pressure can then be measured, as can the pressure gradient across the aortic valve, thereby

TABLE 8–1

Characteristic Hemodynamic Profiles

Diagnosis	Systemic BP	RA Pressure	PA Pressure	PCW	CO	SVR	Treatment
Normal	120/80 mmHg	0–5 mmHg	12–30/5–15 mmHg	8–12 mmHg	5 L/min	800–1200 dynes-sec-cm^{-5}	
Cardiogenic shock	↓	↑	↑	↑	↓	↑↑	Vasopressors, inotropes
Septic shock	↓	↓	Nl or ↓	↓	↑	↓↓	Vasopressors, IV fluids, antibiotics
Hypovolemia	↓	↓	↓	↓	↓	↑	Volume resuscitation
Pulmonary hypertension/ Cor pulmonale	Nl	↑	↑↑↑	Nl	Nl	Nl	Pulmonary vaso-dilators, diuretics
Pericardial tamponade*	↓	↑	↑	↑	↓	↑	Pericardiocentesis

*In pericardial tamponade, the RA, PA diastolic, and PCW pressures are not only elevated, but are equal.

RA: right atrium; PA: pulmonary artery; PCW: pulmonary capillary wedge; CO: cardiac output: SVR: systemic vascular resistance; Nl: normal.

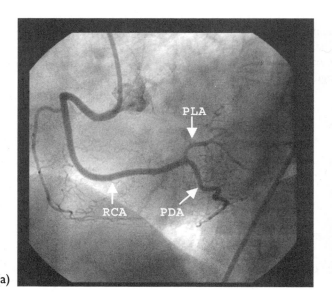

(a)

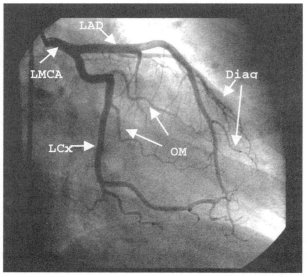

(b)

Figure 8–3 Normal coronary angiogram. (a) Normal right coronary artery (RCA) showing bifurcation into the posterior descending artery (PDA) and the posterolateral artery (PLA). (b) Normal left main coronary artery (LMCA) and its bifurcation into the left anterior descending (LAD) and left circumflex (LCx) arteries. The diagonal branches (Diag) arise from the LAD and the obtuse marginal (OM) branches arise from the LCx.

allowing for the assessment of aortic stenosis (see Figure 29.1). Simultaneous right and left heart catheterization permits measurement of the gradient across the mitral valve (MV), allowing for the assessment of mitral stenosis (MS) (see Figure 30–1).

Coronary angiography

Catheters can be directly placed into the coronary ostia (Figure 8–1a), through which radio-opaque contrast material is injected. The contrast fills the lumen of the coronary arteries and their branches, allowing visualization of the coronary anatomy and identification of stenoses or occlusions (Figure 8–3 and Figure 15–3).

Ventriculography and aortography

The left ventricle can be visualized by injection of contrast directly into the LV cavity. Contractility and wall motion of the ventricle can be assessed and mitral regurgitation can be quantified. Injection into the ascending aorta may help to assess the severity of aortic regurgitation, and may identify an aortic aneurysm or dissection.

INDICATIONS FOR LHC

Left heart catheterization may be performed for diagnostic or therapeutic purposes. Indications for **diagnostic** LHC include the following:

- to define the coronary anatomy in patients with:
  - acute ST elevation myocardial infarction (MI) (with a view to immediate angioplasty)
  - unstable angina or non-ST elevation MI with high-risk markers (especially if elevated troponin or concomitant heart failure)
  - post-infarction angina
  - stable angina refractory to medical therapy or with high-risk stress test result
  - cardiac arrest survivors
  - recurrent chest pain for which noninvasive testing is equivocal or nondiagnostic
- to measure hemodynamics and quantify valvular abnormalities in patients with aortic or mitral valve disease
- to assess left ventricular systolic function
- to evaluate proximal aortic disease (dissection or aneurysm)

- to assess hemodynamics in patients with suspected pericardial constriction or restriction

Therapeutic applications of cardiac catheterization include:

- angioplasty and stent placement for the treatment of coronary artery disease
- intra-aortic balloon pump placement for cardiogenic shock and as a bridge to surgery in patients with refractory ischemia or mechanical complications of MI
- balloon valvuloplasty for valvular stenosis
- percutaneous closure of intracardiac shunts

COMPLICATIONS OF CARDIAC CATHETERIZATION

The most frequent complication of cardiac catheterization is bleeding; this requires transfusion in ~1% of patients. Major complications such as death, MI, stroke, ventricular fibrillation, anaphylactic reactions to contrast, and emergent need for coronary artery bypass graft (CABG) are rare (<1% incidence). Contrast nephropathy occurs in as many as 15% of patients and is much more common in diabetics and patients with pre-existing renal insufficiency. Vascular injury at the access site (arterial laceration, thrombosis, distal embolization, pseudoaneurysm, AV fistula, hematoma, retroperitoneal hemorrhage), renal failure, cholesterol embolization, non-life threatening allergic reactions, infection at the access site, atrial arrhythmias, and heart block are also well recognized complications.

CONTRAINDICATIONS TO CARDIAC CATHETERIZATION

Relative contraindications to catheterization include:

- active infectious processes
- ongoing major organ bleeding
- recent (<1 month) stroke
- worsening renal impairment
- severe anemia
- severe electrolyte and/or acid–base disturbances
- severe active non-cardiac systemic illness
- severe uncontrolled psychiatric illness

- digitalis toxicity
- severe systemic hypertension

◆ KEY POINTS ◆

1. Cardiac catheterization is a safe and effective tool for the diagnosis of cardiovascular diseases.

2. Important information provided by cardiac catheterization includes right and left heart pressures, oxygen saturations, cardiac output, left ventricular function, and coronary artery anatomy.

3. Cardiac catheterization is the gold standard for assessing the severity of valvular heart disease, especially valvular stenosis.

9 Diagnostic Modalities for Arrhythmias

Several diagnostic modalities are available for use in patients with known or suspected arrhythmic disorders. These include tilt table testing, ambulatory ECG monitoring, and electrophysiological study (EPS) with programmed stimulation.

TILT-TABLE TESTING

During this test, a patient is strapped onto a level table and then tilted to an upright position (usually 60° from supine) for 15 to 30 minutes. The patient's blood pressure and heart rate are monitored and the patient is assessed for symptoms of presyncope or syncope.

Indications

The main indication for tilt-table testing is to evaluate patients with suspected neurocardiogenic (vasovagal) syncope. It may also be useful in patients with recurrent syncope of unclear cause.

Pathophysiology of the Response

Theoretically, rapidly assuming the upright position results in a sudden decrease in venous return to the right heart. This evokes a sudden increase in ventricular contractility and stimulates ventricular mechanofibers (C-fibers). A parasympathetic-mediated, paradoxical reflex ensues (Bezold-Jarisch reflex) in which systemic vascular resistance and heart rate both precipitously drop resulting in cerebral hypoperfusion and syncope.

Interpretation of the Test

Three abnormal responses may be seen:

- cardioinhibitory response: sudden heart block and/or drop in heart rate without significant blood pressure change
- vasodepressor response: a dramatic reduction in blood pressure with little change in the heart rate (less common)
- mixed response: a combination of the cardioinhibitory and vasodepressor responses (most common abnormal response)

The test is considered positive if it precipitates a syncopal episode or elicits presyncopal symptoms in the face of a significant reduction in heart rate and/or blood pressure (Figure 9–1). The sensitivity of this test for the detection of vasovagal syncope is approximately 70%. Unfortunately, serial testing of an individual patient may not elicit the same response, and 20–25% of patients without a history of syncope will have an abnormal test.

AMBULATORY ECG MONITORING

An ambulatory ECG monitor (Holter monitor) is a portable telemetric device that allows continuous ECG recording in the outpatient setting. Patients usually wear the device for 24 to 48 hours, during which they

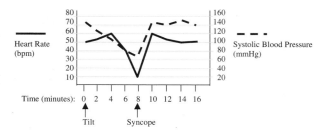

Figure 9–1   Abnormal response to tilt table testing. Following initial tilt to 60°, the patient rapidly developed hypotension and bradycardia (mixed vasodepressor and cardio-inhibitory response), and subsequently lost consciousness. This resolved after lying the patient supine.

perform their usual activities and record any symptoms that they experience. The device is interrogated for the presence of arrhythmias, which can then be correlated with the patient's symptoms. Indications for Holter monitoring include:

- to evaluate for an arrhythmic cause of unexplained syncope, near syncope, or dizziness
- to evaluate for an arrhythmic cause of palpitations
- to assess a patient's response to antiarrhythmic therapy

Twenty-four hour monitoring may be helpful for patients who have frequent symptoms; however, infrequent symptoms are unlikely to occur during the short duration of recording. Loop monitors (or event monitors) are similar to the 24-hour monitors but can be worn for weeks or months at a time and record a person's ECG when the device is activated. This device may be useful for the evaluation of infrequent symptoms. Devices are now available that are implanted under the skin of the chest wall and can remain in place for many months. These may be useful to evaluate very infrequent symptoms.

ELECTROPHYSIOLOGICAL STUDY (EPS)

Electrophysiological studies involve the introduction of multiple catheter-based electrodes through the femoral veins and into the right atrium and ventricle. These electrodes are then strategically positioned in

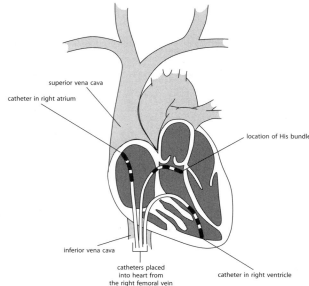

Figure 9–2   Intracardiac position of catheters for electrophysiological studies. The catheters are positioned to allow measurement of electrical activity in the right atrium (RA), right ventricle (RV), and the bundle of His. *Illustration by Shawn Girsberger Graphic Design.*

the heart and used to measure endocardial electrical activity (Figure 9–2). Each segment of the cardiac conduction system (from the sinoatrial node to the His-Purkinje fibers) can be systematically studied to assess its ability to conduct electrical impulses normally. Additionally, the atrial and ventricular myocardium and the conduction system can be evaluated to determine their ability to generate and maintain tachyarrhythmias.

Indications

EP studies are primarily indicated in the evaluation of certain tachyarrhythmias. They may also occasionally be useful in assessing certain bradyarrhythmias. Specific indications include the evaluation of:

- non-sustained ventricular tachycardia (VT) in patients with prior myocardial infarction (MI) and left ventricular ejection fraction (LVEF) <35%
- sustained VT or cardiac arrest in the absence of a precipitating cause (e.g., ischemia, hypokalemia)

- supraventricular tachycardia (SVT) of uncertain mechanism

- wide complex tachycardia of uncertain origin

- heart block of unclear etiology (especially 2nd-degree heart block, type 2)

- unexplained syncope in patients with decreased LVEF

- possibly for risk-stratifying patients with symptomatic hypertrophic cardiomyopathy

Once the EP catheters are in place, attempts are made to induce the tachyarrhythmia by electrically stimulating certain areas of the heart (programmed electrical stimulation). Once the arrhythmia is induced, its conduction sequence can be mapped. In certain arrhythmias, the electrical circuit by which the arrhythmia is perpetuated can be interrupted with the use of radiofrequency (RF) energy. This energy is used to make a focal burn in the endocardium overlying a part of the abnormal circuit. This **ablates** the conductive tissue where the energy was applied, thereby destroying the circuit and preventing recurrences of the arrhythmia (**RF ablation**). Examples of arrhythmias that are frequently amenable to RF ablation include:

- atrioventricular reentrant tachycardia (e.g., Wolff-Parkinson-White)

- AV nodal reentrant tachycardia

- atrial flutter

- certain forms of ventricular tachycardia

Patients who have inducible ventricular tachyarrhythmias during an EP study may be candidates for implantation of a cardioverter-defibrillator.

◆ KEY POINTS ◆

1. Tilt-table testing is indicated for the evaluation of suspected neurocardiogenic syncope.

2. Twenty-four hour ambulatory EKG monitoring may be helpful in identifying arrhythmias that occur on a relatively frequent basis. Event monitors are useful in evaluating less frequent arrhythmias.

3. EP testing may be used to determine the mechanism of both tachy- and bradyarrhythmias, and to localize the source or pathway of a tachyarrhythmia so that RF ablation can be performed.

10

Other Imaging Modalities

Although the vast majority of cardiac imaging is performed with echocardiography, nuclear perfusion imaging, or coronary angiography, several other imaging modalities are currently in clinical use or may be so in the future.

CHEST RADIOGRAPHY
(see Figure 10–1)

Chest radiography provides an image of various cardiac and vascular structures and remains an important tool in the initial evaluation of patients with suspected heart disease. In reviewing a chest x-ray (CXR) for evidence of cardiovascular disease, attention should be focused on the following:

- cardiac size (normally less than ½ the thoracic diameter)
- evidence of individual chamber enlargement (see Table 10–1)
- the pulmonary vasculature (cephalization of pulmonary vessels, Kerley B lines, pulmonary artery enlargement; see Table 10–2)
- aortic and mediastinal size
- evidence of prior cardiothoracic surgery (sternotomy wires, surgical clips, prosthetic rings and/or valves, pacemaker, implantable defibrillator)
- calcification of the vasculature, valves, or pericardium

MULTIPLE GATED BLOOD POOL IMAGING (MUGA)

MUGA, a form of radionuclide ventriculography (RVG), is one of the most reliable methods of quantifying ventricular systolic function. In performing a MUGA, the patient's blood is labeled with a radioactive tracer and the radioactivity subsequently emitted from the heart is measured with a gamma camera. The quantity of radiation emitted at any instant reflects the amount of blood in the heart at that point in time. By "gating" the measurement of radioactivity to the person's ECG, systolic and diastolic radiation emission can be measured separately and compared; the difference reflects the amount of blood ejected from the heart with each contraction (the **ejection fraction**). Both right ventricular and left ventricular ejection fractions can be accurately measured.

Advantages
- high degree of accuracy
- reproducible
- provides information about both right and left ventricular function
- assessment of function not limited by body habitus
- easy to perform (requires less than 30 minutes)

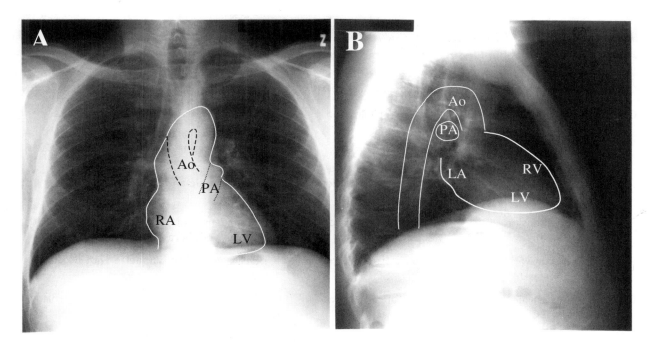

Figure 10–1 Normal chest x-ray and location of cardiac structures. (a) Posterior-anterior view. (b) Lateral view. Ao: aorta; LA: left atrium; LV: left ventricle; PA: pulmonary artery; RA: right atrium; RV: right ventricle.

TABLE 10–1

Characteristic Radiographic Findings of Specific Cardiac Abnormalities

Cardiac Abnormality	Associated Radiographic Finding
Left atrial enlargement	Straightening or lateral bulging of left heart border, widening of the carinal angle to >75°
Right atrial enlargement	Bulging of right heart border
Left ventricular hypertrophy	Rounding of left ventricular apex
Left ventricular enlargement	Downward and lateral displacement of left ventricular apex, globular appearance, loss of retrocardiac air space (on lateral view)
Right ventricular enlargement	Loss of retrosternal air space (on lateral view)

Disadvantages

- radiation exposure
- provides essentially no information about valvular structure and function
- less accurate in patients with arrhythmias

Clinical Utility

MUGA/RVG is frequently used when accurate, serial measurements of ventricular function are needed and slight changes in ejection fraction are clinically significant. Such situations include monitoring for cardiotoxicity in patients receiving chemotherapy, and evaluation

TABLE 10–2

Abnormal Radiographic Findings in Selected Cardiovascular Disorders

Cardiovascular Disorder	Abnormal CXR Finding	Radiographic Appearance
Congestive heart failure	Vascular cephalization	Prominent vessels in upper lung fields
	Kerley B lines	Horizontal, linear densities in the lateral lung fields reflecting engorged lymphatic vessels
	Blunting of the costo-phrenic angle (i.e., pleural effusion)	Concave upward radio-opacity of the costophrenic angle
Pulmonary hypertension	Pruning of the pulmonary vasculature	Prominent central pulmonary arteries with loss of peripheral pulmonary vasculature
Pericardial effusion with or without tamponade	"Water bottle" heart	Enlarged cardiac silhouette with broad inferior diameter
Constrictive pericarditis	Pericardial calcification	Thin, radio-opaque outline of the cardiac silhouette
Aortic aneurysm/dissection	Widened mediastinum	Wide mediastinal shadow
Congenital cardiac shunts (ASD, VSD)	Shunt vascularity	Increased pulmonary vascular markings; atrial enlargement

ASD: atrial septal defect; VSD: ventricular septal defect.

pre- and post-cardiac transplantation to monitor for acute allograft rejection. MUGA is also useful to determine LV and RV systolic function when technical limitations (e.g., extreme obesity, severe COPD) impair the quality of the images obtained by other modalities (e.g., echocardiography).

ELECTRON BEAM COMPUTED TOMOGRAPHY (EBCT)

EBCT, formerly known as **ultrafast** or **cine** CT, provides high-resolution imaging of the heart that is gated to the cardiac cycle. It differs from standard CT in that the imaging source does not need to be rotated around the patient, thus allowing for faster image acquisition. EBCT can provide both anatomic and functional data, including the assessment of ventricular volumes, myocardial mass, ejection fraction, regional cardiac

function, contractility, infarct size, valvular function, and pericardial disease. In addition, it can detect and quantify coronary artery calcification, a surrogate marker of coronary atherosclerosis (see Figure 10–2).

Advantages
- superb image resolution
- not limited by patient's body habitus
- rapid acquisition time
- relatively inexpensive (~$475)

Disadvantages
- provides anatomical not physiological information
- movement during image acquisition can lead to artifact
- patient must breath hold for 20–50 seconds to reduce motion artifact

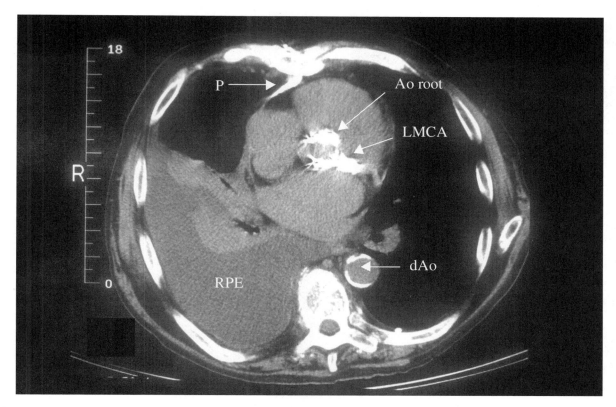

Figure 10–2 Electron beam CT in a patient with severe coronary artery disease and constrictive pericarditis. There is dense calcification of the aortic root (AO root), left main coronary artery (LMCA), descending thoracic aorta (dAo), and the pericardium (P). A large right pleural effusion (RPE) is also noted.

- radiation exposure

- intravenous contrast (typically required for image acquisition) may be nephrotoxic

- 25% of coronary segments can't be imaged owing to respiratory motion artifact, excessive calcification, or small vessel caliber

Clinical Utility

Currently, the main utility of cardiac EBCT is in the evaluation of pericardial diseases and cardiac tumors. It is the test of choice for the visualization of the pericardium in suspected constrictive pericarditis, and for anatomical delineation of invasive cardiac tumors. EBCT may also play a role in the noninvasive assess-

ment of coronary artery disease (CAD). Coronary arterial calcification is an early component of atherosclerotic plaque formation, and its measurement may reflect total atherosclerotic burden. EBCT can accurately detect and quantify coronary calcium, and, as such, it can be used as a screening test to identify CAD in asymptomatic patients. A calcium score can be derived (range from 0 to >400); high scores (>400) have a strong correlation with the presence of obstructive CAD (sensitivity: 80–100%), but have low specificity (40–60%). Nonetheless, the finding of coronary calcification in an asymptomatic patient does not warrant any specific therapy aside from risk factor modification, and controversy exists regarding the appropriate use of this modality in predicting clinical outcome or guiding preventive therapy.

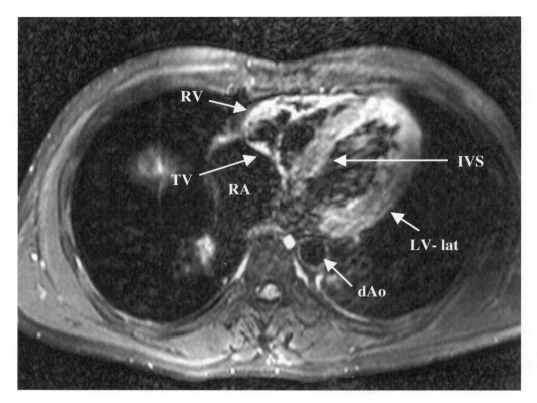

Figure 10–3   Cardiac MRI. IVS: interventricular septum; LV-lat: lateral wall of the left ventricle; RV: right ventricle; RA: right atrium; TV: tricuspid valve. Image courtesy of R. Tello, Dept of Radiology, Boston Medical Center, Boston, Massachusetts.

CARDIAC MRI

Cardiac magnetic resonance imaging (MRI) offers great potential as a new modality for noninvasive cardiac imaging (Figure 10–3); however, its application in clinical medicine has been limited by the complex nature of the technology and its high cost. Images are obtained in the same way as routine MRI, and image acquisition is gated to the person's ECG so that systole and diastole can be distinguished. Patients must be able to hold their breath for 20–50 seconds to eliminate respiratory motion during image acquisition. Cardiac MRI provides a variety of anatomical and functional information including left and right ventricular ejection fraction, myocardial mass, intracardiac volumes, regional wall motion analysis, myocardial ischemia, myocardial viability, coronary anatomy, valvular structure and function, anatomical abnormalities, pericardial diseases, infiltrative disorders of the myocardium, and myocardial wall thickness.

Advantages

- superb image resolution, without interference from lung, bone, or fat
- absence of radiation exposure
- images can be obtained in any orientation or geometric plane
- provides for assessment of almost every aspect of cardiac anatomy and performance

Disadvantages

- not available at all facilities
- costly
- sophisticated technology that requires additional, extensive training

- requires gating of images to the ECG (may be difficult in patients with atrial fibrillation)
- cannot be used in patients with pacemakers, defibrillators, or other metallic foreign bodies
- patients with claustrophobia may not be able to tolerate the study
- motion during image acquisition can result in artifacts
- patients must be able to hold their breath for 20–50 seconds

Clinical Utility

Currently, cardiac MRI is used predominantly for research purposes. In the future, it may become clinically useful for the assessment of myocardial and valvular function, delineation of coronary anatomy, detection of myocardial ischemia, detection of post-infarction complications (e.g., ventricular septal defects, left ventricular aneurysms), assessment of myocardial viability, and for the diagnosis of myocardial and pericardial diseases.

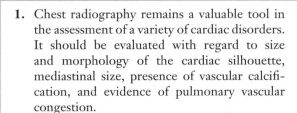

◆ KEY POINTS ◆

1. Chest radiography remains a valuable tool in the assessment of a variety of cardiac disorders. It should be evaluated with regard to size and morphology of the cardiac silhouette, mediastinal size, presence of vascular calcification, and evidence of pulmonary vascular congestion.
2. MUGA scanning provides an accurate and highly reproducible assessment of LV and RV function.
3. Electron beam computed tomography (CT) is the test of choice for visualizing pericardial thickening and invasive cardiac tumors. It may also play a role as a screening test for CAD.
4. Currently, cardiac MRI is mainly investigational; however, it may soon play a role in the diagnostic evaluation of a variety of cardiac disorders.

Part III
Coronary Artery
Disease

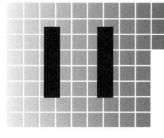

Coronary Artery Disease— Pathophysiology

Coronary artery disease (CAD) is the leading cause of death in the United States, accounting for one half of the nearly one million deaths resulting from cardiovascular disease each year. The term atherosclerosis is derived from the Greek "athero" (gruel) and "sclerosis" (hardening). Atherosclerosis of the coronary arteries is the major cause of CAD; intracoronary thrombosis (atherothrombosis) also plays an important role. CAD is a progressive degenerative process that begins in childhood and manifests in middle to late adulthood as acute coronary syndromes (i.e., unstable angina and acute myocardial infarction [MI]) or chronic ischemic heart disease (e.g., chronic stable angina, ischemic cardiomyopathy). Epidemiological studies have identified multiple risk factors for atherosclerosis and CAD; the modification of these risk factors holds promise for the prevention and treatment of this disease.

NORMAL CORONARY ANATOMY

The heart receives blood through the left and right coronary arteries, which are the first branches of the aorta (Figure 11–1). The right coronary artery (RCA) gives off acute marginal branches to the right ventricle, and, in 85% of people, it also gives off branches to the inferior aspect (posterior descending artery [PDA]) and posterior aspect (posterolateral branches) of the left ventricle. This is referred to as **right dominant circulation**.

The left main coronary artery is quite short and bifurcates into the left anterior descending (LAD) and the left circumflex (LCx) arteries. The LAD gives off diagonal branches that supply blood to the anterior aspect of the left ventricle, and the LCx artery gives off obtuse marginal branches that supply blood to the lateral aspect of the left ventricle. In 10% of people, the LCx gives rise to both the posterior descending and posterolateral arteries (**left dominant circulation**). In 5% of people, the RCA gives rise to the posterior descending artery and the LCx gives rise to the posterolateral arteries (**codominant circulation**).

Small collateral vessels interconnect the coronary arteries. These collaterals are non-functional in the normal setting but provide an alternate route for blood flow if the coronary artery becomes stenosed.

NORMAL CORONARY ARTERY PHYSIOLOGY

The coronary arteries are conductance vessels and offer very little resistance to coronary blood flow in their normal state. They can, however, constrict or dilate in response to vasoactive substances, thereby allowing the heart to maintain a fairly constant level of coronary blood flow despite changes in perfusion pressure. This phenomenon is referred to as **autoregulation** and allows coronary blood flow to increase in the face of increased myocardial oxygen demand (e.g., exercise).

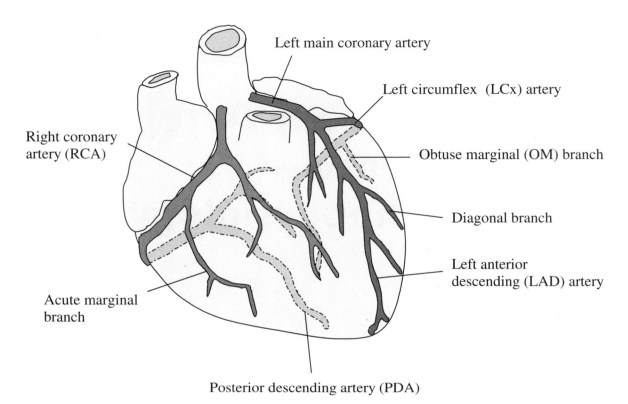

Left main coronary artery

Left circumflex (LCx) artery

Right coronary artery (RCA)

Obtuse marginal (OM) branch

Diagonal branch

Left anterior descending (LAD) artery

Acute marginal branch

Posterior descending artery (PDA)

Figure 11–1   Anatomy of the coronary arteries.

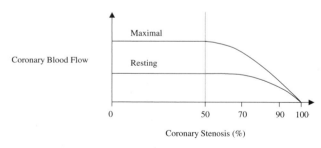

Coronary Blood Flow

Maximal

Resting

0   50   70   90 100

Coronary Stenosis (%)

Figure 11–2   Coronary flow reserve and alterations in coronary blood flow in relation to the degree of coronary artery stenosis present. "Maximal" refers to the maximal coronary blood flow possible in response to increased myocardial oxygen demand. The difference between the maximal and resting flows is the coronary flow reserve. Maximal coronary blood flow is significantly reduced in the face of a stenosis of >70%. Resting coronary blood flow is not significantly affected until the stenosis is >90%.

The difference between the resting coronary blood flow and the maximal coronary blood flow is referred to as the **coronary flow reserve** (Figure 11–2).

The normal arterial wall consists of the endothelium, the intima, the media, and the adventitia. The endothelium plays an important role in autoregulation. It synthesizes and releases powerful vasodilators such as endothelium-derived relaxing factor (nitric oxide) and prostacyclin in response to various stimuli, including platelet-derived factors (acetylcholine, serotonin, and adenosine 5′-diphosphate [ADP]), thrombin, and increased shear stress (**flow-mediated vasodilation**). The endothelium is also intimately involved in the prevention of intravascular thrombosis via its production of antiplatelet (heparan, prostacyclin) and thrombolytic (tissue plasminogen activator) factors. Thus, a normal, intact endothelium is crucial in regulating coronary vascular tone and maintaining adequate coronary blood flow.

PATHOGENESIS OF ATHEROSCLEROSIS

The initiating event of atherosclerosis is an injury to the vascular endothelium; the subsequent response to this injury leads to the development of atherosclerotic lesions. The initial injury can be mechanical (shear stress), biochemical (e.g., lipoproteins, tobacco), and possibly infectious (e.g., viruses, *Chlamydia*). This injury results in alterations in endothelial permeability, increased adhesiveness of leukocytes to the endothelium, and altered release of vasoactive and hemostatic substances from endothelial cells. These changes, collectively referred to as **endothelial dysfunction**, are the earliest measurable changes of atherosclerosis and result in a local prothrombotic state and impaired ability of the endothelium to modify vascular tone.

Following the initial injury, circulating monocytes adhere to the endothelial surface and migrate into the vascular intima where they become macrophages. Low-density lipoprotein (LDL) is transported through the endothelial cells and ingested by the macrophages, thus producing "foam cells." Collections of these foam cells produce the earliest visible lesion of atherosclerosis, a yellowish deposit in the vascular wall known as a "fatty streak."

The activated macrophages produce and release toxic substances (e.g., superoxide anion, oxidized LDL) that result in endothelial denudation and subsequent platelet adhesion to the site of injury. Platelets and activated macrophages also release various cytokines and growth factors resulting in the migration and proliferation of T cells, smooth muscle cells, and fibroblasts. This process eventually creates a neointima with a fibrous cap overlying the lipid core.

THE ATHEROSCLEROTIC PLAQUE

Atherosclerotic plaques may be predominantly fibrotic or may consist of a large lipid core with a thin fibrous cap (Figure 11–3). Fibrotic plaques generally appear during early adulthood, are white in appearance and may progressively protrude into and narrow the lumen of the artery, resulting in decreased coronary blood flow. In response, the vessel distal to the stenosis dilates in the resting state to allow for normalization of resting blood flow. This, however, decreases the vessel's ability to augment flow in response to increased metabolic demands (decreased coronary flow reserve). Once the metabolic demands exceed the maximal coronary blood flow, ischemia and angina develop. In general, a 70% decrease in the diameter of the artery is enough to limit blood flow in the face of increased demand (e.g., exercise) and produce exertional angina. A 90% decrease in the arterial diameter may limit blood flow

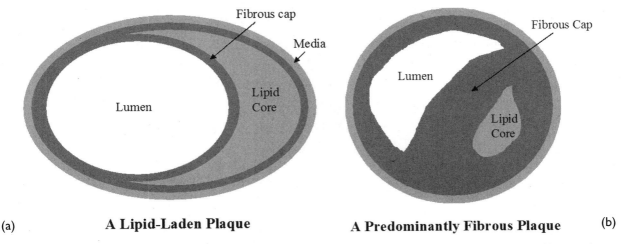

(a) **A Lipid-Laden Plaque**   **A Predominantly Fibrous Plaque** (b)

Figure 11–3 Morphology of atherosclerotic plaques. (a) Lipid-rich plaque. (b) Predominantly fibrous plaque (see text for details).

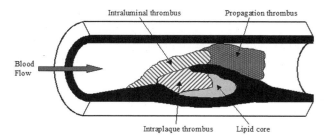

Figure 11–4 A vulnerable plaque with rupture of the shoulder region and subsequent thrombosis of the vascular lumen.

TABLE 11–1

Risk Factors for Atherosclerosis

Positive Risk Factors	Major:
	Hypertension
	Hyperlipidemia
	Smoking
	Diabetes mellitus
	Male gender
	Advanced age
	Family history of premature atherosclerosis
	Minor:
	Obesity
	Physical inactivity
	Hyperhomocysteinemia
	Elevated lipoprotein a (Lpa)
	Elevated fibrinogen levels
	Elevated plasminogen activator inhibitor
Negative Risk Factors	Elevated HDL

and result in angina even in the resting state (see Figure 11–2).

In largely lipid-laden plaques, the accumulating lipid causes necrosis of the macrophages, resulting in the release of digestive enzymes such as collagenase and gelatinase (matrix metalloproteinases). These enzymes weaken the fibrous cap and a "vulnerable plaque" is formed. This type of plaque is prone to fissure or rupture, especially at the edge (or "shoulder") of the lesion (Figure 11–4). Such plaque rupture exposes the lipid core and vascular collagen to the circulating blood, leading to platelet activation and aggregation. A thrombus is then formed at the site of plaque rupture, resulting in partial or complete occlusion of the coronary artery and resulting in the clinical syndromes of unstable angina and acute myocardial infarction (refer to Chapters 14 and 15).

RISK FACTORS

Many epidemiological studies have demonstrated an association between CAD and certain risk factors, some of which clearly play a causal role (e.g., hypertension, hyperlipidemia, diabetes, smoking) (see Table 11–1). High-density lipoprotein (HDL) is a negative risk factor; higher levels of HDL cholesterol (>60 mg/dl) are associated with a decreased risk of CAD. Some risk factors (e.g., diabetes, hypercholesterolemia, smoking, etc.) can be modified, whereas others (age, gender, and family history) cannot. Modification of risk factors decreases the future risk of CAD, stabilizes existing CAD, and potentially stimulates regression of atherosclerotic plaques in patients with established disease.

◆ KEY POINTS ◆

1. Coronary artery disease is the leading cause of death in the United States.

2. Coronary artery disease is caused by atherosclerosis of the coronary arteries and has both acute and chronic manifestations (refer to Chapters 14 and 15).

3. Atherosclerosis is characterized by endothelial injury, inflammation, lipid deposition, plaque formation, and thrombosis.

4. Risk factors for CAD can be identified and modified to reduce the risk of this disease.

12

Dyslipidemia

Dyslipidemia refers to a group of disorders characterized by abnormal circulating levels of lipid or lipoprotein fractions. They are caused by genetic and/or environmental conditions that alter the metabolism of these lipoproteins.

NORMAL LIPID AND LIPOPROTEIN METABOLISM
(see Figure 12–1)

The major plasma lipoproteins are distinguished by their lipid content and density, and their constituent proteins (Table 12–1). **Chylomicrons** (formed within the intestine from dietary fat) and **very-low-density lipoproteins** (VLDL) (produced in the liver) are both rich in **triglycerides** (TG). They are metabolized to **chylomicron remnants** and **intermediate-density lipoproteins** (IDL), respectively, after acquiring apolipoprotein C-II (apo C-II) from **high-density lipoproteins** (HDL) and then undergoing hydrolysis by lipoprotein lipase (LPL) in muscle and adipose tissue. The liver clears chylomicron remnants, and IDL undergoes further conversion to **low-density lipoproteins** (LDL), which can circulate for 3–5 days. LDL accounts for approximately 70% of the total plasma cholesterol and is cleared mainly by the liver.

Lipoprotein (a) [Lp(a)] is secreted by the liver and makes up less than 10% of the total plasma lipoprotein mass. LDL, together with Lp(a), has been shown to be atherogenic, and elevated levels are associated with increased risk of cardiovascular disease. HDL is secreted by both the liver and intestine; it readily accepts cholesterol from cells and other lipoproteins, and is believed to be cardioprotective.

EPIDEMIOLOGY

Approximately 32% of American men and 27% of American women have hypercholesterolemia that requires treatment. More than half of the coronary heart disease in the United States is attributable to lipid abnormalities, predominantly elevated LDL cholesterol. An individual's cholesterol or LDL is, on average, intermediate between that of his parents, reflecting genetic influences.

ETIOLOGY

In the majority of people, elevated lipid levels result from a combination of factors that include obesity, inactivity, a diet high in fats and cholesterol, and genetic predisposition. A minority of patients have dyslipidemia that results purely from genetic mutations in the genes involved in lipid metabolism (primary dyslipidemias). The underlying metabolic defects and

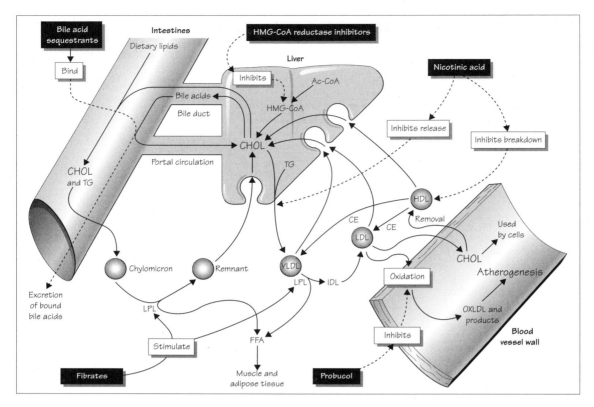

Figure 12–1   Normal metabolism of lipoproteins and sites of action of lipid lowering agents.
(Used with permission from: Aaronson PI, et al. The Cardiovascular System at a Glance.
Oxford: Blackwell Science, 1999: 70.)

TABLE 12–1

Properties of Lipoproteins

Lipoprotein Class	Origin	Major Surface Apoproteins	Major Core Lipid
Chylomicrons	Intestine	B-48, C, E	Dietary TG, cholesterol esters
VLDL	Liver	B-100, C, E	Hepatic TG
LDL	VLDL catabolism	B-100	Cholesterol esters
Lp (a)	Liver	B-100, (a)	Cholesterol esters
HDL	Liver, intestine	A, C	Cholesterol esters

TG: triglyceride; VLDL: very low-density lipoprotein; LDL: low-density lipoprotein; HDL: high-density lipoprotein; Lp (a):
lipoprotein (a).

associated lipid profiles of these primary dyslipidemias
are outlined in Table 12–2. Of these primary dyslipidemias, **polygenic hypercholesterolemia** is the most
common.

A variety of conditions can produce elevated lipoprotein levels in the absence of an underlying genetic defect
(**secondary hyperlipidemia**). These conditions are outlined in Table 12–3.

TABLE 12–2

Classification of Primary Dyslipidemias

Class	Lipid Profile	Phenotypes	Metabolic Defect(s)
I, V	↑ chylomicrons (class I) ↑ VLDL (class V)	Familial LPL deficiency Familial apo CII deficiency	Impairment/absence of LPL Functional deficiency of LPL
IIa	↑ LDL	Familial hypercholesterolemia; Familial defective apoB100; Polygenic hypercholesterolemia	LDL receptor defects (↓ receptor number or ↓ affinity for LDL)
IIb	↑ VLDL, ↑ LDL	Familial combined hyperlipidemia	↑ VLDL secretion +/− LPL defect
III	↑ VLDL, ↑ IDL	Dysbetalipoproteinemia	Defective apoE
IV	↑ VLDL	Familial hypertriglyceridemia	↑ VLDL production or ↓ TG metabolism

VLDL: very low-density lipoprotein; LDL: low-density lipoprotein; LPL: lipoprotein lipase.

TABLE 12–3

Secondary Causes of Hyperlipidemia

Secondary Causes of Hypercholesterolemia	Secondary Causes of Hypertriglyceridemia
High-fat diet	Type II diabetes mellitus
Obstructive liver disease	Obesity
Nephrotic syndrome	Hypothyroidism
Hypothyroidism	Alcohol use
Medications (corticosteroids, anabolic steroids, progestins)	Medications (beta-blockers, diuretics, estrogen)

DETECTION OF DYSLIPIDEMIA

Every adult over the age of 20 years should have a complete fasting lipid profile (total serum cholesterol, HDL-cholesterol [HDL$_c$], and TGs) measured every 5 years. If TG levels are <400 mg/dL, then LDL-cholesterol (LDL$_c$) can be calculated as follows:

$$LDLc = Total\ cholesterol - (HDLc + TG/5)$$

CLINICAL MANIFESTATIONS

History

Most patients with hyperlipidemia are asymptomatic, although patients with severe hypertriglyceridemia (TG > 1,000 mg/dL) may present with acute pancreatitis. Patients should be thoroughly questioned regarding symptoms of cardiovascular disease (angina, claudication, transient ischemic attack [TIA], cerebrovascular accident [CVA]). Measurement of lipid levels should be performed in concert with a search for other major risk factors for coronary artery disease (CAD), including:

- current cigarette smoking
- hypertension (BP > 140/90 mmHg, or on antihypertensive medications)
- age (men ≥45 years, women ≥55 years)
- family history of premature CAD (in males <55 years or females <65 years). A strong family history of dyslipidemia or cardiovascular disease suggests a primary lipid disorder.
- HDL: low HDL (<40 mg/dl) is a risk factor for CAD, whereas high HDL (>60 mg/dl) is considered protective and negates the effect of one other risk factor.

PHYSICAL EXAMINATION

Corneal arcus (a gray ring around the cornea), xanthelasmas (yellowish peri-orbital plaques), xanthomas (subcutaneous nodules on extensor tendons), and hepatosplenomegaly are sometimes present in patients with dyslipidemias. Manifestations of atherosclerosis, including diminished peripheral pulses and arterial bruits should be looked for in patients with, or suspected of having, a dyslipidemia.

TREATMENT

Goals (see Table 12–4)

For the vast majority of hyperlipidemic patients, the goal of therapy is reducing CAD risk by lowering LDL_c. The National Cholesterol Education Program (NCEP) has developed guidelines (Adult Treatment Panel III, or ATP III) for treating hyperlipidemia based on a person's absolute lipid levels, the presence of CAD or CAD equivalents (other atherosclerotic disease, including symptomatic carotid artery disease, peripheral arterial disease, and abdominal aortic aneurysm; and

TABLE 12–4

LDL Treatment Recommendations

Risk Profile	LDL Level at which to Initiate Drug Therapy	Goal LDL
Without CAD, fewer than 2 other risk factors	≥190	<160
Without CAD, 2 or more risk factors	≥160	<130
With CAD or CAD equivalent*	≥130[a]	<100

*CAD equivalent refers to other atherosclerotic disease or diabetes mellitus.

[a] Physician should exercise clinical judgement in patients with LDL of 101–129 mg/dL to determine if drug therapy should be initiated.

diabetes mellitus), and the presence of other coexisting cardiac risk factors (refer to the section on History). In patients without CAD and with fewer than two other cardiac risk factors, the goal of treatment is an LDL_c <160mg/dL; in patients with two or more risk factors, the goal LDL_c is <130mg/dL. Patients with known CAD or CAD equivalents should have an LDL_c of <100mg/dL.

Hypertriglyceridemia (TG ≥150mg/dL) is usually associated with, and responds to treatment of, elevated LDL_c. For persistently elevated TGs, therapy should be instituted to lower the non-HDL cholesterol (total cholesterol – HDL_c) to no greater than 30mg/dL above the respective LDL_c goal.

Nonpharmacological Therapy

Primary treatment for hypercholesterolemia and hypertriglyceridemia involves dietary therapy, in concert with weight loss and regular exercise. These measures are collectively referred to as therapeutic lifestyle changes (TLC) under ATP III. The TLC diet derives less than 7% of total calories from saturated fat and contains <200mg/day of cholesterol. Intake of soluble fiber (10–25 g/day) and plant stanols/sterols (2 g/day) should also be considered as therapeutic options to enhance LDL lowering. On average, dietary therapy lowers lipid levels by about 10–20%. Secondary causes of dyslipidemia should also be corrected or treated.

Pharmacological Therapy (see Table 12–5)

Drug therapy for hypercholesterolemia should be considered when LDL_c level remains above the initiation level for drug therapy despite 3 to 6 months of maximal dietary therapy. Pharmacological treatment may also be considered as initial therapy in addition to diet in patients with elevated lipid levels and known CAD, atherosclerotic vascular disease, or diabetes. The preferred first line agent for hypercholesterolemia is an HMG-CoA reductase inhibitor, or "statin," because of its efficacy in reducing both LDL and cardiovascular events (myocardial infarction [MI] or death). Second line agents include niacin and bile acid sequestrants (e.g., cholestyramine). These agents may also be added to a statin for refractory patients, in which case close monitoring for liver toxicity is required.

TABLE 12–5

Lipid-Lowering Agents

Drug Class	Mechanism of Action	Lipid Effects	Side Effects
Bile-acid sequestrants	↑ Fecal bile acid excretion ↑ LDL-receptor activity	↓↓ LDL ↑ HDL ?↑ TG	Constipation Abdominal bloating ↓ Absorption of other drugs
Nicotinic acid (niacin)	↓ Plasma free fatty acids ↓ Hepatic VLDL synthesis	↓ LDL ↑ HDL ↓↓ TG	Elevated LFTs Increased uric acid GI upset, flushing and pruritis
HMG-CoA reductase inhibitors (statins)	↓ Cholesterol biosynthesis ↑ LDL-receptor activity	↓↓ LDL ↑ HDL ↓ TG	Elevated LFTs Myositis (↑ CK; rare) Mild GI symptoms
Fibric-acid derivatives (fibrates)	↓ Hepatic VLDL synthesis ↑ LPL activity	+/− LDL ↑ HDL ↓↓ TG	Elevated LFTs Cholelithiasis Myositis (rare) Diarrhea, nausea
Probucol	Enhances scavenger pathway removal of LDL	↓ LDL ↓↓ HDL − TG	Prolonged QT Ventricular arrhythmias (rare) Nausea, diarrhea Flatulence

LFTs: liver function tests; CK: creatine kinase.

Drug therapy for hypertriglyceridemia is recommended if TG levels remain high (≥200 mg/dL) for any patient, or borderline high (150–199 mg/dL) for patients with CAD risk factors despite an adequate trial of lifestyle modification. A statin is usually sufficient therapy in patients with borderline elevations of TG; niacin or a fibric-acid derivative (fibrate) may be necessary for patients with higher TG levels. Patients should be monitored closely when statins and fibrates are used in combination, as this regimen is associated with a higher risk of myositis and rhabdomyolysis.

A fasting lipid profile should be obtained 1 to 3 months after starting or changing lipid therapy. If goal lipid levels are not achieved, more aggressive lifestyle modifications or pharmacological therapy should be employed. Liver function tests and serum creatine kinase (CK) level should also be checked several months after initiation of pharmacological therapy to assess for occult toxicity.

◆ KEY POINTS ◆

1. The major serum lipids are LDL, HDL, and triglycerides.

2. Dyslipidemias usually result from the combined effects of diet, inactivity, obesity, and genetic factors.

3. Elevated LDL cholesterol, and to a lesser extent elevated triglycerides, is associated with increased risk of CAD and cardiovascular events.

4. Low HDL (<40 mg/dL) is a risk factor for CAD, whereas increased HDL (>60 mg/dL) is protective.

5. The treatment of dyslipidemias is based on the absolute level of lipids, the presence of other CAD risk factors, and the presence of established cardiovascular disease or diabetes mellitus.

13 Chronic Stable Angina

Angina is the clinical manifestation of myocardial ischemia. It is overwhelmingly the result of a limitation in coronary blood flow induced by atherosclerotic narrowing of the coronary arteries. Angina that is long-standing and reproduced by a predictable amount of exertion is referred to as **chronic stable angina**.

PATHOPHYSIOLOGY

Normal coronary arteries mediate changes in coronary blood flow in response to changes in myocardial oxygen demand (MVO_2). When the demands of the heart increase (such as during exercise), the coronary arteries dilate to allow increased blood flow to meet these demands (see Figure 11–2). This system of autoregulation occurs at the level of the arterioles, requires an intact vascular endothelium, and is mediated by byproducts of metabolism including adenosine, acidosis, low oxygen tension, and high levels of carbon dioxide. When a coronary artery becomes narrowed by greater than 70%, its blood flow is decreased by approximately 90%. In this setting, maximal coronary vasodilation occurs and allows for enough blood flow to meet the metabolic demands of the resting heart. However, during periods of increased myocardial demand (e.g., exercise), the artery is unable to dilate further, resulting in inadequate coronary blood flow and ischemia. Higher grade stenoses (>90% reduction in diameter) may cause ischemia in the resting state. The narrowing

of coronary arteries is overwhelmingly the result of atherosclerosis, the pathogenesis of which is described in Chapter 11.

CLINICAL MANIFESTATIONS

History

The term **angina pectoris** (see also Chapter 1) is used to describe a discomfort in the chest or adjacent areas caused by myocardial ischemia without myocardial necrosis. In chronic stable angina, the discomfort is usually precipitated by physical or emotional stress. It is frequently not painful, but, rather, is described as "pressure-like" or "squeezing." It is usually retrosternal in location but can radiate to the neck and the arms, and can be associated with dyspnea, diaphoresis, nausea, or vomiting.

Typical angina begins gradually and reaches maximal intensity over a few minutes, then gradually subsides with rest or after the administration of nitroglycerin. The resolution of the discomfort with nitroglycerin can be a helpful diagnostic feature of angina; however, it is a relatively nonspecific response — esophageal pain and other syndromes may also be alleviated by nitroglycerin. Characteristics that are not suggestive of angina include fleeting chest pain, discomfort that is brought on or worsened by breathing or arm movement, or discomfort that is reproducible by palpation on examination. Identification of risk factors for atherosclerosis is crucial in the assessment and treatment of patients with chronic stable angina (see Table 11–1).

Physical Examination

The physical examination of patients with coronary artery disease (CAD) and chronic stable angina often is entirely normal. However, evidence of hypertension (elevated blood pressure, retinal changes), hyperlipidemia (xanthomas, xanthalasma), and vascular disease (diminished pulses, vascular bruits) should raise the suspicion of underlying CAD. Examination of the heart is often normal, but in patients with prior myocardial infarction (MI), signs of left ventricular dysfunction (dyskinetic apical impulse, third heart sound, elevated jugular venous pressure, or pulmonary edema) may be present. A transient murmur of mitral regurgitation may be heard during an episode of angina and results from ischemic papillary muscle dysfunction.

DIFFERENTIAL DIAGNOSIS

A wide variety of disorders can mimic anginal chest pain and are outlined in Chapter 1.

DIAGNOSTIC TESTING

The diagnosis of angina (and thus of CAD) can often be made by history alone. Further objective testing may be confirmatory, or may be necessary to clarify the diagnosis when the cause of the patient's symptoms is not clear. In approximately 50% of patients with chronic stable angina the resting electrocardiogram is normal or demonstrates nonspecific ST-T changes. Q waves, conduction abnormalities, or premature ventricular complexes may be present in patients with a prior MI.

Stress testing is frequently used to establish the diagnosis and estimate prognosis of patients with chronic stable angina (see Chapter 6). Exercise-induced ST segment depression is the hallmark of exertional ischemia. Features on stress testing that reflect a poorer prognosis in patients with chronic stable angina include:

- a greater magnitude of ST depression (>2 mm)
- ischemic changes occurring in multiple (>5) ECG leads
- ischemia occurring at a low level of stress
- exercise-induced hypotension

Echocardiography (see Chapter 7) can also be used to identify evidence of a prior MI and assess left ventricle (LV) function in these patients. A definitive diagnosis of CAD can be made by performing coronary angiography. This procedure allows precise determination of the number and severity of coronary stenoses, which can be used to estimate prognosis and to guide therapy.

MANAGEMENT

General Approach

There are several key aspects of the management of chronic stable angina, which are often considered and applied simultaneously.

1. Symptomatic relief of angina can be achieved by either decreasing MVO_2 (with medications) or increasing myocardial oxygen supply/coronary blood flow (with medications or with percutaneous or surgical revascularization).

2. Any concomitant disorders such as anemia, fever, tachycardia, thyrotoxicosis, congestive heart failure (CHF), and infections, increase the metabolic demands on the heart and should be identified and treated.

3. Aggressive risk factor modification (including cholesterol lowering, hypertension control, treatment of diabetes mellitus, smoking cessation, weight loss, dietary changes, and regular exercise) should be undertaken to lower the subsequent risk of future adverse cardiac events (Table 13–1).

Pharmacological Therapy (Table 13–2)

Several different classes of medications are useful as anti-anginal therapy, including nitrates, beta-blockers, calcium-channel blockers and antiplatelet therapy. Nitrates are potent vasodilators that reduce both preload and afterload, thus reducing MVO_2. They also dilate the coronary vasculature to some extent, thereby improving supply. Nitrates can be used either to treat symptoms or as chronic prophylactic therapy; however, it is important to have a nitrate-free period when using long-acting nitrates to prevent the development of tolerance.

Beta-blockers and calcium-channel blockers both reduce MVO_2 by decreasing heart rate, blood pressure, and contractility, and are effective in relieving symptoms of angina and improving exercise tolerance. Beta-

TABLE 13–1

Risk Factors for Coronary Artery Disease and the Goals of Modification

	Risk Factor	Goal of Modification
Modifiable Risk Factors	Hypertension	SBP < 135, DBP < 85
	Diabetes mellitus	FBS < 120, HA1c < 8
	High LDL$_c$	LDL < 160 if no other risk factors
		LDL < 130 if 1–2 risk factors
		LDL < 100 if known CAD or diabetes
	Low HDL$_c$	HDL > 35
	Cigarette smoking	Total cessation
	Physical inactivity	30 minutes of exercise ≥3×/week
	Obesity	<120% ideal body weight
Nonmodifiable Risk Factors	Male gender	—
	Family history of premature CAD	—

FSB: fasting blood sugar; HA1c: hemoglobin A1c; SBP: systolic blood pessure; DBP: diastolic blood pressure; LDLc: low-density lipoprotein cholesterol.

TABLE 13–2

Effect of Anti-anginal Agents on Determinants of Myocardial Oxygen Supply and Demand

	Preload	Afterload	HR	Contractility	MVO$_2$	Supply
Nitrates	↓↓	↓	—	—	↓	↑
Beta-blockers	—	↓	↓↓	↓↓	↓↓↓	—
Calcium blockers	—	↓↓	↓	↓	↓↓	↑

HR: heart rate; MVO$_2$: myocardial oxygen demand.

blockers are the agents of choice for the treatment of patients who have had a prior MI or have known LV dysfunction (refer to Chapters 14, 15, and 19) and produce a significant mortality benefit in these settings. Aspirin inhibits platelet aggregation and prevents thrombosis at the site of a coronary stenosis, an effect that is essential in the treatment of all forms of coronary artery disease. All patients with symptoms of CAD should, therefore, be placed on daily aspirin therapy. Patients who are intolerant of aspirin may be treated with other antiplatelet agents such as clopidogrel.

Revascularization Therapies

When angina persists despite optimal medical management, or when patients with "high-risk" stress tests are identified, cardiac catheterization should be recommended to define the coronary anatomy and determine the feasibility of coronary revascularization. Revascularization may be performed by either percutaneous transluminal coronary angioplasty (PTCA), with or without coronary stenting, or coronary artery bypass grafting (CABG) (see Table 13–3).

TABLE 13–3

Percutaneous Versus Surgical Coronary Revascularization

	PTCA	CABG
Advantages	Less invasive; Shorter hospital stay; Lower initial cost; Easily repeated	Improves survival; More complete revascularization; Improved outcome in diabetic patients
Disadvantages	Less complete revascularization; No clear mortality benefit; Need for repeat procedures	Higher initial morbidity and mortality; Higher initial cost

PTCA: percutaneous transluminal coronary angioplasty; CABG: coronary artery bypass graft.

PTCA has been shown to be more effective than medical therapy in relieving symptoms of angina, but without a clear mortality benefit. CABG can provide complete revascularization, is effective for angina control, and has been shown to be superior to both medical therapy and PTCA in terms of mortality in high-risk patients. Patients in whom bypass surgery is of particular benefit include those with left main CAD, and those who have LV dysfunction and either three-vessel CAD or two-vessel CAD with involvement of the proximal left anterior descending coronary artery. This is especially true for diabetic patients.

PRINZMETAL'S VARIANT ANGINA

In 1959, Prinzmetal described a syndrome of anginal chest pain that occurs almost always at rest, and is associated with ST-segment elevation on the ECG. It may be associated with acute MI, ventricular arrhythmias, or sudden death.

Etiology

Variant angina is caused by coronary artery spasm leading to complete occlusion of the vessel. This tends to occur in areas adjacent to atheromatous plaques, but can also occur in normal arterial segments (pure coronary vasospasm). Cigarette smoking is an important risk factor for variant angina. Cocaine use can precipitate coronary vasospasm even in individuals without a prior history of this syndrome.

Clinical Manifestations

Patients with variant angina tend to be younger than patients with chronic stable angina, and the chest pain with which they present tends to occur at rest rather than with exertion. In contrast to the ST segment depression associated with classic angina, the ECG during episodes of variant angina demonstrates ST-segment elevation. The diagnostic hallmark of variant angina is the finding of spasm of a proximal coronary artery with resultant ischemia during coronary arteriography. Intracoronary infusion of ergonovine or acetylcholine can be used to induce coronary vasospasm in patients with suspected variant angina.

Management

Coronary vasospasm responds very promptly and completely to nitrates. Short-acting nitrates are useful in abolishing acute attacks, while long-acting nitrates can prevent recurrent episodes. Calcium-channel blockers, especially nifedipine, are also very effective. Beta-blockers have a variable effect and may be detrimental owing to the resulting unopposed alpha-adrenergic vasoconstriction. Overall long-term prognosis is good unless there is co-existing CAD, MI, or significant arrhythmias.

◆ KEY POINTS ◆

1. Chronic stable angina is caused by obstructive, flow-limiting, atherosclerotic stenoses within the epicardial coronary arteries.

2. Chronic stable angina is characterized by exertional chest pain that is relieved with rest or after the administration of nitroglycerin.

3. Exercise stress testing is helpful in clarifying the diagnosis and prognosis of patients with suspected angina; cardiac catheterization remains the gold standard for diagnosing CAD.

4. Aspirin, risk factor reduction, and anti-anginal medications are the mainstays of medical therapy; percutaneous or surgical revascularization is indicated for patients with refractory angina or high-risk non-invasive test results.

5. Prinzmetal's angina is the result of coronary artery spasm, usually at the site of an atherosclerotic plaque. It is associated with ST segment elevation on ECG and responds to nitrates or calcium-channel blockers.

6. Beta-blockers are relatively contraindicated in the treatment of vasospastic angina owing to their potential to induce unopposed alpha-adrenergic vasoconstriction.

14

Unstable Angina and Non-ST Elevation Myocardial Infarction

Acute coronary syndromes (ACS) is a term that refers to unstable angina (UA), non ST-elevation myocardial infarction (NSTEMI; previously referred to as non-Q-wave MI), and ST-elevation MI (STEMI; previously referred to as Q-wave MI). The first two of these syndromes (UA and NSTEMI) will be discussed in this chapter and STEMI will be discussed in the next.

EPIDEMIOLOGY

In the United States alone, there are nearly 1.5 million hospital admissions for UA and NSTEMI each year. Additionally, NSTEMI accounts for 30–40% of all MIs.

Etiology (see also Chapter 11)

Slowly progressive, high-grade coronary stenoses can cause angina and may progress to complete occlusion; however, they rarely precipitate ACS because of the development of collateral circulation. Rather, most ACS result from rupture of lipid-laden atherosclerotic plaque with subsequent intravascular thrombosis (see Figure 11–4). If the thrombus is flow-limiting but not occlusive, or is only transiently occlusive, UA or NSTEMI results. In addition to atherosclerosis, several other disorders may result in myocardial ischemia and infarction. These include:

- coronary vasospasm (of normal coronary arteries or at the site of an atherosclerotic plaque)
- severe hypertension
- disorders that increase myocardial oxygen demand (MVO_2) (e.g., hyperthyroidism, pheochromocytoma, sepsis) or decrease oxygen delivery (anemia)

CLINICAL MANIFESTATIONS

History

Unstable angina encompasses a broad range of anginal presentations that include:

- crescendo angina superimposed on chronic stable angina
- new onset angina (within 2 months) brought on by minimal exertion
- rest angina of >20 minutes in duration
- post-MI angina (occurring >24 hours after MI)

An NSTEMI presents with features similar to UA except that the anginal symptoms tend to be more severe and prolonged. Congestive heart failure (CHF) may accompany UA or NSTEMI if severe ischemia or underlying left ventricle (LV) dysfunction is present. Ischemic-induced arrhythmias (sinus tachycardia, premature ventricular complexes [PVCs], non-sustained ventricular tachycardia [VT]) may also occur (see Chapter 16).

Physical Examination

Physical examination during an ACS may demonstrate:

- tachycardia
- hypertension
- transient S_3 or S_4
- transient or increased murmur of mitral regurgitation (papillary muscle ischemia)

angina but normalized after resolution of angina), whereas they persist or evolve following an NSTEMI.

Cardiac enzymes (creatine kinase-MB isoenzyme [CK-MB] and troponins) are highly sensitive and specific markers of myocardial necrosis, and distinguish NSTEMI (elevated enzymes) from UA (normal enzyme levels). Serial measurements (on admission and every 8 hours for 24 hours) of CK-MB are usually performed to differentiate between UA and NSTEMI, and to estimate infarct size. Serum CK levels begin to normalize after 24–48 hours whereas troponin levels remain elevated for 7–10 days; the latter provides a useful test for diagnosing MI several days after the event (see Figure 14–2).

DIAGNOSIS

The diagnosis of UA is primarily based on clinical symptoms and confirmed by ancillary tests. The electrocardiogram (ECG) obtained during chest pain typically demonstrates ST segment depression or symmetric T wave inversions (Figure 14–1); however, it may be normal in approximately 5% of patients. These ECG changes are often labile during UA (present during

DIFFERENTIAL DIAGNOSIS

The complete differential diagnosis of chest pain is reviewed in Chapter 1. The most important diagnoses to consider include:

- pulmonary embolism
- aortic dissection
- pneumothorax

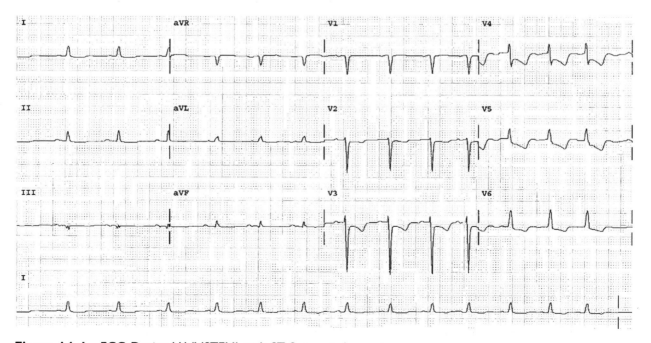

Figure 14–1   ECG During UA/NSTEMI with ST Segment depression.

- pneumonia
- pericarditis
- gastrointestinal disorders (gastroesophageal reflux disease, cholelithiasis, pancreatitis)

PROGNOSIS

Unstable angina progresses to MI in about 10% of cases and to death in about 5%. The presenting symptoms,

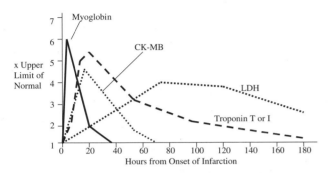

Figure 14–2   Serum markers of myocardial injury.

ECG findings, and serum markers of myocardial necrosis all affect the risk of MI or death in patients with UA and NSTEMI. Factors that identify a patient as being at high risk are summarized in Table 14–1. The presence of one or more of these factors suggests the need for more aggressive therapy.

TREATMENT

The primary goals of treatment are to control symptoms and preserve myocardial function. These goals are accomplished by:

- administration of analgesia
- reduction of myocardial oxygen demand
- improvement in coronary blood flow
- prevention of intracoronary thrombosis

Additionally, long-term prevention of recurrent ischemic events through risk factor modification is essential.

Liberal use of anxiolytics (benzodiazepines) and analgesia (morphine) helps to relieve pain and anxiety, thus

TABLE 14.1

Risk Categories of Patients with Unstable Angina

High Risk	Intermediate Risk	Low Risk
At least one of the following features must be present:	No high-risk feature but must have any of the following:	No high or intermediate risk features but any of the following:
Prolonged (>20 min) ongoing rest pain	Resolved prolonged rest pain	Increased angina frequency, severity, or duration
Pulmonary edema	Rest angina (>20 min) relieved with SL NTG	Angina provoked at lower than usual threshold
Rest angina with dynamic >1 mm ST changes	Angina with dynamic T wave changes	Normal or unchanged ECG
Angina with new MR murmur	New-onset Class III to IV angina within past 2 weeks	New onset angina within past 2 months
Angina with S3 or rales	Nocturnal angina	
Angina with hypotension	Q waves or resting ST depression <1 mm in multiple leads	
Positive cardiac troponin*	Age >65 years	

Risk refers to the risk of progression of MI or death.

*May be classified as NSTEMI.

decreasing heart rate and blood pressure and reducing MVO_2.

Antiplatelet therapy should be initiated as soon as the diagnosis of UA or NSTEMI is suspected. At least 160 mg of aspirin should be given acutely, followed by 81–325 mg daily. The first dose should be chewed to ensure rapid absorption. Clopidogrel (300 mg initial dose followed by 75 mg daily) appears to decrease morbidity when added to aspirin, and is an alternative antiplatelet agent for patients with an aspirin allergy.

Antithrombotic therapy with either unfractionated heparin or low-molecular-weight heparin (LMWH) (enoxaparin or dalteparin), should be administered for 48–72 hours to patients with intermediate or high risk features. LMWHs are more effective than unfractionated heparin but are contraindicated in the setting of renal insufficiency. Glycoprotein IIb–IIIa inhibitors, which block platelet activation and aggregation, have been shown to be of benefit in the treatment of UA and NSTEMI, and should be used in patients with high risk clinical features.

Beta-blockers decrease MVO_2 and are thereby effective in controlling ischemia. They should be used in all patients with UA/NSTEMI unless contraindicated. Non-dihydropyridine calcium channel antagonists may be used in patients without heart failure and with preserved LV systolic function, and may prevent recurrent infarction in this setting. Nitrates, in oral, transdermal, or intravenous forms, are effective in relieving anginal symptoms and for prophylaxis against further ischemic episodes, but they do not affect mortality. Angiotensin converting enzyme (ACE) inhibitors appear to decrease morbidity and mortality in some patients with UA/NSTEMI, and should be added if hemodynamically tolerated.

Thrombolytic therapy has no role in the treatment of UA and NSTEMI, as it is associated with higher mortality due to intracranial hemorrhage in these patients.

After the patient with UA or NSTEMI has been stabilized, cardiac catheterization and coronary revascularization should be considered. Initial studies comparing **conservative therapy** (medications, risk stratification with exercise tolerance test [ETT]) to an **early invasive strategy** (cardiac catheterization and revascularization) found a higher morbidity in the invasive group. More recent studies using intracoronary stenting have favored the early invasive strategy. Thus, the decision to proceed to cardiac catheterization is made on a case-by-case basis, based on an individual patient's risk profile, comorbidities, and patient/physician preference. A generally accepted approach follows:

- low-risk patients: noninvasive stress testing for further risk stratification (may be done off medications if diagnosis is uncertain)
- intermediate-risk patients: noninvasive stress testing after stabilization with medications
- high-risk patients: cardiac catheterization and revascularization if anatomically indicated

Patients who undergo noninvasive testing and have moderate to severe ischemia should undergo cardiac catheterization and revascularization, either percutaneously (PTCA with or without stent implantation) or surgically (CABG) depending on their anatomy.

RISK FACTOR MODIFICATION

Risk factor modification is a key component of long-term therapy. Goals of risk factor modification are outlined in Table 13–1.

◆ KEY POINTS ◆

1. Acute coronary syndromes (ACS) refers to unstable angina, non-ST elevation MI, and ST elevation MI.

2. Acute coronary syndromes result from atherosclerotic plaque rupture and intracoronary thrombosis.

3. Initial treatment of UA/NSTEMI includes analgesia, antiplatelet agents, heparin, beta-blockers, and nitrates.

4. Low and intermediate risk patients should undergo risk stratification with stress testing, and cardiac catheterization if the test is very abnormal. High-risk patients should undergo cardiac catheterization and revascularization.

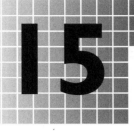

15

ST-Elevation Myocardial Infarction

ST-elevation myocardial infarction (STEMI; previously referred to as **Q-wave** or **transmural** MI) is an acute coronary syndrome in which there is persistent, complete occlusion of the involved coronary artery.

PATHOPHYSIOLOGY
(see Chapters 11 and 14)

STEMI is overwhelmingly the result of atherosclerotic plaque rupture with subsequent coronary thrombosis. Rarely, STEMI may be the result of another disorder including:

- coronary emboli (from intracardiac thrombi or valvular vegetation)
- *in situ* thrombosis (due to a hypercoagulable state)
- vasculitis (e.g., Kawasaki's disease)
- coronary artery dissection (either primary or as a result of aortic dissection)

CLINICAL MANIFESTATIONS
(see also Chapter 1)

The majority of patients with STEMI report severe, persistent, substernal chest pain that is commonly associated with nausea, vomiting, diaphoresis, dyspnea, and apprehension. Approximately 25% of patients are asymptomatic or have atypical symptoms. Large infarctions may present as congestive heart failure (CHF) or cardiogenic shock. Patients with an inferior MI may present with hypotension from right ventricular infarction. Ventricular tachyarrhythmias are common and account for most of the deaths during the first hours following a STEMI (see Chapter 16).

DIAGNOSIS

The hallmark of STEMI is ST segment elevation on the ECG (Figure 15–1). Serial 12-lead ECGs should be performed to confirm the diagnosis and localize the area of infarction. A characteristic evolution of ECG changes occurs (Figure 15–2). ST-elevation is present initially; this is followed sequentially by loss of R wave height, development of Q waves, T wave inversion, and finally, return of the ST segments to baseline. Patients with extensive anterior wall MI may present with a new left bundle branch block.

Cardiac enzymes have a similar pattern of elevation in STEMI as they do during non-ST elevation MI (see Figure 14–2); however, the absolute increase tends to be greater. Echocardiography during an STEMI demonstrates hypokinesis or akinesis of the left ventricle (LV) in the distribution of the occluded vessel. This finding can be helpful in the assessment of patients with suspected acute MI (AMI) but with a non-diagnostic or borderline electrocardiogram (ECG).

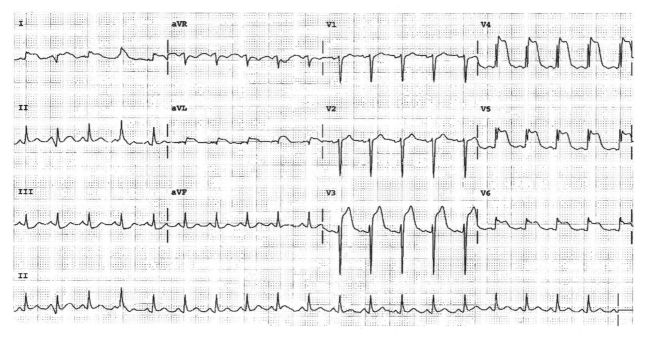

Figure 15–1   Electrocardiogram during an acute ST elevation myocardial infarction. Note the marked ST segment elevation in leads V₃–V₆, I, and aVL.

MANAGEMENT

Acute Therapy

Time is a key factor during an STEMI, because therapies are more beneficial when administered early. Therefore, rapid assessment and treatment should be the goal. Initial management should include:

1. a brief, targeted history
2. directed physical examination to identify complications and comorbid conditions
3. 12-lead ECG to confirm the diagnosis (within 10 minutes of presentation)
4. institution of analgesia, oxygen, antiplatelet agents, antithrombotic agents, and beta-blockers
5. determination of the need for reperfusion therapy

The initial management of STEMI is similar to that of UA/NSTEMI. Antiplatelet therapy (aspirin) and antithrombotic therapy (unfractionated or low-molecular-weight heparin) should be started as soon as STEMI is diagnosed. The first dose of aspirin should be chewed

to ensure rapid absorption. Oxygen should be administered by nasal cannula or facemask. Analgesia and anxiolytics are important for pain control and to decrease heart rate and blood pressure. Sublingual nitroglycerin should be administered and intravenous nitroglycerin should be started if ischemic chest pain persists. Beta-blockers decrease mortality and reinfarction after an STEMI and should be administered to all patients unless contraindications exist (e.g., hypotension, bradycardia, bronchospasm). Calcium channel blockers are generally not indicated in this setting.

If the patient has evidence of persistent ischemia (continued angina, persistent ST elevation) after initial medical treatment, reperfusion therapy with thrombolysis or primary angioplasty should be considered. Eligibility and exclusion criteria for thrombolytic therapy are outlined in Table 15–1. Time is a key issue, because thrombolysis is of minimal benefit beyond 6 hours after onset of symptoms.

Thrombolytic therapy with tissue plasminogen activator (tPA) establishes patency of the infarct-related artery in 75–80% of cases, and has been proven to decrease mortality, decrease infarct size, improve LV

Finding		Timing after onset of transmural ischemia
Normal		
"Hyperacute" T waves		Immediately
ST segment elevation		Within minutes
Loss of R wave height, development of Q wave, T wave inversion		Within hours
ST segment returns to baseline		24 – 48 hours
Normalization of T waves		Days to weeks

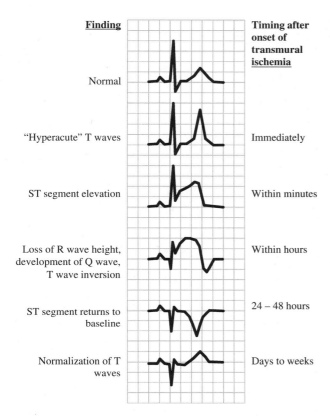

Figure 15–2 Evolution of ECG changes after an STEMI.

TABLE 15–1

Criteria for Thrombolysis in Acute MI

Indications

1. Chest pain consistent with AMI, and
2. ST-elevation >0.1 mV in >2 contiguous leads or new LBBB, and
3. <6 hours from onset of symptoms (consider if 6–12 hours)

Absolute Contraindications

1. Active internal bleeding (excluding menses)
2. Suspected aortic dissection
3. Prior hemorrhagic stroke at any time; other CVA within one year
4. Known intracranial neoplasm

Relative Contraindications

1. Uncontrolled HTN on presentation (BP > 180/110 mmHg)
2. History of prior CVA
3. INR >2–3; known bleeding diathesis
4. Recent trauma (within 2–4 weeks)
5. Noncompressible vascular punctures
6. Recent (within 2–4 weeks) internal bleeding
7. Pregnancy
8. Active peptic ulcer
9. History of chronic severe hypertension
10. For streptokinase/anistreplase: prior exposure (especially within 5 days to 2 yrs) or prior allergic reaction

AMI: acute myocardial infarction; LBBB: left bundle branch block; CVA: cerebrovascular accident; HTN: hypertension; INR: international normalized ratio.

function, and reduce heart failure in patients suffering an STEMI. Other thrombolytic agents (rPA, TNK-tPA) yield similar results and are easier to administer. Streptokinase is somewhat less effective but is associated with a lower rate of intracranial hemorrhage.

Primary angioplasty offers an alternative reperfusion technique (Figure 15–3). It is more effective at restoring flow in the affected coronary artery (>95% success rate) than is thrombolytic therapy, and it has a lower risk of intracranial hemorrhage. Comparative trials have demonstrated superiority of primary angioplasty with regard to mortality, reinfarction, recurrent ischemia, and stroke. The main limitation to primary angioplasty is its lack of widespread availability. At institutions where primary percutaneous transluminal coronary angioplasty (PTCA) is available, it is the preferred strategy. At hospitals where primary PTCA is not available, thrombolytic therapy should be administered; patients with contraindications to thrombolytic therapy and

those failing to reperfuse after attempted thrombolysis should be transferred to a nearby hospital with angioplasty facilities for either primary or rescue angioplasty.

Post-MI Management

After thrombolytic therapy, patients should be continued on heparin for an additional 24–48 hours. Following an anterior MI, some patients develop mural thrombi in the LV cavity; these patients require continued anticoagulation with coumadin for 3–6 months.

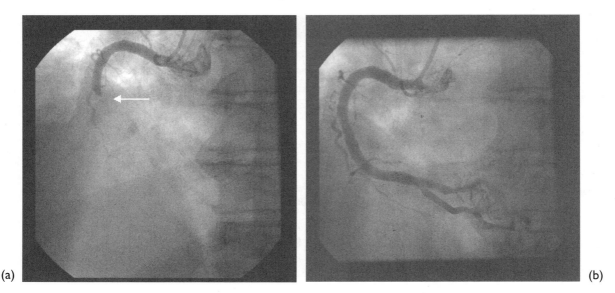

(a)   (b)

Figure 15–3   Coronary angiogram during an acute inferior myocardial infarction. (a) Initial angiogram reveals an occluded right coronary artery (arrow). (b) Same artery after angioplasty and placement of an intracoronary stent at the site of occlusion.

Aspirin is continued indefinitely. Beta-blockers should be continued and increased to the highest dose tolerated; angiotensin converting enzyme (ACE) inhibitors should be initiated, especially if significant LV systolic dysfunction is present. Lipid levels should be checked within 24 hours of admission and appropriate lipid-lowering therapy with HMG-CoA reductase inhibitors ("statins") should be started. As with NSTEMI, aggressive risk factor modification should be undertaken.

Echocardiography is generally performed several days after AMI to assess LV function. It can also identify LV mural thrombi, valvular disease (mitral regurgitation), ventricular septal defects, and ventricular aneurysms.

Patients who have undergone primary PTCA with successful reperfusion, have no residual high-grade stenoses, and have had an uncomplicated course, are usually discharged home 3–4 days after admission without further testing. Patients who are managed conservatively, including those who received thrombolytic therapy, should undergo low-level exercise tolerance testing (ETT) 3–5 days after infarction to assess for

ischemia and for risk stratification. A symptom-limited ETT is recommended 3–6 weeks after discharge. If either of these tests reveals significant inducible ischemia or the patient develops recurrent angina, cardiac catheterization and revascularization should be performed. Treatment for complications of MI is described in Chapter 16.

◆   **KEY POINTS**   ◆

1. STEMI results from atherosclerotic plaque rupture and subsequent coronary thrombosis.

2. Initial therapy for STEMI includes analgesia, oxygen, aspirin, heparin, nitrates, and beta-blockers.

3. Patients with persistent angina and ST elevation should undergo reperfusion therapy with angioplasty, if available. If angioplasty is not available, thrombolytic therapy should be administered.

16

Complications of Myocardial Infarction

Despite recent major advances in its treatment, an acute myocardial infarction (AMI) is still associated with significant morbidity and mortality. This is, in large part, a result of infarct-related complications including:

- heart failure (both left and right ventricular dysfunction)
- cardiogenic shock
- arrhythmias
- mechanical complications (ventricular free wall rupture, ventricular septal defect [VSD], papillary muscle rupture)

HEART FAILURE

Pathophysiology

Ischemic heart disease can result in heart failure through a variety of mechanisms. Acute ischemia results in an immediate rise in left ventricular diastolic pressure owing to impairment of myocardial relaxation. Continued ischemia results in reversible systolic dysfunction, thereby decreasing cardiac output and further elevating intracardiac pressure. Both the systolic and diastolic dysfunction may precipitate heart failure during an acute ischemic event.

Myocardial infarction (MI) results in myocardial necrosis with a resultant loss of left ventricular systolic function. Following the acute phase of an MI, ventric-ular remodeling occurs and results in LV dilation. This altered ventricular morphology produces a further fall in LV systolic function. These factors contribute to the development of both acute and chronic heart failure in this setting. The development of congestive heart failure (CHF) following an MI also relates to the infarct size (the larger the infarction, the more severe the degree of left ventricular dysfunction), and infarct location (an anterior wall MI results in more severe dysfunction than does an inferior or lateral wall MI).

Diagnosis

Patients with significant LV dysfunction following an MI may have symptoms and signs of CHF, including dyspnea, orthopnea, tachypnea, tachycardia, pulmonary rales, and an S_3 or S_4 gallop. Chest x-ray frequently demonstrates pulmonary vascular congestion and cardiomegaly. An echocardiogram will demonstrate hypo- or akinesis of the effected areas of the LV, and allows for estimation of the overall left ventricular ejection fraction. Invasive assessment of intracardiac pressures with a pulmonary artery catheter can definitively establish the diagnosis of CHF, but is required in a minority of patients with an acute MI (e.g., patients with CHF complicated by hemodynamic instability).

Treatment

The management of mild to moderate heart failure in the acute MI setting includes treatment of the underlying ischemia, as well as diuresis, afterload reduction, and avoidance of hypoxia. Preload reduction with diuretics (e.g., furosemide) and nitrates is effective in reducing symptoms of pulmonary congestion, whereas afterload reduction with angiotensin converting enzyme (ACE) inhibitors improves both symptoms and mortality. Beta-blockers reduce long-term mortality in CHF, and should be given to most post-MI patients irrespective of LV function; however, they must be used with caution in patients with decompensated heart failure in the acute setting.

Care must be taken to avoid overdiuresis in these patients. Most patients presenting with an acute MI and mild CHF are not volume overloaded. In fact, they are frequently somewhat volume-depleted owing to tachypnea, diaphoresis, and vomiting. Aggressive diuresis in this setting can result in intravascular volume depletion and can precipitate hypotension.

CARDIOGENIC SHOCK

The most severe form of acute heart failure is referred to as **cardiogenic shock**. It affects approximately 7% of patients with AMI.

Definition

Cardiogenic shock is characterized by:

- reduced cardiac output (cardiac index <2.2 L/kg/min)
- hypotension (SBP <90 mmHg)
- elevated pulmonary capillary wedge pressure (PCWP >18 mmHg)
- organ hypoperfusion

Pathogenesis

Approximately 80% of MI patients with cardiogenic shock have an extensive infarction with severe LV dysfunction (~40% of the LV must be infarcted to result in cardiogenic shock); the remaining patients have mechanical complications (see below) or hypovolemia. Patients with advanced age, prior infarction, diabetes mellitus, large infarction size, and known pre-existing LV dysfunction are at increased risk of developing cardiogenic shock after an infarction.

Diagnosis

Patients with cardiogenic shock are hypotensive, have signs of pulmonary edema, and have poor organ perfusion (e.g., mental status changes, decreased urine output, cold extremities). ECG frequently demonstrates signs of acute (ST elevation or depression) or chronic (pathological Q waves) ischemic heart disease. The hemodynamic abnormalities can be confirmed with invasive monitoring (Swan-Ganz catheterization).

Treatment

Management of cardiogenic shock requires continuous hemodynamic monitoring as a guide to optimizing left ventricular filling pressure and cardiac output. Medical management includes the use of vasopressors (such as dopamine) to maintain adequate blood pressure, inotropes (such as dobutamine) to augment cardiac output, and diuretics to decrease pulmonary congestion. Patients who develop cardiogenic shock within 24 hours of presentation of an AMI have improved survival if they undergo revascularization by either percutaneous transluminal coronary angioplasty (PTCA) or coronary artery bypass graft (CABG), and should be considered for emergent cardiac catheterization. Placement of an intra-aortic balloon pump (IABP) is sometimes necessary to augment systemic blood pressure, improve organ perfusion, augment diastolic coronary artery perfusion, and improve heart failure. Despite aggressive therapy, the mortality of cardiogenic shock resulting from an AMI approaches 70%.

RIGHT VENTRICULAR INFARCTION

Right ventricular infarction (RVI) usually occurs in association with an inferior LV infarction because both these territories are supplied by the right coronary artery. Isolated RV infarction is rare.

Clinical Manifestations

Patients with significant RVI have signs of RV failure, namely elevated jugular venous pressure (JVP), hepatic congestion, and hypotension. Kussmaul's sign (an inspiratory increase in JVP) may be present. Pulmonary congestion is usually absent unless there is concomitant LV dysfunction.

Diagnosis

The diagnosis can frequently be made on a 12-lead ECG with right-sided precordial leads. This may show >1mm ST-elevations, particularly in lead V_4R. This finding may be transient and usually resolves within 12 to 24 hours after infarction. Echocardiogram will demonstrate RV hypokinesis, and usually reveals an associated inferior wall motion abnormality. Right heart catheterization demonstrates a low cardiac output, low pulmonary capillary wedge pressure (PCWP), and elevated right heart pressures. The differential diagnosis of RVI includes pulmonary embolism and cardiac tamponade.

Treatment

Acute treatment of an RVI includes reperfusion therapy (thrombolysis or angioplasty) for the associated inferior MI. Hypotensive patients require volume resuscitation (to maintain adequate RV preload) and inotropic support with dobutamine.

MECHANICAL COMPLICATIONS OF AMI (Figure 16–1)

Following an AMI, disruption of necrotic myocardium may occur and result in left ventricular free wall rupture,

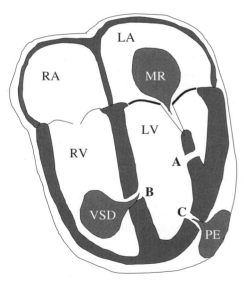

Figure 16–1 Mechanical complications of AMI. (a) Papillary muscle rupture results in acute, severe mitral regurgitation (MR). (b) Rupture of the interventricular septum produces an acute ventricular septal defect (VSD) resulting in left-to-right shunt flow. (c) Ventricular free wall rupture causes the rapid development of a pericardial effusion (PE) that results in pericardial tamponade. RA: right atrium. RV: right ventricle. LA: left atrium. LV: left ventricle.

VSD, or rupture of a papillary muscle with resultant acute mitral regurgitation. These conditions are summarized in Table 16–1.

Clinical History

Mechanical complications usually occur 3–5 days after an acute MI. Patients suffering from free wall rupture may present with recurrent chest pain, pericardial tamponade, or sudden death. Patients with an acute VSD or papillary muscle rupture usually have a new, harsh systolic murmur associated with a precordial thrill, and rapidly develop pulmonary edema and hemodynamic collapse.

Diagnosis

The diagnosis of a mechanical complication following an AMI can be confirmed by echocardiography and pulmonary arterial catheterization (see Table 16–1).

Treatment

The treatment of LV free wall rupture includes pericardiocentesis (if in tamponade) and emergent surgery and LV repair. Treatment of an acute VSD or papillary muscle rupture includes inotropic agents, vasodilators, and placement of an intra-aortic balloon pump as temporizing measures while awaiting emergent surgical intervention. Despite rapid surgical intervention, survival after LV free wall rupture is rare. Survival after an acute VSD or papillary muscle rupture is generally <50%, but depends on their rapid recognition and initiation of therapy.

ARRHYTHMIAS

A wide variety of arrhythmias may occur during an acute MI. Some are relatively benign, but many are life threatening and account for the majority of infarct associated sudden cardiac deaths. The advent of coronary care units and continuous telemetry monitoring has allowed for the early recognition and treatment of these arrhythmias, and has resulted in a significant reduction in mortality in the peri-infarct period. The genesis, diagnosis, and treatment of these arrhythmias are more fully discussed in Chapters 22–24. The specific etiology and treatment of various rhythm disturbances as related to the specific setting of AMI are listed in Table 16–2.

TABLE 16–1

Mechanical Complications of Myocardial Infarction

Variable	Free Wall Rupture	Ventricular Septal Defect	Papillary Muscle Rupture
Days post-MI	3–6	3–5	3–5
New murmur	25%	90%	50%
Palpable thrill	No	Yes	Rare
Previous MI	25%	25%	30%
Echo findings	Pericardial effusion	Shunt flow across septal defect	Flail or prolapsing mitral valve leaflet with severe regurgitation
Swan-Ganz catheterization	Equalization of diastolic pressures (tamponade)	Oxygen saturation step-up in RV	Prominent V waves seen on pulmonary capillary wedge tracing
Mortality			
- Medical	90%	90%	90%
- Surgical	Case reports	50%	40–90%

Modified from *Heart Disease*, 5th edition, Braunwald, p. 1241, W.B. Saunders, 1998.

OTHER COMPLICATIONS OF ACUTE MI

Pericarditis (see Chapter 33) frequently occurs in the peri-infarct period as a result of pericardial inflammation adjacent to regions of myocardial necrosis. An autoimmune pleuro-pericarditis associated with fever and an elevated erythrocyte sedimentation rate can also occur, usually weeks after the initial infarction (Dressler's syndrome). Treatment is with aspirin or non-steroidal anti-inflammatory agents. Anticoagulants should be avoided owing to an increased risk of developing hemorrhagic pericarditis.

Ventricular aneurysms are areas of focal myocardial dilation that occur as a result of ventricular remodeling following an AMI. They are readily detected by echocardiography and may produce persistent ST-segment elevation on the surface ECG. **True aneurysms** are made up of scar tissue, rarely rupture, and require no specific therapy. False aneurysms, or **pseudo-aneurysms**, represent ventricular wall rupture with containment by the pericardium, and have a high risk of spontaneous rupture. Surgical repair is the treatment of choice.

Both arterial and venous emboli may occur in patients with AMI. Venous emboli result from the hypercoagulable state as well as physical inactivity, manifest as deep venous thromboses or pulmonary emboli, and can be prevented by early ambulation or administration of prophylactic anticoagulants. Arterial emboli originate from left ventricular mural thrombi and can result in stroke, renal failure, mesenteric infarction, or limb ischemia. These occur more frequently following anterior wall infarctions, especially with associated aneurysm formation. Mural thrombi may be identified by echocardiography and require systemic anticoagulation with warfarin for 3 to 6 months to lower the thromboembolic risk.

TABLE 16–2

Arrhythmias in Acute Myocardial Infarction

Arrhythmia	Mechanism	Goal of Treatment	Therapy
Ventricular premature beats	Electrical instability	Correct electrolyte abnormalities Reduce sympathetic tone	Potassium, magnesium repletion; beta-blockers.
Ventricular tachycardia	Electrical instability	Restore sinus rhythm Prophylaxis against VF	Cardioversion/defibrillation acutely. Consider anti-arrhythmic agents if prolonged or recurrent.
Ventricular fibrillation	Electrical instability	Restore sinus rhythm	Immediate defibrillation
Accelerated idioventricular rhythm	Electrical instability	Restore sinus rhythm	Observation unless hemodynamically unstable. Increase sinus rate (atropine or atrial pacing) if symptomatic. Avoid anti-arrhythmic agents.
Sinus tachycardia	↑ sympathetic tone	Correct underlying cause Control heart rate	Antipyretics, analgesics, volume repletion, diuretics, or transfusion if needed. Beta-blockers unless CHF present.
Atrial fibrillation or atrial flutter	↑ sympathetic tone, pericarditis	Control heart rate Restore sinus rhythm	Beta-blockers, calcium blockers, or digoxin for rate control. Consider cardioversion.
Supraventricular tachycardia	↑ sympathetic tone	Control heart rate Restore sinus rhythm	Vagal maneuvers, beta-blockers, or calcium blockers. Consider cardioversion.
Sinus bradycardia	↑ vagal tone SA nodal ischemia	↑ HR if hemodynamically unstable	Observe if stable. Atropine or atrial pacing if hemodynamically unstable.
Atrioventricular (AV) block	↑ vagal tone AV node ischemia	Treatment dependent on severity of block and hemodynamic compromise	1st degree block and Wenckebach: observe if stable. Higher degrees of block: atropine. Consider temporary pacemaker (especially if anterior MI).
Intraventricular block (e.g., left or right bundle branch block)	Ischemia/infarction of conduction tissue	Observe	Consider temporary pacemaker for new left bundle branch block.

◆ KEY POINTS ◆

1. Congestive heart failure in the setting of acute myocardial ischemia or infarction results from both diastolic and systolic dysfunction. It is treated with afterload reduction (ACE inhibitors), preload reduction (nitrates), and diuresis.

2. Most patients with mild to moderate CHF complicating an acute MI are not volume overloaded. Overly aggressive diuresis in this setting may precipitate hypotension.

3. Cardiogenic shock is characterized by systemic hypotension (SBP <90 mmHg), low cardiac output (CI <2.2 L/kg/min), elevated pulmonary capillary wedge pressure (>18 mmHg), and evidence of organ hypoperfusion.

4. Treatment of cardiogenic shock includes pressors, inotropes, and diuretics. Patients with cardiogenic shock complicating an AMI should be considered for emergent cardiac catheterization and coronary reperfusion.

5. Right ventricular infarction is characterized by hypotension, elevated neck veins, and lack of pulmonary congestion. It usually occurs in conjunction with an inferior left ventricular infarction. Treatment consists of volume expansion, inotropic support, and reperfusion therapy for the associated inferior MI.

6. Mechanical complications following an acute MI include ventricular free wall rupture, VSD, and papillary muscle rupture. These are all surgical emergencies and are associated with excessive mortality.

7. True aneurysms of the LV rarely rupture, whereas pseudo-aneurysms are prone to rupture and require surgical resection.

Part IV
Heart Failure

17

Cardiovascular Hemodynamics

The four cardiac chambers comprise two separate pumps (the right and left sides of the heart) that function together in series. The efficiency of these pumps depends in part on their inherent contractile properties (contractility), as well as on the rate at which the pumps fill (preload) and the resistance against which they must pump (afterload). These and other hemodynamic variables are important measures of cardiac function and are altered in characteristic ways in the setting of heart failure. Assessment of the hemodynamic status of the failing heart allows for the recognition of specific disease states, quantification of disease severity, tailoring of specific therapy, and evaluation of the therapeutic response. Thus, an understanding of basic cardiovascular hemodynamics is essential to the understanding and management of heart failure.

HEMODYNAMIC PARAMETERS

Intracardiac Pressures

The assessment of intracardiac pressure is discussed at length in Chapter 8, but will briefly be reviewed here with regard to the assessment of heart failure. The normal pressure in each of the cardiac chambers is shown in Figure 17–1. Changes in these pressures may reflect alterations in a person's volume status or the functional state of their heart. Most of these pressures can be directly measured by placing a catheter into the chamber of interest.

The pressure required to fill the left ventricle (the **filling pressure**) is an important measure of ventricular function. It can be measured directly via placement of a catheter within the left ventricular cavity (**left ventricular end-diastolic pressure** or LVEDP), or it can be indirectly assessed by measurement of the pulmonary capillary wedge pressure (PCWP). In the absence of pulmonary vascular disease the PCWP reflects left atrial pressure. Furthermore, in the absence of mitral stenosis, the left atrial (LA) pressure reflects LVEDP. Thus, the PCWP can be used as an accurate surrogate for LVEDP.

Cardiac Output

The cardiac output (CO) is the volume of blood that is pumped by the heart in one minute and is the product of the heart rate (HR) and the stroke volume (SV, the amount of blood the heart pumps with each beat):

$$CO = HR \times SV (units: \ L/min)$$

The cardiac index (CI) is a method of normalizing the CO to body size and is obtained by dividing the CO by the body surface area (BSA, in meters squared [m^2]):

$$CI = CO/BSA (units: \ L/min/m^2)$$

The normal CO is approximately 4 to 6 liters per minute; however, this may increase greater than five-fold as a result of increases in heart rate and stroke volume. The heart rate (also referred to as **chronotropy**) is largely controlled by the autonomic

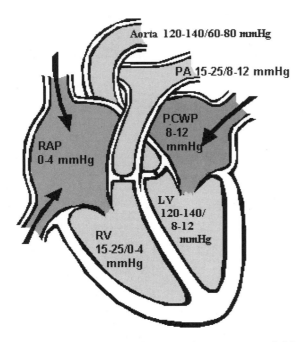

Figure 17–1   Normal intracardiac pressures. RAP: right atrial pressure; RV: right ventricle; PA: pulmonary artery; PCWP: pulmonary capillary wedge pressure; LV: left ventricle. Note that the PCWP is an indirect measure of left atrial pressure.

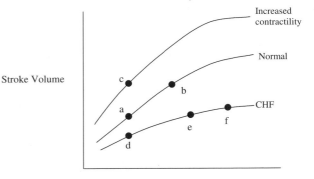

Figure 17–2   Frank Starling curve in various hemodynamic settings. In the normal setting, as filling pressure (preload) increases, stroke volume (SV) increases (point a → point b). Increased contractility (i.e., infusion of inotropic agents) is associated with an increased SV at any level of preload (point a → point c). In contrast, decreased contractility (i.e., heart failure) is associated with a decrease in SV at a given level of preload (point a → point d). In this setting, an increased preload is required to maintain the same SV (point a → point e). Additionally, further increases in preload (point e → point f) result in relatively minimal augmentation of stroke volume at the expense of a marked elevation in filling pressure.

nervous system. The stroke volume depends on three hemodynamic factors: preload, afterload, and contractility.

Preload

Preload refers to the volume of blood in the left ventricle just prior to systole (**LV end diastolic volume**). This volume, however, cannot easily be measured, and left ventricular filling pressure (LVEDP, LA pressure, or mean PCWP) is, therefore, used as a surrogate.

Afterload

Afterload is the force against which the left ventricle must pump. According to the law of LaPlace, afterload is directly proportional to blood pressure and left ventricular diameter, and inversely proportional to left ventricular thickness. Clinically, however, systolic blood pressure alone is often used as a measure of afterload. Afterload can also be quantified by assessment of the systemic vascular resistance (SVR), which can be calculated as:

$$SVR = [(MAP - CVP)/CO] \times 80$$
$$(units: dynes - sec - cm^{-5})$$

MAP is the mean arterial pressure and CVP is the central venous pressure. In general, as afterload increases, stroke volume and cardiac output decrease.

Contractility

Contractility (also referred to as **inotropy**) is the inherent strength of ventricular contraction independent of preload and afterload. Contractility can be augmented by increased activity of the sympathetic nervous system, and by sympathomimetic medications (e.g., dopamine or dobutamine). Contractility can be decreased by beta-blocking agents and calcium channel antagonists.

Pressure-Volume Relationships

The relationship between left ventricular filling pressure and stroke volume is described by the Frank-Starling curve (Figure 17–2). As can be seen, over a

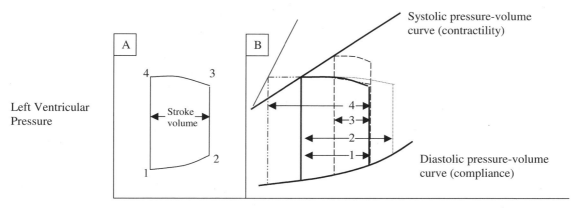

Figure 17–3   Left ventricular pressure-volume loops. (a) Normal pressure volume loop. The mitral valve opens at point 1 followed by left ventricle (LV) filling. The LV reaches a maximum volume at point 2 (LV end diastolic pressure/volume, or **preload**) followed by isovolumic contraction (line 2–3). The aortic valve opens at point 3, allowing for LV ejection (line 3–4). The volume of blood ejected represents the stroke volume. Maximum pressure is generated at point 4 (LV end systolic pressure, or **afterload**) and is followed by aortic valve closure and isovolumic relaxation (line 4–1). (a) Effect of changing hemodynamic parameters on stroke volume. (1) Normal stroke volume. (2) Increasing preload results in increased stroke volume. (3) Increasing afterload results in decreased stroke volume. (4) Increasing contractility results in increased stroke volume.

wide range of volumes, an increase in preload results in an increase in stroke volume. At extremely high preload (not shown in figure) the relationship fails and stroke volume falls (likely the result of over-stretching of myocardial contractile elements).

As can be seen in Figure 17–2, heart failure is associated with decreased contractility resulting in a lower stroke volume for a given preload. In an attempt to augment stroke volume, the preload increases substantially. This increased pressure is transmitted to the pulmonary vasculature, resulting in pulmonary edema.

The relationship between left ventricular pressure and volume can be represented graphically by a pressure-volume loop (Figure 17–3a). As can be seen, left ventricular stroke volume (i.e., LV performance) is affected by changes in preload, afterload, and contractility (Figure 17–3b). Abnormalities in any of these factors can result in impaired myocardial performance and alterations of normal cardiac filling pressures.

The end-diastolic pressure-volume curve defines the **compliance**, or distensibility, of the ventricle. A highly compliant ventricle is one that can accommodate a large volume of blood with only a small rise in pressure (as occurs with chronic aortic insufficiency). In contrast, a

poorly compliant ventricle (as occurs with ventricular hypertrophy or acute ischemia) is one in which a small increase in volume results in a significant increase in pressure.

Ejection Fraction

The overall systolic function of the heart is reflected in the ejection fraction. This is the proportion of blood that is in the ventricle at the end of diastole that is subsequently ejected during systole. The normal ejection fraction is approximately 60%, and can be measured by echocardiography, nuclear scanning, or contrast ventriculography.

Normal hemodynamic values are summarized in Table 17–1.

ALTERATIONS OF HEMODYNAMIC PARAMETERS IN HEART FAILURE

Most forms of heart failure are associated with a fall in cardiac output, frequently as a result of a decrease in contractility (systolic dysfunction). Systolic blood pressure (BP) may also fall since BP is proportional to

TABLE 17–1

Summary of Normal Cardiac Hemodynamic Values

Hemodynamic Parameter	Range of Normal Values
Heart rate	60–80 bpm (at rest)
Cardiac output	4–6 L/m
Cardiac index	2.5–4.0 L/min/m^2
Systemic vascular resistance	800–1200 dynes-sec-cm^{-5}
Pulmonary capillary wedge pressure	8–12 mmHg
Ejection fraction	60%

the product of the CO and SVR. Vasoconstriction occurs as a compensatory mechanism to maintain an adequate BP, and accounts for the increase in SVR that is usually present in patients with heart failure (frequently >1500 dynes-sec-cm^{-5}). However, this increase in afterload results in a further fall in stroke volume (see Figure 17–3b).

Heart failure is also associated with an increase in left ventricular preload. The increased LVEDP is transmitted back to the pulmonary vasculature resulting in a rise in the PCWP. A PCWP of >18 mmHg may alter the local Starling forces such that fluid enters the extravascular space, and pulmonary edema develops. Chronic elevation in the PCWP results in pulmonary vasoconstriction, thereby elevating the pulmonary vascular

resistance, and resulting in pulmonary hypertension. This results in right ventricular pressure overload, and, eventually, right ventricular failure with elevation of right atrial and central venous pressures.

The therapy of heart failure is aimed at correcting these hemodynamic abnormalities, specifically, decreasing afterload, decreasing preload, and increasing contractility.

 KEY POINTS

1. The cardiac output is the volume of blood that is pumped by the heart in one minute and is the product of the heart rate and the stroke volume.

2. The pulmonary capillary wedge pressure is an indirect measure of left ventricular end diastolic pressure, and, thus, is a measure of preload.

3. Afterload is proportional to blood pressure and is estimated by the systemic vascular resistance.

4. Over a wide range of volumes, increases in preload result in increases in stroke volume.

5. Heart failure is associated with a fall in stroke volume, frequently resulting from a decrease in contractility. A compensatory increase in preload and afterload helps to maintain stroke volume and blood pressure, but results in pulmonary vascular congestion.

18

Mechanisms of Heart Failure

Clinically, heart failure can be defined as the inability of the heart to pump sufficient blood to meet the metabolic demands of the body. The term **cardiomyopathy** refers to a disorder of the myocardium that may or may not be associated with clinical heart failure.

CLASSIFICATIONS

Heart failure may be classified as systolic or diastolic, right-sided or left-sided, high-output or low-output, and acute or chronic. These classifications reflect either the underlying pathophysiology of heart failure or the pattern of the patient's symptoms.

Systolic heart failure is characterized by impaired myocardial contractility. The heart becomes weakened and cannot pump blood effectively during systole. Consequently, blood backs up into the pulmonary system resulting in pulmonary vascular congestion. This is the primary mechanism of heart failure in both ischemic and non-ischemic dilated cardiomyopathies. The severity of left ventricle (LV) systolic dysfunction can be assessed by echocardiography, contrast ventriculography, or nuclear imaging, and can be quantified by calculation of the left ventricular ejection fraction (LVEF):

- normal LVEF: ≥50%
- mildly reduced LVEF: 40–50%
- moderately reduced LVEF: 30–40%
- severely reduced LVEF: <30%

Diastolic heart failure is characterized by impaired ventricular relaxation (i.e., decreased ventricular compliance). In this setting, any given volume of blood that enters the LV cavity will result in a higher than normal LV pressure. This results in impairment of diastolic ventricular filling and an increase in left ventricular end-diastolic pressure (LVEDP). The increased pressure is transmitted to the pulmonary system resulting in pulmonary vascular congestion. This is the primary mechanism of congestive heart failure (CHF) in hypertensive, hypertrophic, and infiltrative heart diseases.

Many heart failure patients, particularly those with advanced disease, have both systolic and diastolic heart failure. Advanced systolic dysfunction results in a rise in LVEDP, resulting in diastolic dysfunction. Many patients with diastolic dysfunction develop systolic dysfunction late in their disease (see Table 18–1).

Left-sided heart failure results from disorders that predominantly affect the left ventricle (e.g., myocardial infarction [MI], hypertension, valvular heart disease) or produce global myocardial dysfunction (i.e., nonischemic cardiomyopathy). Left-sided heart failure produces symptoms of pulmonary venous congestion (dyspnea, orthopnea, and paroxysmal nocturnal dyspnea).

Right-sided heart failure is most commonly the result of left-sided heart failure but can occur independently (e.g., right ventricle [RV] infarction, acute pulmonary embolism), and produces signs of systemic venous congestion (edema, ascites, congestive

TABLE 18.1

Common Causes of Heart Failure and Their Major Pathophysiological Abnormalities

Cause of Heart Failure	Major Pathophysiological Abnormality	
	Systolic Dysfunction	Diastolic Dysfunction
Acute ischemia	+	++
Ischemic cardiomyopathy	++	+
Nonischemic cardiomyopathy	++	+
Aortic stenosis	With advanced disease	++
Mitral regurgitation	++	With advanced disease
Hypertension	With advanced disease	++
Infiltrative heart disease (i.e., amyloid, sarcoid)	+	++
Hypertrophic cardiomyopathy	With advanced disease	++

hepatomegaly, jugular venous distension). Right-sided heart failure resulting from primary lung disease (e.g., pulmonary hypertension, chronic obstructive pulmonary disease [COPD]) is referred to as **cor pulmonale**. Both right- and left-sided heart failure frequently coexist (**biventricular heart failure**).

Low-output heart failure results when the heart is unable to pump enough blood to meet the body's normal metabolic demands, and can be seen with various forms of both systolic and diastolic failure. **High-output heart failure** results when a relatively normally functioning heart is unable to keep up with the body's abnormally increased metabolic demand, as may occur with thyrotoxicosis, anemia, and arteriovenous fistulas.

Acute heart failure refers to the sudden development of heart failure symptoms in a person who was either previously asymptomatic or whose heart failure was well controlled. It commonly occurs in the setting of:

- myocardial ischemia or infarction
- severe hypertension
- sudden valvular dysfunction (e.g., ischemic mitral regurgitation, ruptured mitral or aortic valve).

Chronic heart failure is that which has existed for a period of time. The patient may be chronically symptomatic or have well-controlled symptoms on medical therapy.

Frequently, several classifications can be used to describe heart failure in a single individual. For example, a person may have chronic, left-sided, systolic heart failure.

COMPENSATORY MECHANISMS

In response to the decreased cardiac output that accompanies CHF, several adaptive processes occur that help to maintain adequate cardiac output and tissue perfusion by augmenting stroke volume and heart rate. These include:

- Activation of the renin-angiotensin-aldosterone system results in improved blood pressure and tissue perfusion through angiotensin-induced vasoconstriction and aldosterone-induced sodium and water retention.
- Increased activity of the sympathetic nervous system results in vasoconstriction, increased ventricular contractility, and increased heart rate.
- Vasopressin and natriuretic peptides are released and result in fluid retention, increased preload, and, thereby, increased stroke volume.
- Endothelin is also released and produces further vasoconstriction.

Although these responses are initially adaptive, they eventually have deleterious effects (see Table 18–2). The

TABLE 18.2

Compensatory Responses to Heart Failure

Compensatory Mechanism	Beneficial Effect	Detrimental Effect
Renin-angiotensin activation	↑ SVR to maintain BP and tissue perfusion	↑ SVR results in ↓ CO
↑ Aldosterone	Volume retention leads to ↑ preload, ↑ SV, and ↑ CO	Volume overload
↑ Sympathetic tone	↑ HR and contractility result in ↑ CO; ↑ SVR maintains BP	May induce ischemia; ↑ SVR results in ↓ CO
Natriuretic peptides	Volume retention leads to ↑ preload, ↑ SV, and ↑ CO	Volume overload
Endothelin	↑ SVR to maintain BP and tissue perfusion	↑ SVR results in ↓ CO

SVR: systemic vascular resistance; BP: blood pressure; CO: cardiac output; SV: stroke volume.

increased afterload induced by angiotensin, norepinephrine, and endothelin may decrease stroke volume and result in a further decline in cardiac output. The volume expansion results in fluid overload and elevated intracardiac pressure. If the LVEDP (and, therefore, the mean pulmonary capillary wedge pressure [PCWP]) acutely exceeds ~18–20 mmHg, pulmonary edema develops. In patients with chronic heart failure, increased pulmonary lymphatic drainage partially compensates for the increased intrapulmonary pressure and may allow patients to remain relatively asymptomatic despite a PCWP of >25 mmHg.

The failing heart also undergoes structural changes in response to myocyte loss (i.e., myocardial infarction), increased afterload, or chronic volume overload. As a first response, the left ventricle initially hypertrophies; this may be followed by left ventricular dilation. These changes help to normalize the wall stress and lower the LVEDP. However, the progressive hypertrophy and dilation eventually alter the shape of the heart, producing a spherical LV cavity. This process is known as

ventricular remodeling and eventually results in a further increase in wall stress and LVEDP, and a decrease in LV systolic function.

◆ **KEY POINTS** ◆

1. Heart failure may be classified as systolic or diastolic, left-sided or right-sided, low-output or high-output, and acute or chronic.

2. Systolic heart failure is characterized by impaired ventricular contraction, whereas diastolic heart failure is characterized by impaired ventricular relaxation.

3. Vasopressin, endothelin, aldosterone, natriuretic peptides, the renin-angiotensin system, and the sympathetic nervous system all contribute to the compensatory response to heart failure.

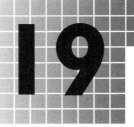

Clinical Manifestations and Treatment of Heart Failure

EPIDEMIOLOGY

Heart failure (HF) affects nearly 500,000 Americans, is the leading discharge diagnosis for persons over the age of 65, and accounts for almost $20 billion in health care costs annually. It is expected these numbers will continue to rise as the population ages.

ETIOLOGIES

In the United States, the most common cause of systolic HF is ischemic heart disease. However, heart failure may also result from a variety of other primary cardiac disorders, including congenital or acquired valvular abnormalities, hypertension, and infiltrative or inflammatory diseases of the myocardium (Table 19–1). A variety of metabolic abnormalities and several toxins may also result in heart failure. A thorough evaluation will usually implicate one of these disorders in the etiology of congestive heart failure (CHF); however, the exact cause cannot be determined in a significant number of cases. In such cases, the etiology is referred to as **idiopathic**. The major causes of diastolic heart failure include systemic hypertension, acute ischemia, hypertrophic cardiomyopathy, and the restrictive cardiomyopathies.

CLINICAL MANIFESTATIONS

History

Dyspnea is the most common symptom of left-sided heart failure. It may occur at rest or with exertion, may worsen immediately after lying down as a result of a sudden increase in venous return (orthopnea), or may occur several hours after the patient lies down to sleep as a result of central redistribution of extravascular fluid (paroxysmal nocturnal dyspnea). Wheezing and nocturnal cough may also result from CHF. Fatigue, lethargy, and poor exercise tolerance are frequent symptoms of heart failure and reflect poor cardiac output. Right-sided heart failure classically produces lower extremity edema that is exacerbated by prolonged standing and improved by elevation of the legs. Right-sided heart failure may also result in abdominal discomfort and nausea as a result of intestinal edema and may produce ascites. Chest pain or tightness is common in heart failure, may result from elevated intracardiac or intrapulmonary pressures, or may reflect underlying coronary artery disease.

Physical Examination

Signs of heart failure are the same regardless of its cause. Signs of left-sided CHF include:

TABLE 19–1

Etiologies of Heart Failure

Etiologic Category	Examples
Ischemia	Acute ischemia Ischemic cardiomyopathy (CMP)
Valvular heart disease	Aortic stenosis or regurgitation Mitral stenosis or regurgitation
Hypertensive heart disease	Acute hypertension Hypertensive cardiomyopathy
Toxins	Alcohol, cocaine, adriamycin
Metabolic abnormalities	Hyper- or hypo-thyroidism Thiamine deficiency (Beri-beri) Selenium deficiency (Keshan's disease)
Infiltrative diseases	Amyloidosis Hemachromatosis Sarcoidosis
Infectious diseases	Viral myocarditis
High-output failure	Arteriovenous shunts Paget's disease Beri-beri Anemia
Idiopathic CMP	Cause unknown (presumed viral)
Hypertrophic CMP	Various genetic mutations

- pulmonary rales (fine inspiratory crackles)
- dullness at the lung bases (resulting from pleural effusions)
- left-sided third heart sound (S_3) (systolic dysfunction)
- left-sided fourth heart sound (S_4) (diastolic dysfunction)
- left ventricular heave

Signs of right ventricular CHF include:

- elevated jugular venous pressure
- ascites
- hepatomegaly
- edema

Patients who have symptoms or signs of vascular congestion or organ hypoperfusion are said to have decompensated heart failure, whereas patients without these features are said to be compensated.

DIFFERENTIAL DIAGNOSIS

The main differential diagnosis of left-sided heart failure includes pneumonia, pulmonary embolism, and chronic obstructive pulmonary disease. The differential diagnosis of right-sided heart failure includes cirrhosis, nephrotic syndrome, pericardial disease, venous stasis, and deep venous thrombosis.

DIAGNOSTIC EVALUATION

The evaluation of the patient with CHF should include a search for the cause and an assessment of the severity of the heart failure. Routine laboratory examination should include a hematocrit and a measure of thyroid function. A chest x-ray may reveal pulmonary vascular congestion (vascular redistribution, Kerley B lines, etc.), cardiomegaly, or pleural effusions. An electrocardiogram (ECG) should be performed to evaluate for evidence of underlying coronary artery disease or left ventricular hypertrophy (LVH).

An echocardiogram is essential and allows for the accurate determination of biventricular systolic and diastolic function. With systolic heart failure, echocardiography demonstrates a depressed left ventricular ejection fraction. With pure diastolic heart failure, echocardiography usually demonstrates LVH, a normal LV ejection fraction, and evidence of abnormal diastolic ventricular filling on Doppler evaluation. Echocardiography can also identify valvular abnormalities that may have caused the heart failure or may reveal evidence of underlying CAD.

Placement of a pulmonary arterial (PA) catheter (Swan-Ganz catheter) allows for the direct measurement of intracardiac pressures, can confirm the diagnosis of heart failure when the diagnosis is in doubt, and can help to guide therapy. If the cause of the CHF is thought to be CAD, coronary angiography is indicated and will define the extent of the coronary disease and the feasibility of revascularization.

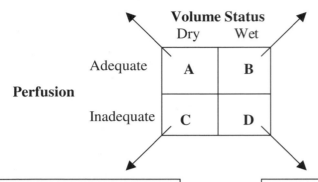

Clinically compensated.
Treatment: vasodilators, β-blockers
+/- diuretics, digoxin

Congested without hypoperfusion.
Treatment: diuretics

Volume Status
Dry   Wet

Adequate | A | B |

Perfusion

Inadequate | C | D |

Hypoperfused without congestion.
Treatment: vasodilators and
inotropes.

Congested and hypoperfusion.
Treatment: vasodilators, inotropes,
and diuretics

Figure 19–1   Hemodynamic profiles based on clinical signs in patients with decompensated heart failure, and the associated therapies. Adequate perfusion is indicated by normal mentation, adequate urine output, and warm extremities.

TREATMENT OF HEART FAILURE

General Approach

All patients with heart failure should limit their ingestion of salt. Patients with mild-to-moderate heart failure can accomplish this aim by eating low-salt foods and not adding extra salt to prepared foods. Patients with more severe heart failure may need to limit their salt intake to <2 grams of sodium per day. Restriction of fluid intake is usually not necessary except in the most severe cases. Patients with heart failure should be encouraged to exercise regularly, and all potentially modifiable risk factors for atherosclerosis should be addressed, including smoking cessation, lipid control, and weight loss. Avoidance of alcohol and illicit drugs are also important aspects of heart failure therapy.

The management of the individual patient with heart failure depends, in part, on the etiology of their disease and the acuity of their symptoms. Potentially reversible causes should be sought out and specific treatment initiated. Treatment of the patient with acutely decompensated heart failure is aimed at improving systemic perfusion, decreasing congestion, and establishing a stable hemodynamic state. The goals of long-term therapy of the compensated heart failure patient are the control of symptoms, prevention of decompensation, and reduction of mortality.

The choice of specific therapy for the decompensated patient should be directed by their clinical presentation, i.e., whether they present with signs of congestion, hypoperfusion, or both. The hemodynamic status of these patients (i.e., congested with adequate perfusion, hypoperfused, or congested and hypoperfused) and the most appropriate regimen for their treatment can often be determined by answering two simple questions (see Figure 19–1):

- Is the patient wet (i.e., volume-overloaded with pulmonary and peripheral congestion) or dry?

- Is the patient adequately or inadequately perfused (i.e., normal mentation, adequate urine output, warm extremities)?

Invasive hemodynamic monitoring with a PA catheter is occasionally required and allows for a more precise determination of the severity of heart failure. The PA catheter can also be used to guide therapy in an effort to normalize a patient's hemodynamics (so-called "tailored therapy"). Ideal hemodynamic parameters in patients with chronic heart failure include a pulmonary capillary wedge pressure (PCWP) ~15–18 mm Hg, right atrial pressure ≤8 mm Hg, cardiac index ≥2.2 L/min/m², and a systemic vascular resistance (SVR) of 1000–1200 dynes/sec/cm⁻⁵.

Treatment of Systolic Heart Failure

Pharmacological Therapies

The pharmacological therapy of systolic heart failure centers around the control of excess body water, reduction of afterload, and augmentation of contractility. These hemodynamic changes help to normalize cardiac pressure-volume relationships (see Figure 19–2). Acutely decompensated patients frequently require intravenous medications (Table 19–2); whereas compensated patients can be managed with oral therapy (Table 19–3).

In patients with pulmonary congestion or signs of volume overload, diuretics will usually improve their symptoms. Furosemide, which acts in the loop of Henle, is the most common diuretic used for treating HF, but has not been shown to decrease mortality. Thiazide diuretics, which act in the distal convoluted tubule, are less frequently used; however, the addition of a thiazide (i.e., metolazone) to furosemide can be remarkably effective for inducing diuresis. This combination may also result in renal potassium and magnesium wasting; electrolyte levels need to be checked regularly when using these medications. Spironolactone, an aldosterone inhibitor, is a relatively weak diuretic but has recently been shown to decrease symptoms as well as improve mortality in patients with NYHA (New York Heart Association) class III–IV heart failure.

In patients with either asymptomatic left ventricular systolic dysfunction or symptomatic systolic heart, vasodilators are clearly beneficial. These agents decrease systemic vascular resistance, thereby decreasing afterload and improving cardiac output. Angiotensin converting enzyme (ACE) inhibitors and angiotensin receptor blockers (ARBs) are the most effective oral vasodilators. ACE inhibitors decrease the progression of heart failure, improve symptoms, and decrease mortality in patients with HF. ARBs may be equally effective but are less well studied. Hydralazine is a less effective vasodilator, but still a useful agent in those

patients who cannot take ACE inhibitors or ARBs because of renal dysfunction or medication intolerance. In patients with acutely decompensated heart failure, afterload reduction can be accomplished rapidly with intravenous nitroprusside or nitroglycerin.

Digoxin is a cardiac glycoside that inhibits the Na⁺-K⁺ ATPase, resulting in higher intracellular calcium levels and thereby augmenting contractility. Digoxin improves symptoms in patients with heart failure and decreases their need for hospitalization; however, it does not improve mortality. Many other oral inotropic agents have been studied and all have shown either no benefit or increased mortality in HF patients. Dobutamine and dopamine are beta-agonists, and are effective intravenous inotropic agents especially useful for patients with decompensated HF. These agents augment cardiac output, improve tissue perfusion, and may result in brisk diuresis.

Nitrates are venodilators, and, as such, result in decreased preload. They are useful for the control of

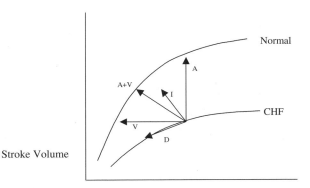

Figure 19–2 Frank Starling curve in heart failure and the effects of specific agents on stroke volume and preload. In the normal setting, as filling pressure (preload) increases, stroke (SV) increases. In heart failure, the SV is decreased, and an increased preload is required to maintain the same SV. Diuretics (D) and venodilators (V) decrease filling pressures without significantly improving stroke volume. Arterial vasodilators (A) and inotropes (I) improve stroke volume without significantly affecting filling pressures. Combination therapy with venodilators and arterial vasodilators (A + V) both improves cardiac performance and lowers filling pressures.

TABLE 19–2

Intravenous Agents Used in the Treatment of Patients with Decompensated Heart Failure

Drug	Hemodynamic Effect	Mechanism of Action	Dose Range	Side Effects
Dobutamine	↑CO, ↓SVR, ↓PCWP	α- and β-adrenergic agonist properties	2–15 µg/kg/min	Tachycardia, ventricular arrhythmias
Dopamine (low dose)	↓SVR, ↔CO, ↔PCWP	Renal and splanchnic vasodilation	1–2 µg/kg/min	Higher doses result in adrenergic stimulation and vasoconstriction
Milrinone	↑↑CO, ↓↓SVR, ↓↓PCWP	Phosphodiesterase inhibitor increases cAMP levels	Bolus: 25–50 µg/kg Infuse: 0.25–0.5 µg/kg/min	Hypotension, tachyarrhythmias
Nitroprusside	↓↓SVR, ↑CO, ↓↓PCWP	NO donor, potent arterial and venous vasodilation	10 µg/min, titrating by 20 µg/min every 15 minutes until HD goals met or hypotension	Coronary "steal," cyanide thiocyanate toxicity, hypotension
Nitroglycerin	↓SVR, ↔CO, ↓PCWP	Decreases ventricular filling pressures and myocardial oxygen demand, arterial and venous vasodilation	50–400 µg/min	Headache, hypotension
Furosemide	↓PCWP	Loop diuretic; stimulates salt (and water) loss	Intermittent bolus (10–400 mg) or continuous infusion	Volume depletion, hypotension, electrolyte abnormalities

CO: cardiac output; SVR: systemic vascular resistance; PCWP: pulmonary capillary wedge pressure; HD: hemodynamic; ↔: no significant effect.

congestive symptoms, and for control of angina in patients with concurrent CAD. They do not improve mortality.

Beta-blocking agents were long thought to be contraindicated in patients with systolic HF, owing to their negatively inotropic effects. However, recently, several beta-blockers (carvedilol, metoprolol) have been shown to be both safe and effective in the treatment of heart failure; they improve symptoms and substantially decrease mortality. Nonetheless, these agents can lead to an initial worsening of congestive symptoms. Therefore, it is important to start these agents at low doses (e.g., carvedilol 3.125 mg twice daily, metoprolol 25 mg daily), increase slowly (titrate upward every 2–4 weeks as tolerated), and use diuretics for control of congestive symptoms. A general approach to the outpatient management of chronic heart failure is summarized in Figure 19–3.

Surgical Therapies

Coronary artery revascularization, either surgically or percutaneously, should be considered in patients with heart failure and evidence of ischemic disease. Successful revascularization may improve contractile function, alleviate symptoms, and attenuate the remodeling process.

Ventricular assist devices (VADs) are mechanical pumps that are surgically implanted into the heart and can temporarily sustain a patient's circulation until the heart recovers or the patient receives a heart transplant. Presently, VADs are being used only as temporizing measures; however, in the future these devices may become a more permanent form of therapy.

Cardiac transplantation provides a definite survival advantage over medical therapy in patients with advanced heart failure, and is associated with a one-year survival rate approaching 80% and a 5-year survival rate of approximately 65%. Unfortunately, because of a

TABLE 19–3

The Beneficial Effects of Oral Agents Used in the Management of Heart Failure

Drug	Improve Symptoms	Decrease Mortality	Prevent Recurrent CHF
Diuretics	Yes	No	No
Digoxin	Yes	No	+/−
Inotropes	Yes	↑mortality	No
Direct vasodilators	Yes	Yes	No
ACE inhibitors	Yes	Yes	Yes
Beta-blockers	Yes	Yes	Yes
Spironolactone	Yes	Yes	No

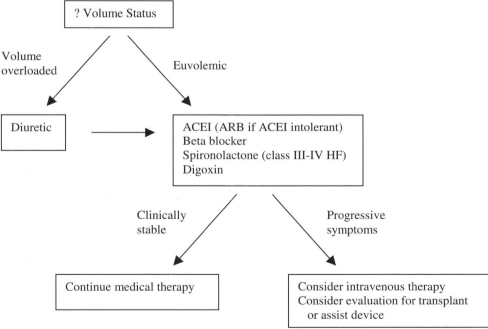

Figure 19–3 Algorithm for the outpatient management of chronic systolic heart failure. Initial evaluation of patients with left ventricular dysfunction should include an assessment of volume status. If signs or symptoms of volume overload are present, initial management should include diuresis. In the asymptomatic, euvolemic patient, initial therapy should consist of an ACE inhibitor followed by the cautious addition of a beta-blocker. Spironolactone should be initiated in patients with moderate to severe symptoms. Digoxin should be reserved as a second line agent for those patients who remain symptomatic despite the above therapy. If symptoms persist despite optimal medical therapy, assist device or transplant should be considered.

shortage of donor hearts, most patients die while waiting for a transplant. Approximately 40,000 people die each year from chronic heart failure, while only 2500 donor hearts become available. As a result of this shortage, attempts have been made to develop a totally artificial heart. These self-contained, mechanical devices have been implanted in just a few patients as part of experimental trials, and have had short-term success. With further technical advances, these devices may offer long-term support for patients with severe heart failure. Currently, the only absolute contraindications to cardiac transplantation are other medical conditions independent of the patient's heart failure that would limit his or her life expectancy.

Treatment of Diastolic Heart Failure

The management of pure diastolic dysfunction is problematic, as much less is known about the treatment of diastolic HF than of systolic HF. Management is aimed at treating the underlying cause, alleviating congestive symptoms, and attempting to improve diastolic function with the use of negatively inotropic agents. Both beta-blockers and calcium channel blockers appear to be equally effective in this regard, but may need to be used in high doses. Diuretics should be used cautiously to control pulmonary or systemic congestion. Patients with diastolic dysfunction are very preload-dependent; overdiuresis may result in hypotension, tachycardia, and worsened diastolic function.

◆ KEY POINTS ◆

1. Heart failure is an increasingly prevalent disease that accounts for billions of health care dollars.

2. Initial management of patients with decompensated heart failure should be aimed at normalizing volume status and improving systemic perfusion.

3. Therapies that have been shown to decrease mortality in all patients with systolic heart failure include ACE inhibitors and beta-blockers. Spironolactone improves mortality in patients with class III–IV symptoms.

4. Digoxin, nitrates, and diuretics are used primarily for symptom control.

5. Patients with progressive symptoms despite optimal medical therapy should be considered for cardiac replacement therapy (VAD or transplant).

6. The management of diastolic heart failure primarily consists of treatment with negative inotropes and limited diuresis. These therapies are, however, of unproven benefit.

20 Myocarditis

Myocarditis is an inflammatory disease of the myocardium that results from a variety of underlying disorders. Its manifestations range from asymptomatic left ventricle (LV) dysfunction to fulminant congestive heart failure (CHF).

EPIDEMIOLOGY

The true incidence of myocarditis is uncertain owing to the high frequency of asymptomatic cases. It is estimated that the myocardium becomes involved in 1–5% of patients presenting with an acute viral illness.

ETIOLOGY

Causes of myocarditis include:

- viral infections (e.g., Coxsackie B, adenovirus, influenza, HIV)
- acute rheumatic fever
- Lyme disease (*Borrelia burgdorferi*)
- Chagas' disease (*Trypanosoma cruzi*)
- toxins (e.g., cocaine, anthracyclines, catecholamines),
- systemic diseases (collagen vascular, autoimmune, or granulomatous diseases)
- hypersensitivity reactions to a variety of antibiotics, antihypertensives, and anticonvulsants

The vast majority of cases are the result of viral infections.

PATHOGENESIS

The offending agent or toxin may cause direct myocyte damage or necrosis. More importantly, an immune response is stimulated, in which macrophages and T-lymphocytes infiltrate the myocardium and release pro-inflammatory cytokines such as tumor necrosis factor and interleukin-1. This reaction may proceed for months and eventually result in left ventricular dysfunction.

CLINICAL MANIFESTATIONS

History

The typical patient with acute myocarditis is an otherwise healthy, young adult. The clinical presentation varies widely. Most cases are probably minimally symptomatic and never come to medical attention. Symptomatic patients usually present with heart failure of recent onset. Other presenting symptoms include palpitations, chest pain, syncope, and sudden cardiac death. Patients may recall a preceding viral syndrome.

Physical Examination

The physical examination is similar to that of other patients with heart failure. Most patients are tachycardic and moderately dyspneic. A pericardial friction rub may be present if the pericardium is also inflamed. Signs of systemic disease should be sought, including lymphadenopathy (suggests sarcoidosis), rash (suggests hypersensitivity reaction), and features of acute rheumatic fever (see Chapter 28).

DIAGNOSTIC EVALUATION

Abnormal laboratory findings in acute myocarditis include:

- elevated creatine kinase and troponin (elevated only in the acute phase)
- elevated erythrocyte sedimentation rate
- abnormal ECG that may show transient ST elevation, diffuse T wave inversions, atrial and ventricular arrhythmias
- elevated acute viral titers

Echocardiography typically demonstrates ventricular systolic dysfunction that may be either global or regional. Intracardiac thrombi, valvular regurgitation, and pericardial effusions may also be seen. Nuclear scanning and contrast-enhanced magnetic resonance imaging (MRI) can detect the degree and extent of inflammation in myocarditis, but are of uncertain utility.

Endomyocardial biopsy can definitively establish the diagnosis of myocarditis; demonstration of an inflammatory myocardial infiltrate with associated myocyte damage confirms the diagnosis. However, a negative biopsy does not exclude the diagnosis, because the histological changes may be short-lived and the involvement of the myocardium may be heterogeneous. Biopsy should be considered if the clinical evaluation suggests a specific disorder for which treatment is available; however, its routine use remains controversial.

DIFFERENTIAL DIAGNOSIS

Acute myocarditis can mimic acute myocardial infarction (AMI) (chest pain, ST-T wave changes, myocardial enzyme elevation, and regional wall motion abnormalities). A careful history must be obtained to distinguish between the two entities. One distinguishing feature is the pattern of cardiac enzyme elevation. Following an AMI, the creatine kinase MB isoenzyme (CK-MB) rises within hours, peaks within the first day, and slowly

returns to normal over the next several days. With myocarditis, the CK-MB may remain persistently elevated for days to weeks.

PROGNOSIS

Given the variability in presentation and diagnosis of this disease, prognostication is difficult. In general, approximately one-third of patients presenting with acute myocarditis and LV dysfunction will regain normal cardiac function; one-third will have persistent, mild left ventricular dysfunction; and one-third will develop progressive symptomatic left ventricular dysfunction.

TREATMENT

The treatment of acute myocarditis is largely supportive including restricted activity, monitoring for arrhythmias, and institution of routine therapy for heart failure (see Chapter 19). In certain forms of myocarditis (e.g., Lyme disease, Chagas' disease, acute rheumatic fever) specific therapy may be of some value; however, in most forms of myocarditis (i.e., viral myocarditis) immunosuppressive and immunologic therapy is of no proven benefit. Nonsteroidal anti-inflammatory agents have been shown to increase myocyte damage in animal models and are contraindicated in the early phase of myocarditis.

Patients with fulminant myocarditis may develop cardiogenic shock and require inotropic support or mechanical assist devices (see Chapter 19). Although many of these patients improve with aggressive medical therapy, patients with severe, progressive myocardial dysfunction should be considered for heart transplantation.

◆ KEY POINTS ◆

1. Viral infections are the most common cause of myocarditis.

2. Myocarditis can result in diffuse or patchy involvement of the myocardium.

3. Anti-inflammatory and immunosuppressive therapy do not have proven benefit for the treatment of acute myocarditis.

21 The Cardiomyopathies

The cardiomyopathies (CMPs) are primary diseases of the myocardium. They may result from a variety of conditions, but can largely be classified into **dilated**, **hypertrophic**, and **restrictive** forms.

CLASSIFICATION

These three classes of CMP may be distinguished by their morphological appearance and LV function (Figure 21–1).

- **Dilated cardiomyopathy (DCM)** is characterized by left ventricular dilation and systolic dysfunction. Often, four-chamber dilation is present. Regional wall motion abnormalities may be present even in the absence of significant coronary artery disease (CAD).
- **Hypertrophic cardiomyopathy (HCM)** is characterized by marked thickening of the ventricular myocardium, small left ventricular cavity size, and hyperdynamic systolic function.
- **Restrictive cardiomyopathy (RCM)** is characterized by normal LV size and systolic function, and impaired diastolic function. Mild ventricular thickening may be present.

There is significant overlap among classes, and features of more than one type may be present in the same individual. Diastolic dysfunction is a prominent feature of all three.

DILATED CARDIOMYOPATHY

Epidemiology

The reported incidence of DCM is 5 to 8 cases per 100,000 people per year. It is more common in males than in females, and in African Americans than in their caucasian counterparts.

Etiology

A wide variety of disorders can result in DCM, including:

- viral infections (e.g., adenovirus, enterovirus, HIV)
- immunologic/inflammatory diseases (e.g., systemic lupus erythematosus [SLE], rheumatoid arthritis, scleroderma)
- toxins (e.g., alcohol, anthracyclines)
- metabolic disorders (hyper- or hypothyroidism, beri-beri, selenium deficiency)
- pregnancy (post-partum CMP)
- tachycardia (atrial fibrillation, atrial flutter)

In addition, genetic factors may also play a role. In approximately one-quarter of cases of DCM, the cause

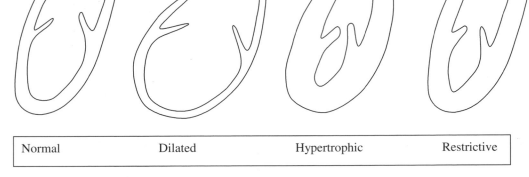

| Normal | Dilated | Hypertrophic | Restrictive |

Figure 21–1 Schematic representation of left ventricular size and shape among the various cardiomyopathies (CMPs). Dilated CMP results in a large ventricular cavity with thin ventricle walls. Hypertrophic CMP is associated with a markedly thickened ventricle with a small ventricular cavity. Restrictive myocardial disease is associated with a normal LV cavity size and mildly thickened ventricular walls.

remains unknown; most of these "idiopathic" cases are likely the result of prior viral myocarditis.

Clinical Manifestations of DCM

History and Physical Examination
(see also Chapter 19)
Most patients with DCM present between the ages of 20 and 50 with symptoms of left-sided heart failure. Other manifestations include arrhythmias (atrial and ventricular tachyarrhythmias), thromboembolic events (from atrial or ventricular thrombi), syncope, and sudden cardiac death. The physical examination of patients with DCM is indistinguishable from that of patients with other forms of systolic heart failure.

Diagnostic Evaluation

Echocardiography is the main diagnostic modality in DCM and usually reveals four-chamber dilation with depressed LV systolic function. Other routine diagnostic studies in a patient with CMP should include electrolytes, complete blood count, thyroid function tests, and iron studies. ECG often demonstrates an interventricular conduction delay and left axis deviation. Chest x-ray reveals cardiomegaly and may demonstrate pulmonary congestion.

Patients should be questioned about occupational exposures, alcohol consumption, illicit drug use, and family history of CMP. Stress testing and coronary angiography are useful in patients in whom the history suggests underlying CAD. Myocardial biopsy is not routinely performed.

Treatment

The treatment of DCM is the same as for other forms of systolic dysfunction (see Chapter 19).

HYPERTROPHIC CARDIOMYOPATHY

HCM is an inherited disorder of the cardiac sarcomere and is characterized by marked ventricular hypertrophy. It is a heterogeneous disease with varied morphologic, clinical, and hemodynamic manifestations resulting in a variety of descriptive subtypes, including hypertrophic obstructive cardiomyopathy (HOCM), idiopathic hypertrophic subaortic stenosis (IHSS), and asymmetric septal hypertrophy (ASH).

Epidemiology

Patients with HCM typically present in adolescence or early adulthood. There is an increased risk of sudden cardiac death (1–6% per year), with the following factors associated with the highest risk:

• younger age at diagnosis (≤14 years)

- history of syncope or nonsustained ventricular tachycardia
- family history of sudden death

Ten to 15% of patients with HCM progress to left ventricular dilation and systolic dysfunction.

Etiology

At least 50% of cases of HCM are familial, usually with autosomal dominant inheritance. Over 70 genetic alterations of at least 9 different genes on 4 chromosomes (1, 11, 14, 15) have been identified in familial forms of HCM. These genes encode various proteins of the cardiac sarcomere, including myosin heavy and light chains, troponin T and I, tropomyosin, and myosin-binding protein C. The etiology of sporadic cases of HCM remains unknown.

Pathophysiology

Marked ventricular hypertrophy (wall thickness > 15 mm, with normal being <11 mm) is the hallmark of HCM; most patients demonstrate asymmetric septal involvement. On myocardial biopsy, myocyte hypertrophy, myofibrillar disarray, and fibrosis are characteristic findings.

Asymmetric septal hypertrophy causes a narrowing of the left ventricular outflow tract (LVOT) that worsens during systole. The resulting increase in flow velocity in the LVOT pulls the anterior mitral leaflet toward the interventricular septum (Venturi effect); this results in further obstruction to LV outflow by the mitral valve leaflet and also can result in mitral regurgitation.

Diastolic dysfunction, mitral regurgitation, and myocardial ischemia also contribute to the symptoms of HCM. Myocardial ischemia may occur despite normal epicardial coronary arteries as a result of increased muscle mass, elevated diastolic filling pressure, increased wall stress, and decreased capillary density.

Physical Examination

Patients with HCM often have a prominent fourth heart sound and a hyperdynamic precordial impulse. The dynamic left ventricular obstruction often found in this disorder produces a coarse, crescendo-decrescendo, systolic murmur over the left sternal border that increases during expiration or during the strain phase of Valsalva (see Table 4–2). This feature, and the lack of radiation to the carotids, distinguishes the murmur of HCM from that of aortic stenosis.

Diagnostic Evaluation

ECG usually reveals marked left ventricular hypertrophy, left atrial enlargement, and left axis deviation. Echocardiography is the diagnostic test of choice and demonstrates marked left ventricular (and frequently right ventricular) thickening. Systolic anterior motion of the mitral apparatus, mitral regurgitation, and a dynamic gradient are other characteristic echocardiographic features.

Cardiac catheterization may also aid in the diagnosis of HCM by demonstrating a pressure gradient within the ventricle. This gradient may be quite labile and not apparent at rest, but may be brought out by the Valsalva maneuver.

Treatment (see Figure 21–2)

High-dose beta-blockers and calcium antagonists (primarily verapamil) are the mainstays of medical therapy. These drugs are negatively inotropic, resulting in decreased LV contractile force, and, thereby, reduce the LVOT obstruction. They frequently improve both symptoms and exercise tolerance. Disopyramide may also be effective if these agents fail. Diuretics, if clinically indicated, should be used cautiously, as the cardiac output in HCM is dependent on adequate preload.

Septal myomectomy (with or without mitral valve replacement) should be considered for patients with severe HCM (LVOT gradient >50 mmHg) who do not respond to medical therapy. This procedure significantly reduces the LVOT gradient in over 90% of patients, and results in clinical improvement. Alcohol infusion into the septal arteries is an alternative to myomectomy and produces an infarction of the septum with resulting thinning of the septal myocardium and relief of the LVOT obstruction.

The role of dual-chamber pacing (may reduce the LVOT obstruction) and implantable defibrillators (for prevention of sudden cardiac death) is unclear in HCM.

Atrial arrhythmias are common in HCM. Loss of organized atrial contraction owing to atrial fibrillation can result in significant hemodynamic compromise. Thus, attempts should be made to restore and maintain sinus rhythm in these patients.

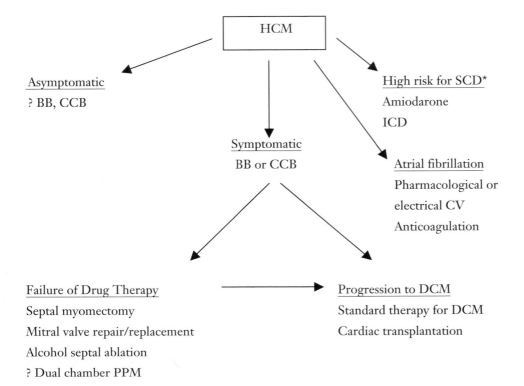

Figure 21–2 Treatment strategy for HCM.

RESTRICTIVE CARDIOMYOPATHY

Pure RCM is characterized by diastolic dysfunction in the absence of a dilated or hypertrophic LV.

Etiology

Restrictive cardiomyopathy may be a primary disorder (idiopathic) or be secondary to another disease:

- idiopathic (endomyocardial fibrosis, hypereosinophilic syndrome)
- infiltrative disorders (amyloidosis, sarcoidosis, hemochromatosis, glycogen storage disease)
- scleroderma
- carcinoid heart disease

Clinical Manifestations

The presentation of RCM is similar to that of severe constrictive pericarditis (see Chapter 35). Evidence of biventricular failure is usually present, although signs and symptoms of right heart failure predominate. The jugular venous pulsations classically demonstrate rapid X and Y descents (see Figure 4–1)

Differential Diagnosis

RCM may mimic other forms of heart failure; however, the main differential lies in the distinction between restrictive cardiomyopathy and constrictive pericarditis (see below).

Diagnostic Evaluation

In primary RCM, echocardiography demonstrates normal ventricular size and systolic function and abnormal diastolic function. In secondary RCM, myocardial thickening and LV and RV systolic dysfunction are often present.

The distinction between constrictive pericarditis and RCM is often aided by their hemodynamic profiles. Both restrictive cardiomyopathy and constrictive peri-

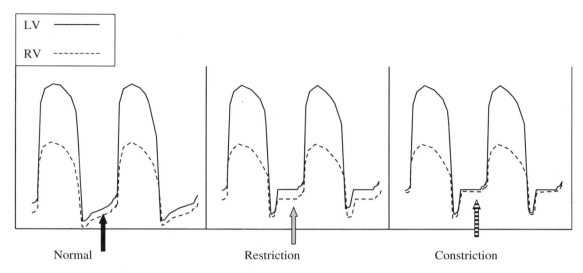

Figure 21–3 Left (LV) and right (RV) ventricular pressure tracings in a normal heart, in restrictive cardiomy-opathy, and in constrictive pericarditis. In the normal setting, diastolic pressure in the LV exceeds that in the RV; both rise gradually during diastole (black arrow). In restriction, the ventricles are poorly compliant; diastolic pressures are elevated and ventricular filling results in a rapid rise in pressure followed by diastasis (the **dip and plateau pattern**, or **square root sign**). Pressure in the LV still exceeds that in the RV owing to a greater effect of the restrictive process on the LV (gray arrow). In constriction, a similar pattern is seen, but the LV and RV pressures are identical owing to the homogeneous effect of the constricting pericardium (striped arrow).

carditis demonstrate elevated venous pressures and a rapid rise and then plateau of diastolic ventricular pressure (square root sign) (Figure 21–3). However, in constriction the restraining effect of the pericardium affects both ventricles equally; therefore, the RV and LV diastolic pressures remain equal throughout the respiratory cycle, even after volume loading. Most restrictive diseases affect the LV in excess of the RV and the diastolic pressures dissociate with inspiration or volume loading. The presence of pericardial calcification on chest x-ray, CT, or MRI also suggests constrictive disease.

Treatment

The treatment of primary RCM does not differ dramatically from the treatment of other forms of diastolic heart failure (see Chapter 19). In secondary forms of RCM, specific therapy (when available) should be directed at the underlying cause. Venous congestion should be managed with cautious diuresis, as ventricular underfilling can result in decreased cardiac output,

hypotension, and hypoperfusion. Atrial fibrillation is a common occurrence, and restoration and maintenance of sinus rhythm should be the goal. Malignant ventricular arrhythmias can be seen in certain restrictive cardiomyopathies, particularly sarcoidosis, and may require implantable defibrillator placement. Cardiac transplantation should be considered for patients with refractory symptoms.

DIFFERENTIAL DIAGNOSIS OF THE CARDIOMYOPATHIES

Other cardiovascular diseases may result in depressed left ventricular systolic function, abnormal diastolic function, and/or myocardial thickening, and can thereby mimic the cardiomyopathies. These conditions include valvular heart disease, hypertensive heart disease, and ischemic heart disease. It is important to identify these underlying causes, as correction of the primary abnormality may restore cardiac function.

◆ KEY POINTS ◆

1. Dilated cardiomyopathy, hypertrophic cardiomyopathy, and restrictive cardiomyopathy all result in congestive heart failure, but do so through different mechanisms.

2. Dilated cardiomyopathy is characterized by left ventricular (and frequently four-chamber) dilation, resulting in predominantly systolic dysfunction.

3. Hypertrophic cardiomyopathy is characterized by severe left and right ventricular thick-ening resulting in predominantly diastolic dysfunction. LV systolic function is usually preserved.

4. Restrictive cardiomyopathy is characterized by impairment of diastolic function and frequently results from infiltrative disease.

5. Dilated cardiomyopathy is treated with afterload reduction, diuretics, and beta-blockers. Hypertrophic cardiomyopathy is treated with negatively inotropic medications (calcium channel blockers, beta-blockers).

Part V
Arrhythmias

22

Mechanisms of Arrhythmogenesis

Before approaching specific arrhythmias, we shall discuss the mechanisms of their production. Specialized cells in the right atrium, known collectively as the sinoatrial (SA) node, rhythmically generate electrical impulses and thereby function as the pacemaker of the heart. These electrical impulses are propagated through specialized conduction pathways (the His-Purkinje system) resulting in the orderly and sequential depolarization of the atria and then the ventricles (see Figure 5–1). Abnormal production or propagation of these electrical impulses produces arrhythmias, whereas abnormal conduction of the electrical impulses produces heart block (see Table 22–1).

PHYSIOLOGY OF THE ACTION POTENTIAL

Although a comprehensive review of the cardiac action potential (AP) is beyond the scope of this text, some basic knowledge of cardiac electrophysiology is necessary to understand fully the mechanisms of arrhythmias. The action potential is the summation of the electrical activity of a cardiac myocyte (Figure 22–1). In the resting state, the inside of the myocyte is maintained at approximately $-80\,mV$ relative to the outside by the active accumulation of potassium ions (K^+) in the cell and the active expulsion of sodium ions (Na^+) from the cell. When the myocyte is depolarized to $-60\,mV$ (threshold potential), it becomes highly permeable to

Na^+ and calcium (Ca^{2+}). The subsequent ion fluxes result in rapid cellular depolarization (phase 0 of the AP), which is represented by the QRS complex on the surface electrocardiogram (ECG). Phases 1, 2, and 3 of the AP represent stages in cellular repolarization, and are represented on the surface ECG by the ST segment and T wave. During these later phases, the myocyte gradually returns to its resting membrane potential, primarily as a result of K^+ efflux from the cell (Figure 22–1, first panel). During phase 4 of the AP, the membrane potential gradually, and spontaneously, depolarizes toward threshold potential, at which time a new action potential is generated. This property is known as automaticity. The slope of phase 4 in SA nodal tissue is steeper that that of other cardiac tissue (Figure 22–1, second panel); hence, the SA node reaches threshold potential more quickly than the rest of the myocardium, and thereby determines the rate of depolarization of the heart (the heart rate). Knowledge of these fundamental principles will be helpful in understanding the mechanisms of arrhythmia production and the rationale for antiarrhythmic drug use.

MECHANISMS OF TACHYARRHYTHMIAS

A tachyarrhythmia is a cardiac rhythm that produces a heart rate greater than 100 beats per minute (bpm). Most tachyarrhythmias are produced by one of three

TABLE 22–1

Mechanism of Various Types of Arrhythmias

	Mechanism of Arrhythmia	Examples
Tachy-arrhythmias	Increased automaticity	Atrial, junctional, and ventricular premature complexes Accelerated junctional rhythm Accelerated idioventricular rhythm Ectopic atrial rhythm Some forms of ventricular tachycardia
	Triggered activity	Some forms of VT Torsade de Pointes, Bradycardia-dependent VT, long QT syndrome (early afterdepolarizations) Digoxin toxicity (late afterdepolarizations)
	Reentry	AV nodal reentrant tachycardia AV reentrant tachycardia (i.e., WPW) Atrial fibrillation Atrial flutter Most forms of ventricular tachycardia
Brady-arrhythmias	Disorders of impulse formation	Sinus bradycardia Sinus node dysfunction (sick sinus syndrome) Junctional and ventricular escape rhythms
	Disorders of impulse conduction (heart block)	Sinus nodal exit block 1st, 2nd, and 3rd degree AV block Infranodal (His-Purkinje) block

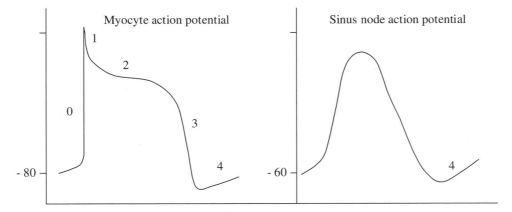

Figure 22–1   The action potential of ventricular myocardium and sinus nodal tissue. The slope of phase 4 repolarization is steeper in SA nodal tissue and accounts for its faster rate of spontaneous depolarization. See text for details.

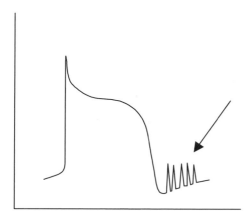

Figure 22–2 Delayed afterdepolarizations. Oscillations of the membrane potential (arrow) may reach threshold potential and trigger recurrent depolarization.

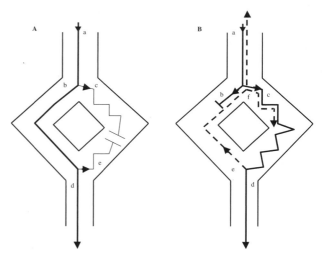

Figure 22–3 The mechanism of reentry. A: In the normal setting, the atrial impulse enters the superior aspect of the reentrant loop (a) and then travels down both the fast (b) and slow (c) pathways. Upon reaching the inferior aspect of the loop, the impulse travels distally (d) and retrograde up the slow pathway (e) where it is extinguished. B: A premature impulse enters the loop (a) and finds the fast path refractory (b). It then proceeds down the slow path (c) and then both distally (d) and retrograde up the fast pathway (e), where it then reenters the loop (f).

mechanisms: increased automaticity, triggered activity, or reentry. Almost all cardiac tissue demonstrates automaticity. The SA node's automaticity results in an inherent heart rate of 60–100 bpm. Other cardiac tissue has slower automaticity and, thus, is suppressed by the SA node activity. Occasionally an area of the myocardium develops abnormally increased automaticity (steeper slope in phase 4 of AP) and thereby stimulates a tachyarrhythmia. The abnormal focus of depolarization may arise in the atrial tissue (e.g., atrial premature complexes, ectopic atrial tachycardia), the AV node (e.g., junctional tachycardia), or the ventricular myocardium (e.g., ventricular premature complexes, idioventricular rhythm).

In normal cardiac tissue, low-amplitude oscillations of the transmembrane potential occur during (early afterdepolarizations) or at the end of (delayed afterdepolarizations) electrical repolarization (Figure 22–2). In abnormal myocardium, higher-amplitude oscillations may develop and cause the membrane potential to reach threshold prematurely, thereby "triggering" another action potential. Examples of triggered automaticity include digitalis-induced arrhythmias and some forms of ventricular tachycardia (e.g., Torsade de Pointes).

Reentry is a common mechanism of arrhythmogenesis and reflects the formation of an abnormal electrical circuit in the heart. Two distinct electrical pathways in the myocardium, each with differing electrical properties, form this circuit. One pathway conducts rapidly but repolarizes slowly, whereas the other pathway conducts slowly and repolarizes rapidly (Figure 22–3). These characteristics allow an electrical loop to be formed and an impulse to reenter the loop in a continuous fashion. The reentrant circuit can occur in a small focus of myocardium (a micro-reentrant circuit) or can involve anatomically distinct pathways (a macro-reentrant circuit). Examples of reentrant arrhythmias include atrioventricular nodal reentrant tachycardia (AVNRT), atrioventricular reentrant tachycardia (AVRT) (using a bypass tract; i.e., Wolff-Parkinson-White [WPW] syndrome), atrial flutter, atrial fibrillation, and most ventricular tachycardias.

MECHANISMS OF BRADYARRHYTHMIAS

A bradyarrhythmia is a rhythm that produces a heart rate of less than 60 bpm. Bradyarrhythmias may arise as a result of abnormally slow impulse formation by the sinus node, or as a result of impaired conduction of an impulse to the remainder of the myocardium. When the sinus node slows its rate of depolarization (sinus bradycardia) or fails to depolarize altogether (sinus arrest), the area of the heart with the next fastest inherent depolarization rate (usually the AV node) will take over as the pacemaker of the heart. The AV node will then beat at a rate of 40–60 bpm (junctional rhythm). If the AV node fails, the ventricular myocardium will beat at a rate of 20–30 bpm (idioventricular rhythm). Rhythms such as these, which are unmasked by failure of a faster pacemaker site, are referred to as "escape rhythms."

Bradycardia may also result from failure of a normal impulse to be propagated through the conduction system. This is termed **heart block**. Heart block can occur anywhere along the conduction system, although it most commonly occurs at the AV node. The block can be partial (1st or 2nd degree block) or complete (3rd degree block), and can be intermittent or persistent.

◆ KEY POINTS ◆

1. Tachyarrhythmias produce heart rates of >100 bpm; bradyarrhythmias produce rates of <60 bpm.

2. Specific ion fluxes result in depolarization and repolarization of the myocyte and generate the cellular electrical activity known as the action potential.

3. Automaticity refers to the inherent ability of cardiac tissue to produce spontaneous action potentials.

4. The SA node normally has the fastest automaticity and, thus, functions as the pacemaker of the heart.

5. Three mechanisms that produce tachyarrhythmias include increased automaticity, triggered activity, and reentry.

6. Mechanisms of bradycardia include delayed or abnormal impulse formation and impaired impulse conduction.

23 Tachyarrhythmias

Tachycardias are defined as arrhythmias that produce heart rates of ≥100 beats per minute (bpm).

ETIOLOGY

The three main mechanisms that produce tachyarrhythmias, enhanced automaticity, triggered activity, and reentry, are discussed in detail in Chapter 22 and will be referred to here in the context of specific arrhythmias. Tachyarrhythmias are more likely to occur in patients with underlying structural heart disease, including:

- prior myocardial infarction (MI)
- left ventricular aneurysm
- cardiomyopathy
- valvular disease
- hypertrophic heart disease
- arrhythmogenic right ventricular dysplasia

However, even a structurally normal heart may develop tachyarrhythmias in certain circumstances, including in the setting of:

- increased catecholamines (e.g., fear, pain, anxiety)
- metabolic abnormalities (e.g., hyper- or hypokalemia, hypomagnesemia, hypocalcemia, hyperthyroidism)
- drugs (e.g., caffeine, cocaine, ethanol)
- medications (e.g., beta-agonists, theophylline, antiarrhythmic agents, thyroid hormone replacement).

CLINICAL MANIFESTATIONS

History

Patients with tachycardias may be asymptomatic, mildly symptomatic, or in fulminant hemodynamic collapse. Additionally, the same type of tachyarrhythmia occurring at the same rate can produce vastly different symptoms in different patients. The symptoms of tachyarrhythmias may be intermittent or persistent and may include:

- palpitations
- lightheadedness or dizziness
- syncope
- chest pain
- dyspnea

Many of these symptoms relate to a fall in cardiac output resulting from decreased time for ventricular filling during tachycardia.

Physical Examination

It is essential to measure the blood pressure of a patient with tachycardia in order to assess the hemodynamic significance of the arrhythmia. Arrhythmias that result in hypotension (systolic blood pressure [SBP] <90 mmHg) require urgent treatment. Palpation of the arterial pulse will reveal the regularity and rate of the rhythm and examination of the jugular venous pulsations may demonstrate cannon A waves suggesting atrioventricular (AV) dissociation (see below), a sign that is highly suggestive of ventricular tachycardia. Variability of the first heart sound (S_1) and an intermittent S_3 and S_4 may also suggest AV dissociation. Auscultation of the lung fields may reveal rales (crackles) consistent with pulmonary vascular congestion, a finding that indicates either underlying left ventricular dysfunction or a more hemodynamically significant arrhythmia.

DIFFERENTIAL DIAGNOSIS

Tachycardias can arise from any part of the heart, including the sinus node, atria, AV node, His-Purkinje system, or ventricles. The most frequently encountered tachyarrhythmias are outlined in Table 23–1.

DIAGNOSTIC EVALUATION

The electrocardiogram (ECG) is the primary tool for differentiating among various tachyarrhythmias. Determining the exact type of tachyarrhythmia present can be difficult, but it is essential for selecting appropriate therapy. The most important aspect of diagnosing a tachyarrhythmia is determining whether it is a supraventricular tachycardia (SVT) that arises from the atria or AV node, or a ventricular tachycardia (VT) that arises from the ventricular myocardium. The QRS morphology helps to distinguish these arrhythmias; those with a narrow QRS complex (<0.120 seconds) are almost always SVTs, whereas those with a wide QRS complex (>0.120 seconds) may be VT or SVT with aberrant conduction. Two other diagnostically helpful features on the ECG are the regularity of the rhythm and the presence or absence of P-waves (see Table 23–1).

TREATMENT OF TACHYARRHYTHMIAS

In general, the goals of therapy of SVT are to control the ventricular rate and to terminate and prevent recurrences of the arrhythmia. The following methods are available:

- vagal maneuvers (e.g., carotid sinus massage) or adenosine to block AV nodal conduction transiently
- AV node-blocking drugs (e.g., calcium channel blockers, beta-blockers, digitalis) to slow the conduction of the arrhythmia to the ventricles

TABLE 23–1

Differential Diagnosis of Tachyarrhythmias

QRS Morphology	Pattern	Examples
Narrow complex	Regular	Sinus tachycardia Ectopic atrial tachycardia Atrial flutter Junctional tachycardia AV nodal reentrant tachycardia (AVNRT) Orthodromic AV reentrant tachycardia (AVRT)
	Irregular	Atrial fibrillation (P waves absent) Multifocal atrial tachycardia (≥3 different P waves present) Atrial flutter with variable conduction (flutter waves present)
Wide complex	Regular	Ventricular tachycardia Supraventricular tachycardia with aberrancy, including antidromic AVRT
	Irregular	Atrial fibrillation with aberrancy

- antiarrhythmic medications to restore and maintain normal sinus rhythm

- synchronized electrical countershock (cardioversion) to restore normal sinus rhythm

- radiofrequency ablation with catheters to modify or destroy reentrant circuits (atrioventricular nodal reentrant tachycardia [AVNRT], atrioventricular reentrant tachycardia [AVRT], atrial flutter).

Ventricular tachyarrhythmias are frequently hemodynamically unstable rhythms that require urgent/emergent therapy. Vagal maneuvers and AV node-blocking drugs are not effective in this setting. The mainstays of treatment are electrical defibrillation to emergently convert hemodynamically unstable rhythms, and antiarrhythmic medications to convert hemodynamically stable VT back to sinus rhythm, as well as to prevent recurrences. Placement of an implantable defibrillator/cardioverter (ICD) may be indicated to prevent sudden death when these ventricular tachyarrhythmias recur.

FEATURES OF SPECIFIC TACHYCARDIAS

Sinus Tachycardia

Sinus tachycardia almost always occurs as a response to some physiological stimulus (e.g., fever, exercise, volume depletion, thyrotoxicosis, hypotension). The ECG demonstrates normal-appearing P waves (inverted in lead aVR, upright in lead II), and the rate rarely exceeds 200 bpm. If the increased heart rate is causing symptoms, it can be slowed with the AV nodal-blocking drugs mentioned above; however, in general, the treatment of sinus tachycardia should be directed toward correcting the underlying cause.

Ectopic Atrial Tachycardia

Atrial tachycardias originate from an area of the atria distinct from the AV node, have similar triggers as does sinus tachycardia, but may occur in the absence of an identifiable precipitant. Frequently the ECG demonstrates P waves that are inverted in the inferior leads (leads II, III, aVF) and upright in lead aVR, reflecting the origin of this arrhythmia from the inferior aspect of the atria. Treatment is similar to the treatment of sinus tachycardia. Chronic treatment with beta-blockers or calcium-channel blocking drugs may be required to prevent recurrences.

Multifocal Atrial Tachycardia (MAT) (Figure 23–1)

MAT is a form of atrial tachycardia in which multiple areas of the atria generate impulses. It is most commonly seen in patients with severe lung disease. The ECG demonstrates an irregularly irregular rhythm with ≥3 different P-wave morphologies and ≥3 different PR intervals. The heart rate is usually difficult to control, although verapamil may be effective. The mainstay of therapy involves treatment of the underlying lung disease.

Atrial Fibrillation (Figure 23–2)

Atrial fibrillation (AF) is one of the most common types of SVT. The risk factors for AF include rheumatic heart disease, hypertension, congestive heart failure, and advanced age. During AF the atria fibrillate at ~400–600 bpm but produce no effective atrial contraction. This predisposes to the formation and subsequent embolization of atrial clots, and accounts for the almost five-fold increase in stroke risk in patients with AF compared with those in normal sinus rhythm. The loss of atrial contraction decreases atrial filling and can significantly reduce cardiac output, especially in patients with reduced LV systolic function. The ECG in atrial fibrillation demonstrates no P-waves, and an irregularly irregular ventricular rhythm, usually at a rate of 100–170 bpm.

There are three goals of treatment for AF:

- rate control

- stroke prevention

- restoration and maintenance of sinus rhythm

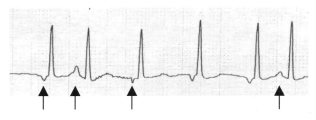

Figure 23–1 Multifocal atrial tachycardia. Note the irregular rhythm and various p wave morphologies (arrows).

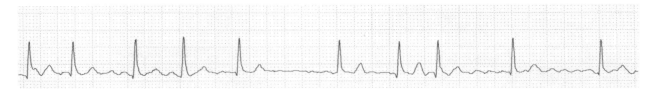

Figure 23–2 Atrial fibrillation.

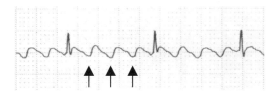

Figure 23–3 Atrial flutter. Note the coarse flutter waves (arrows).

The ventricular rate can usually be controlled with AV nodal-blocking medications (ideal heart rate: <80 bpm). The risk of stroke in patients with chronic or paroxysmal AF can be decreased with the use of warfarin to maintain an international normalized ratio (INR) of ~2–3. Younger patients (age <60) without underlying heart disease, diabetes mellitus, or hypertension (so-called **lone atrial fibrillation**) may be treated with aspirin instead of warfarin, as their risk of embolic event is quite low. AF may be converted to normal sinus rhythm electrically or with antiarrhythmic agents (class IA or class III). Unless required because of hemodynamic compromise, cardioversion should be avoided until the patient has been therapeutically anticoagulated for at least three weeks, or has been shown to be free of atrial thrombi by transesophageal echocardiography.

Atrial Flutter (Figure 23–3)

Atrial flutter is caused by a macro-reentrant circuit in the atrium. Most individuals with this rhythm tend to revert spontaneously to sinus rhythm or develop atrial fibrillation. The ECG demonstrates "flutter waves," which have a "sawtooth" appearance in leads II, III, and aVF, and occur at a rate of 250–350 bpm. However, the usual ventricular rate is one-half of this (2 : 1 block), because of the inability of the AV node to conduct at such rapid rates (decremental conduction). Predisposing factors and treatment are the same as for atrial fibrilla-

tion. In addition, radiofrequency ablation (see Chapter 9) may cure this rhythm.

AV Nodal Reentrant Tachycardia (Figure 23–4)

AVNRT results from a small reentrant loop (micro-reentrant circuit) within the AV node itself. AVNRT is usually initiated by a premature atrial beat and propagates at a rate of 170–220 bpm. The ECG demonstrates a regular tachycardia, either without discernable P-waves, or with P-waves occurring after the QRS complex ("retrograde P-waves"). AV nodal-blocking drugs are the treatment of choice and stop the arrhythmia by slowing conduction through the reentrant circuit. Radiofrequency ablation may be curative.

Atrioventricular Reentrant Tachycardia

AVRT involves a large reentrant loop (macro-reentrant circuit) with one limb of the circuit including the AV node and the other being an abnormal connection between the atria and ventricles (an accessory bypass tract). The most common type of bypass tract occurs in the Wolff-Parkinson-White syndrome (WPW). The ECG in this syndrome demonstrates a delta wave in normal sinus rhythm owing to partial preexcitation of the ventricles via rapid conduction of the atrial impulse through the bypass tract (Figure 23–5). AVRT is usually initiated by a premature beat and may be associated with a narrow QRS complex if the circuit proceeds down the AV node and up the bypass tract (orthodromic AVRT). If the circuit proceeds in the opposite direction (antidromic AVRT), a wide QRS complex occurs. Treatment is the same as for AVNRT. Care must be taken when patients with bypass tracts develop atrial arrhythmias (e.g., atrial fibrillation or flutter). If AV nodal blocking agents are given in this situation, the impulses will be preferentially shunted rapidly down the bypass tract and can precipitate hemodynamic collapse.

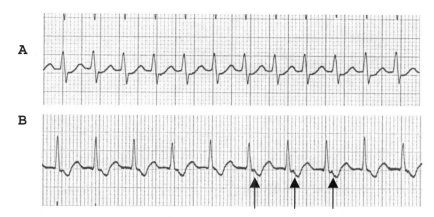

Figure 23–4 AV nodal reentrant tachycardia. (a) No P wave is seen (hidden in QRS). (b) Retrograde P waves are seen in the ST segment (arrows).

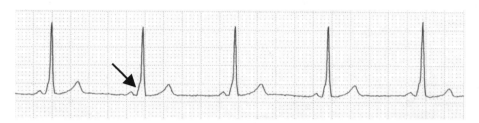

Figure 23–5 Wolff-Parkinson-White syndrome. Note the slurred upstroke of the QRS (delta wave) and the short PR interval.

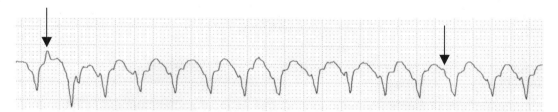

Figure 23–6 Ventricular tachycardia. Note the wide QRS and evidence of AV dissociation (P waves marked by arrows).

Ventricular Tachycardia (Figure 23–6)

Ventricular tachycardia (VT) is usually associated with symptoms and may cause sudden death. It is usually produced by a reentrant circuit located in either ventricle, and is seen most often in the following circumstances:

- acute cardiac ischemia resulting from coronary artery disease (CAD)

- prior myocardial infarction
- cardiomyopathy (ischemic or non-ischemic)
- electrolyte abnormalities (e.g., hypokalemia, hypomagnesemia)
- drug toxicity (e.g., digitalis)
- congenital abnormalities (e.g., right ventricular dysplasia)

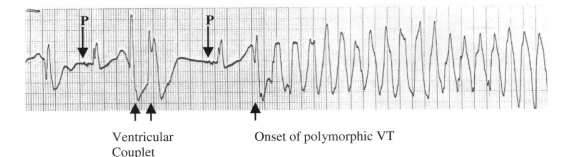

Ventricular Couplet   Onset of polymorphic VT

Figure 23–7 Polymorphic ventricular tachycardia (**Torsade de Pointes**). The underlying rhythm is sinus (note P waves) with a long QT. Multiple premature ventricular complexes are present and induce a ventricular couplet and then polymorphic VT.

The ECG in VT manifests a regular, wide-QRS-complex tachycardia. Occasional P waves may be seen but have no relation to the QRS complexes. This lack of association between the electrical activity of the atria and ventricles, referred to as **AV dissociation**, is a hallmark of VT.

Torsade de pointes is a specific form of VT in which the axis of the QRS complex constantly changes, causing a "waxing and waning" QRS amplitude on ECG (Figure 23–7). This type of VT is frequently the result of drug toxicity and can also be seen in patients with an abnormally prolonged QT interval (congenital long QT syndrome). Treatment of VT includes direct current countershock if it is hemodynamically unstable, and pharmacologic therapy with antiarrhythmic drugs including lidocaine and amiodarone. Recurrences of VT may be prevented by antiarrhythmic medications or treated by implantation of a cardioverter-defibrillator. Torsade de pointes may be treated with magnesium or by pacing the ventricle at a faster rate (overdrive pacing).

DIFFERENTIATION OF WIDE-COMPLEX TACHYCARDIAS

Most wide-complex tachycardias (QRS complex duration >0.12 second) are ventricular in origin (i.e., VT). However, at times, SVT may present as a wide complex tachycardia due to aberrant electrical conduction through the His-Purkinje system. Distinguishing VT from SVT with aberrancy is crucial to pursuing the most appropriate therapy. Some key features on history, physical, or ECG **favor VT** as the diagnosis:

- history of CAD and/or recent or prior MI
- ECG or physical evidence of AV dissociation
- shift in QRS axis from baseline ECG
- QRS duration >0.160 second

Although these signs are not conclusive for VT, if noted they can aid in the diagnosis.

◆ KEY POINTS ◆

1. The most important aspect of arrhythmia management is identifying the particular arrhythmia present. The presence of P waves, the morphology of the QRS complex, and the regularity of the rhythm are key features in this regard.

2. The main goals of treating supraventricular tachyarrhythmias are control of the ventricular rate, restoration of sinus rhythm, and prevention of arrhythmia recurrences.

3. Ventricular tachyarrhythmias are frequently hemodynamically unstable rhythms that require urgent/emergent cardioversion to restore sinus rhythm.

4. Wide complex tachyarrhythmias may be ventricular in origin or may originate in the atria but conduct aberrantly to the ventricles. Features that favor VT over SVT in this setting include a history of CAD or cardiomyopathy, QRS duration >160 milliseconds, evidence of AV dissociation, and a shift in the QRS axis from baseline.

24

Bradyarrhythmias (Bradycardia and Heart Block)

When an individual's heart rate (HR) falls below 60 bpm, the rhythm is termed a bradycardia. When the normal conduction from the atria to the ventricles is delayed or interrupted, heart block is present. Bradycardia may occur with or without heart block, and heart block may occur with or without bradycardia. In general, bradycardia is a benign rhythm unless it produces symptoms, whereas heart block is usually more ominous.

ETIOLOGY

Although the causes for bradyarrhythmias are varied, it is useful to think of them in terms of functional or structural abnormalities (see Table 24–1). Functional abnormalities produce bradycardia by depression of impulse generation and can result in heart block by slowing (and eventually preventing) conduction through the atrioventricular (AV) node and His-Purkinje system. In general, functional abnormalities are the result of autonomic (predominantly increased vagal tone) or pharmacological influences, and are reversible upon treating the precipitating cause. Structural abnormalities, on the other hand, reflect inherent conduction system disease and are frequently progressive and require definitive treatment.

CLINICAL MANIFESTATIONS

History

The clinical importance of bradycardia rests almost entirely on the symptoms it produces; nonetheless, many individuals are asymptomatic despite very slow heart rates. If symptoms do develop, they usually reflect decreased cardiac output/low blood pressure and include:

- syncope or near-syncope
- angina pectoris
- dizziness and lightheadedness
- congestive heart failure
- confusion
- fatigue

Patients may also experience palpitations, the pattern of which depends on the type of arrhythmia present.

It is essential to obtain a thorough medication history to exclude possible medication-induced bradyarrhythmias, and to perform a review of systems aimed at identifying underlying disorders or precipitating causes (e.g., headaches, nausea, pain, etc., resulting in increased vagal tone).

TABLE 24–1

Causes of Bradycardia and Heart Block

Category		Examples	Treatment
Functional	Autonomic influences	Increased vagal tone (fear, GI disorders, acute IMI, increased ICP, CSS)	Atropine for vagal episodes
		Decreased sympathetic tone (hypothyroidism)	Thyroid replacement
	Medications	Beta-blockers Calcium channel blockers Digoxin Antiarrhythmic agents	Stop medications; Specific antidotes for overdose*
Structural		Fibrosis of SA and/or AV node Infiltration of SA and/or AV node (amyloidosis, sarcoidosis) Ischemia or infarction Congenital complete heart block	Pacemaker is usually indicated, especially if symptomatic

*Glucagon for beta-blocker overdose, intravenous calcium for calcium channel blocker overdose, digoxin antibodies for digoxin overdose.
GI: gastrointestinal; IMI: inferior myocardial infarction; ICP: intracranial pressure; CSS: carotid sinus sensitivity.

Physical Examination

Aside from revealing a slow heart rate, the examination of patients with bradyarrhythmias may be unremarkable. It is essential to measure the blood pressure to exclude hypotension (SBP < 90 mmHg) and to determine the hemodynamic significance of the rhythm and the urgency of therapy. In patients with AV dissociation (e.g., complete heart block), cannon A waves may be seen in the jugular venous pulsations, and cardiac auscultation may demonstrate a variable intensity of S_1 and an intermittent S_3 or S_4. Palpation of the carotid arteries may provoke further slowing of the heart rate in patients with carotid sinus hypersensitivity.

DIFFERENTIAL DIAGNOSIS

The term bradyarrhythmias encompasses a variety of rhythm abnormalities. In general, these rhythms can be distinguished through close inspection of the surface electrocardiogram (ECG). Occasionally, electrophysiological testing is required to clarify the nature of the arrhythmia (see Chapter 9).

Sinus Bradycardia

Sinus bradycardia is marked by a heart rate less than 60 bpm and a normal-appearing P-wave preceding each QRS complex. It is generally a benign rhythm caused by medications or increased vagal tone. The latter mechanism accounts for the sometimes marked bradycardia (HR < 50 bpm) that occurs during sleep and is seen in many athletes. Other conditions associated with sinus bradycardia include hypothyroidism, hypothermia, advanced liver disease, and intrinsic disease of the sinoatrial (SA) node.

Sinus Node Dysfunction (SND)

This condition may result from infiltration (e.g., amyloid) or fibrosis (e.g., normal aging) of the SA node and can result in sinus bradycardia, intermittent prolonged sinus pauses (Figure 24–1), or complete sinus arrest. It reflects failure of the SA node to generate an electrical impulse (sinus pause or arrest) or failure of the impulse to propagate beyond the region of the node (sinus exit block). If the SA node slows or pauses long enough, junctional or ventricular escape rhythms will supervene. **Sick sinus syndrome (SSS)** refers to the

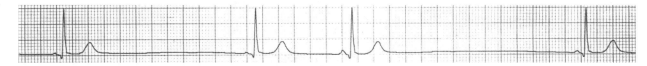

Figure 24–1   A prolonged sinus pause.

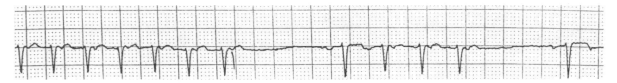

Figure 24–2   Tachy-brady syndrome. There is a run of supraventricular tachycardia followed by a moderate pause.

association of SND with symptomatic bradycardia. In a subset of patients with SSS intermittent tachyarrhythmias (e.g., atrial fibrillation) alternate with bradyarrhythmias (**tachycardia-bradycardia syndrome**) (Figure 24–2).

AV Node Conduction Disorders (Heart Block)

Even in the presence of normal SA node function and a normal rate of impulse formation, bradycardia can still develop if the impulse cannot propagate (i.e., is "blocked") through the AV node. This may occur as a result of functional or structural influences (see Table 24–1). Varying degrees of heart block can occur and can be intermittent or persistent. The degree of block can be diagnosed on a 12-lead ECG by observing the relationship between depolarization of the atria (the P-wave) and ventricles (the QRS complex). In 1st degree AV block there is fixed prolongation of the PR interval (>200 msec) representing slowed conduction through the AV node (Figure 24–3).

Higher degrees of AV block (2nd and 3rd degree) are associated with the failure of atrial impulses to conduct to the ventricles (a P-wave occurs without a resultant QRS complex). In 2nd degree heart block the failure of AV conduction is intermittent and may occur in two different patterns:

- Mobitz I (Wenckebach)
- Mobitz II

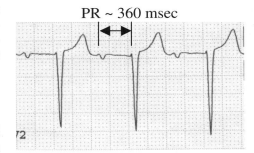

Figure 24–3   First degree AV block.

In the Wenckebach type, the PR interval progressively prolongs until a P wave fails to conduct and the subsequent QRS complex is "dropped" (Figure 24–4). This may occur sporadically or in a fixed pattern (e.g., every 3rd or 4th beat), is usually the result of increased vagal tone, and is a relatively benign rhythm. In Mobitz II heart block, the PR interval remains constant for all conducted beats; however, occasionally one or more P-waves fail to conduct to the ventricles (Figure 24–5). This form of 2nd degree heart block is usually the result of structural disease, is frequently associated with symptoms, and may progress to higher degrees of block.

The most severe form of AV nodal block is 3rd degree heart block (complete heart block). This is characterized by complete inability of any atrial impulse to pass through the AV node. Thus, the ECG demonstrates normal P-

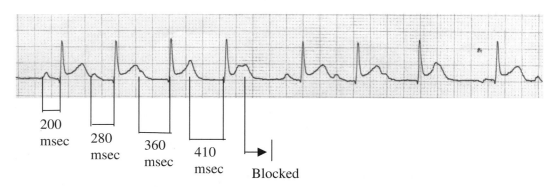

Figure 24–4 Mobitz I, second degree heart block (Wenckebach). Note the progressively prolonged PR interval preceding the non-conducted P wave.

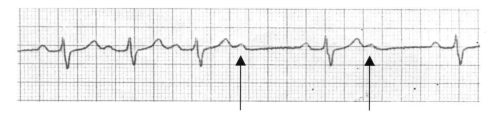

Figure 24–5 Mobitz II, second degree heart block. Note the non-conducted P waves (arrows) in the absence of progressive PR prolongation.

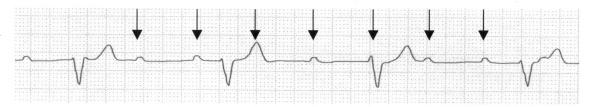

Figure 24–6 Complete heart block. Note that the P waves (arrows) march out faster than and independent of the QRS complexes.

waves without associated QRS complexes (AV dissociation) (Figure 24–6). When complete heart block occurs, the AV node (junctional escape rhythm) or ventricular myocardium (ventricular escape rhythm) takes over as the heart's pacemaker; their intrinsic rates are slower than that of the SA node, and, thus, bradycardia ensues.

DIAGNOSTIC EVALUATION

The most important diagnostic test in the evaluation of bradyarrhythmias is the 12-lead ECG. Careful inspec-

tion for the presence and pattern of P-waves and their relationship to the QRS complexes will usually allow recognition of the specific arrhythmias noted above. Owing to the intermittent nature of these conduction disturbances, prolonged monitoring with Holter monitors or event recorders (see Chapter 9) is sometimes required to identify these arrhythmias in patients with suggestive symptoms. Rarely, the mechanism of bradycardia or heart block cannot be determined on ECG and electrophysiological study is required. An evaluation of thyroid function is warranted in patients with bradycardia, and a thorough review of medications is necessary.

TREATMENT

In the absence of symptoms, bradycardia itself does not generally require treatment. Similarly, 1st degree heart block and Wenckebach block are generally benign rhythms with little clinical implications. In many instances, correcting the underlying cause (e.g., hypothyroidism, hypothermia) may restore a normal heart rate. Drugs that slow conduction should be discontinued and ischemia or infarction should obviously be treated. In patients with symptomatic bradycardia, and in most patients with higher degrees of heart block (2nd degree Mobitz type II and 3rd degree), treatment is warranted. Atropine may increase the heart rate acutely when the cause of the arrhythmia is functional, but can worsen heart block that occurs on a structural basis. Patients with persistent symptomatic bradycardia despite removal of aggravating causes, and those with SND or higher degrees of heart block, generally require implantation of a permanent pacemaker.

◆ KEY POINTS ◆

1. Sinus bradycardia is usually a benign rhythm caused by medication or increased vagal tone.

2. Sick sinus syndrome refers to the association of sinus node dysfunction with symptomatic bradycardia.

3. Second degree heart block, type I (Wenckebach) is associated with progressive prolongation of the PR interval until a nonconducted P wave occurs. Second degree heart block, type II, is associated with a nonconducted P wave in the absence of preceding progressive PR prolongation.

25
Syncope

Syncope is the sudden, transient loss of consciousness and postural tone followed by spontaneous recovery. Presyncope is the sensation of impending syncope without loss of consciousness.

EPIDEMIOLOGY

Syncope is a common clinical entity, accounting for approximately 3% of emergency room visits and 6% of all hospital admissions. The incidence of syncope increases with advancing age, and approximately one-third of the population will suffer an episode of syncope at some point in their lifetime.

PATHOPHYSIOLOGY

Syncope can result from a variety of cardiovascular or non-cardiovascular causes. The common physiological link among all cardiovascular causes of syncope is a transient decrease in cerebral blood flow. This usually results from a sudden fall in blood pressure, producing bilateral cortical or brainstem hypoperfusion. Unilateral carotid artery disease is unlikely to cause syncope. Non-cardiovascular causes of syncope produce loss of consciousness by inducing diffuse brain dysfunction via electrical or metabolic derangement.

DIFFERENTIAL DIAGNOSIS

The cardiovascular causes of syncope can be separated into those that are reflex-mediated, and those resulting from a structural cardiac problem (Table 25–1). The most common type of reflex-mediated syncope is vasovagal syncope (also known as neurocardiogenic syncope) in which various stimuli trigger the sudden development of vasodilation ("vaso") and bradycardia ("vagal"), resulting in hypotension. Vasovagal syncope precipitated by a specific trigger (such as coughing or micturition) is referred to as situational syncope. A similar reflex can be provoked in some people by applying gentle pressure over the carotid artery (carotid sinus hypersensitivity). This may result in vasodilation (vasodepressor response), bradycardia, or both. Orthostatic hypotension resulting from volume depletion or antihypertensive medication is another frequent cause of syncope.

Structural cardiac disease and arrhythmias account for approximately 15–20% of all syncope. Common mechanical causes include aortic stenosis and hypertrophic obstructive cardiomyopathy (HOCM); mitral stenosis, pulmonary hypertension, and cardiac tamponade are less common causes. Both bradyarrhythmias (sick sinus syndrome, atrioventricular [AV] node blockade, etc.) and tachyarrhythmias (ventricular [VT] or supraventricular [SVT] tachycardia) can result in a fall in cardiac output, thereby precipitating syncope. It is noteworthy that SVT rarely causes syncope in the

TABLE 25–1

Cardiovascular Causes of Syncope

Reflex-Mediated (Neurocardiogenic)
Situational (vasovagal)
- Micturition
- Tussive
- Valsalva
- Post-prandial
Orthostasis
- Volume depletion
- Medications
Carotid sinus hypersensitivity

Structural
Cardiac
- Aortic stenosis
- Mitral stenosis
- Hypertrophic cardiomyopathy
- Atrial myxoma
- Myocardial infarction
- Pericardial tamponade
Vascular
- Pulmonary embolism
- Pulmonary hypertension
- Vertebrobasilar insufficiency

Arrhythmic
- Supraventricular tachycardia
- Ventricular tachycardia
- Sinus node dysfunction
- AV nodal block

TABLE 25–2

Non-cardiovascular Causes of Syncope

Central Nervous System
- Cerebrovascular accident
- Seizure
Metabolic Abnormalities
- Hypoglycemia
Psychiatric
- Anxiety
- Pseudo-seizure

absence of underlying structural heart disease or a bypass tract.

Non-cardiovascular causes of syncope (Table 25–2) include neurological and metabolic causes. Psychiatric causes are uncommon.

CLINICAL MANIFESTATIONS

History

The history is the most important aspect of evaluating a patient with syncope and frequently gives clues to the underlying cause. It is important to obtain the history not only from the patient, but also from any witnesses, and to ask the following questions:

1. What was the patient doing at the time of the syncopal episode?
2. Were there any symptoms (e.g., chest pain, palpitations) that preceded the event?
3. Is the patient on any medications?
4. Does the patient have a history of heart disease?
5. Was there any sign of seizure activity? Any incontinence, or tongue biting?
6. How long did the patient remain unconscious?
7. When the person awoke, was he/she confused?

It is important to identify patients who have a cardiac cause of their syncope, as their prognosis is much worse than if they have a non-cardiac cause. Cardiac syncope is always sudden in onset, may be preceded by chest pain or palpitations, and resolves spontaneously (usually in less than 5 minutes). The following findings on history suggest true cardiac syncope:

- syncope following chest pain (suggests myocardial ischemia/infarction)
- syncope preceded by palpitations (suggests an arrhythmic cause)
- exertional syncope (suggests coronary artery disease, aortic stenosis, HOCM)
- syncope without warning or aura (consider arrhythmia)

Table 25–3 outlines important historic features of syncope and the diagnoses they suggest.

TABLE 25–3

Historical Features of Syncope and Suggested Etiologies

Historical Feature of Syncopal Episode	Suggested Cause(s)
Exertional	Aortic or mitral stenosis, HCM, pulmonary hypertension
Associated with chest pain	Myocardial ischemia, pulmonary embolism, aortic dissection
Associated with palpitations	Tachy- or bradyarrhythmias
Patient with history of CAD or cardiomyopathy	Ventricular tachyarrhythmia
Family history of syncope or sudden death	Hereditary long QT syndrome, HCM
Associated with emotional stress, pain, unpleasant auditory or visual stimuli	Vasovagal episode
Following cough, micturition, or defecation	Situational syncope (form of vasovagal syncope)
After arising from lying or sitting position	Orthostatic hypotension, hypovolemia
After turning head; during shaving	Carotid sinus sensitivity
Associated with certain body position	Atrial myxoma or "ball valve" thrombus
Diuretic medication use	Hypovolemia
Antiarrhythmic or anti-psychotic medication use	Ventricular tachyarrhythmias
Parkinson's disease	Autonomic insufficiency
Premonitory aura, tonic-clonic movements, incontinence, or tongue-biting	Seizure
History of CVA or head trauma	Seizure

HCM: hypertrophic cardiomyopathy; CAD: coronary artery disease; CVA: cerebrovascular accident.

Physical Examination

The physical examination should be directed at identifying potential causes of syncope. It is important to evaluate the patient for orthostatic changes in blood pressure and for signs of volume depletion, as well as to listen for the murmurs of aortic stenosis, mitral stenosis, or hypertrophic obstructive cardiomyopathy. Carotid sinus massage should be performed if the history is suggestive, but care must be taken first to exclude carotid vascular disease (i.e., listen for bruits).

DIAGNOSTIC EVALUATION

Many procedures are available to aid in determining the etiology of syncope (Table 25–4); however, the use of these ancillary tests should be guided by results of the history and physical examination. In at least one-third

of cases of syncope, a specific diagnosis cannot be determined; however, in approximately half of cases in which a diagnosis is made, it is suggested by the history or physical examination.

A 12-lead ECG should be obtained in all patients with syncope unless the history clearly suggests a noncardiac cause. The ECG may reveal the actual cause (i.e., heart block, tachyarrhythmias), or suggest potential causes (i.e., evidence of ischemic heart disease, bypass tracts, etc.). In patients in whom an arrhythmia is suspected but not documented on ECG, prolonged monitoring with a 24-hour Holter monitor, event recorder, or implantable recorder may be helpful. An echocardiogram is indicated in patients suspected of having underlying structural heart disease, and may reveal the cause of the syncope (i.e., aortic or mitral stenosis), or demonstrate evidence of prior infarction, thereby raising the suspicion of an arrhythmic cause. If

TABLE 25–4

Diagnostic Modalities in the Evaluation of Syncope

Diagnostic Procedure	Syncope Types in Which it May Be Helpful
ECG	Arrhythmias, heart block, conduction disease
Tilt-table testing	Neurocardiogenic syncope (vasovagal)
Electrophysiological testing	VT, some SVT, some bradycardias
24-hour Holter monitor	Arrhythmias that occur frequently
Event monitor	Infrequent arrhythmias (can monitor for ~ 1 week)
Implantable loop monitor	Very infrequent arrhythmias (can monitor up to 18 mo)
EEG, CT scan	Seizure disorder
Carotid sinus massage	Carotid sinus hypersensitivity

VT: ventricular tachycardia; SVT: supraventricular tachycardia; EEG: electroencephalogram.

the history, physical examination, or initial diagnostic tests suggest an arrhythmic cause for syncope, an electrophysiological study (EPS) may be indicated (see Chapter 9), especially if the patient is also suspected of having coronary artery disease. During EPS, the arrhythmia that caused the syncope can frequently be reproduced or heart block can be identified. In patients without underlying heart disease, EPS rarely identifies the cause of syncope.

Most patients without structural heart disease or clinical evidence of arrhythmias have a reflex cause of syncope (usually vasovagal), and further invasive diagnostic studies are usually not indicated. In such patients who have recurrent syncope, the diagnosis of neurocardiogenic syncope can be confirmed with tilt table testing (see Chapter 9). Patients who are suspected of having seizures or a psychiatric cause of syncope warrant neurologic or psychiatric evaluation, respectively.

PROGNOSIS

Young patients (< age 60) with syncope but without underlying heart disease have an excellent prognosis. Syncope patients with a normal ECG have a low probability of an arrhythmic cause and a low risk of sudden

TABLE 25–5

Treatment for Some Specific Causes of Syncope

Type of Syncope	Possible Therapies
Vasovagal/neurocardiogenic	Avoid provoking stimuli, beta-blockers, volume repletion
Orthostasis	Volume repletion, avoid anti-hypertensive drugs; mineralocorticoid supplementation for primary autonomic insufficiency
VT	Implantable defibrillator, antiarrhythmic drugs
SVT	Rate controlling medications, antiarrhythmic drugs, radiofrequency ablation
Bradycardia	Pacemaker
Aortic or mitral stenosis	Valve replacement
Hypertrophic cardiomyopathy	Myomectomy
Situational	Avoid precipitating factor

VT: ventricular tachycardia; SVT: supraventricular tachycardia.

cardiac death. Patients who have a cardiac cause of syncope have an annual mortality rate as high as 30%.

TREATMENT

The treatment of syncope depends entirely on its cause (Table 25–5). Most types of situational or vasovagal syncope require no specific therapy. Recurrent reflex-mediated syncope in the absence of triggering factors (i.e., neurocardiogenic syncope) may respond to treatment with beta-blockers. Arrhythmias require specific therapy based on the type of arrhythmia present (see Chapters 23 and 24). In general, SVTs can be treated with rate-lowering medications (e.g., beta-blockers, calcium channel blockers, digoxin), antiarrhythmic drugs, or occasionally radiofrequency ablation, whereas VT almost always requires treatment with antiarrhythmic drugs and/or implantation of a cardioverter/defibrillator. Syncope resulting from bradyarrhythmias requires placement of a pacemaker unless a reversible cause is identified (e.g., medications, metabolic abnormalities).

Syncope resulting from underlying heart disease requires correction of the structural abnormality.

For example, aortic and mitral stenosis requires valve replacement, and ischemic heart disease (ischemia or infarction) requires coronary revascularization with percutaneous balloon angioplasty or coronary artery bypass surgery.

◆ KEY POINTS ◆

1. Syncope refers to the sudden, transient loss of consciousness, and can arise as a result of cardiac or non-cardiac disorders.

2. Cardiac syncope is always sudden in onset, may be preceded by chest pain or palpitations, is short-lived, and resolves spontaneously.

3. The most common type of syncope is vasovagal (i.e., neurocardiogenic syncope).

4. Structural heart disease and arrhythmias account for approximately 15–20% of syncopal episodes.

5. A thorough history is the most important aspect of the evaluation of a patient with syncope.

26

Sudden Cardiac Death

The term "sudden cardiac death" (SCD) refers to the unexpected natural death from a cardiac cause occurring within one hour of the onset of symptoms in a patient without a preexisting fatal condition.

EPIDEMIOLOGY AND RISK FACTORS

In the United States, sudden cardiac death (SCD) leads to 300,000 to 400,000 deaths annually, accounting for almost half of all death from cardiac causes. Over 80% of patients with SCD have coronary artery disease (CAD); as a result, the risk factors for SCD closely parallel those for CAD. These include:

- tobacco use
- high cholesterol
- advanced age
- male gender
- hypertension

Other noted risk factors for SCD include:

- left ventricular hypertrophy
- intraventricular conduction block
- depressed left ventricular systolic function

In patients with a prior myocardial infarction (MI), the strongest predictor of SCD is a left ventricular ejection fraction of ≤30%. Frequent ventricular ectopy, espe-

cially nonsustained ventricular tachycardia (NSVT), is also a strong predictor of SCD in post-infarction patients, especially in those with depressed left ventricular systolic function.

The incidence of SCD is highest from birth until 6 months of age due to sudden infant death syndrome (SIDS) and some congenital cardiac anomalies. The incidence declines during adolescence and young adulthood, then rises sharply during middle and advanced age owing to the development of CAD. Approximately 75% of all cases of SCD occur in males. This gender predisposition is even more marked with advancing age; the male:female ratio is approximately 7:1 in the middle-aged and elderly population.

ETIOLOGY AND PATHOPHYSIOLOGY

Most cases of SCD result from cardiac disorders, predominantly CAD. Over 75% of patients who suffer SCD have pathological evidence of a prior MI, and, in as many as 25% of patients with CAD, SCD is the first manifestation of their disease. Other cardiac causes of SCD are outlined in Table 26–1.

Although the specific mode of death in SCD may be difficult to ascertain, many cases are attributed to malignant arrhythmias such as ventricular tachycardia (VT) and ventricular fibrillation (VF). Bradyarrhythmias are a much less common mechanism of SCD. The mecha-

TABLE 26–1

Cardiac Causes of Sudden Death

Cause	Examples
Coronary artery disease	Atherosclerosis, congenital anomalies, coronary aneurysms, coronary embolism, coronary spasm
Valvular heart disease	Aortic stenosis
Hypertrophic heart disease	Hypertrophic cardiomyopathy, hypertensive heart disease
Dilated cardiomyopathy	Ischemia, idiopathic, post-viral, alcohol-associated, myocarditis, arrhythmogenic right ventricular dysplasia
Infiltrative heart disease	Amyloidosis, hemochromatosis, Chagas' disease
Prolonged QT syndrome	Congenital (with or without deafness), drug effect (antiarrhythmics, phenothiazines), electrolyte abnormalities (hyper- or hypokalemia, hypocalcemia, hypomagnesemia)
Congenital heart disease	Aortic stenosis, Eisenmenger's syndrome
Pre-excitation syndromes	Wolff-Parkinson-White syndrome
Cardiac tumors	Atrial myxoma

nisms that produce the VT and VF in SCD include reentry, increased automaticity, and triggered activity (see Chapter 22), and may depend on factors such as autonomic tone.

Patients with long QT syndrome as noted on the surface electrocardiogram (ECG) (corrected QT interval greater than 0.44 second) may develop a type of polymorphic VT known as *Torsade de Pointes* (see Chapter 23) that can cause death by degenerating to VF. Long QT syndrome may be a congenital condition, but more commonly is the result of various drugs or metabolic disturbances including:

- class Ia, Ic, and some class III antiarrhythmics
- antihistamines (e.g., terfenadine)
- antimicrobials (mostly antifungals)
- tricyclic antidepressants
- phenothiazines
- electrolyte abnormalities (hypokalemia, hypomagnesemia, hypocalcemia)

The congenital forms of QT prolongation have been recently attributed to genetic defects that lead to abnormal myocyte potassium and sodium channels. The resultant alterations in ionic fluxes result in abnormal ventricular repolarization, thereby predisposing to the development of **Torsade de Pointes**, possibly through the generation of abnormal afterdepolarizations.

Several factors may predispose to the development of SCD in patients with underlying cardiac disease. These include:

- electrolyte imbalances (potassium, magnesium, calcium)
- transient myocardial ischemia
- hypoxia

PROGNOSIS

The vast majority of patients (>80%) who suffer an episode of SCD do not survive, and the incidence of recurrent SCD among initial survivors is as high as 30% in the first year following the event. The most common causes of death in survivors of SCD relate to neurological injury at the time of the event or infectious complications as a result of prolonged intubation. Among survivors of SCD who survive to hospital discharge, over one-third suffer persistent neurological deficits.

CLINICAL MANIFESTATIONS

History

Among the survivors of SCD, the history should be geared toward identifying potential causes, and should include a review of:

- prior cardiac disease
- concomitant medical conditions
- medication usage

If available, the patient's activities and symptoms immediately preceding the event may offer insight into the etiology.

Physical Examination

The physical examination of survivors of SCD should similarly be geared toward identifying potential causes. Although absolute signs of CAD cannot be discerned on physical examination, evidence of cardiomyopathy (S_3, displaced point of maximal impulse [PMI], etc.) or valvular heart disease (e.g., murmur of aortic stenosis) should be noted. In addition, a thorough neurological examination should be performed to determine the physiological consequences of the event.

DIAGNOSTIC EVALUATION

The initial evaluation in SCD survivors includes an ECG and a few basic laboratory tests. The ECG may reveal evidence of CAD (old or evolving MI, active ischemia), electrical predisposition to ventricular tachyarrhythmias (pre-excitation, long QT), ventricular irritability (frequent ventricular premature complexes, NSVT), or evidence of heart block. Initial laboratory tests should include an electrolyte panel and tests for myocardial injury (creatine kinase, troponin). If the initial ECG suggests an acute MI, cardiac catheterization to define the coronary anatomy and feasibility of revascularization should be considered.

Once stabilized, all survivors of SCD should undergo echocardiography to seek evidence of CAD or valvular heart disease, and to determine left ventricular ejection fraction. Patients with normal left ventricular function but with risk factors for CAD should undergo diagnostic exercise stress testing. In patients with a depressed ejection fraction, cardiac catheterization may be warranted to exclude significant underlying CAD, and electrophysiological studies (EPS) are indicated for risk stratification and guidance of therapy.

TREATMENT

The treatment of survivors of SCD depends on the cause of the event. If a reversible cause is identified (e.g., medication toxicity or electrolyte abnormality), treatment involves correcting the underlying problem. However, the vast majority of SCD survivors do not have a reversible cause, rather, they have CAD. If the patient is thought to have suffered an acute ischemic event as the basis for SCD, then cardiac catheterization and percutaneous (angioplasty) or surgical (coronary artery bypass grafting) revascularization should be performed if possible. In patients with an old MI or underlying cardiomyopathy who are felt to have had an arrhythmic event, EPS is warranted to determine the inducibility of ventricular tachyarrhythmias. Many of these patients will require treatment with an antiarrhythmic agent, such as amiodarone, and most will require implantation of a cardioverter-defibrillator (ICD) to monitor for and treat recurrent tachyarrhythmias. Patients with long QT syndrome require removal of offending medications, correction of metabolic abnormalities, and, frequently, ICD placement.

The primary prevention of SCD is difficult because many patients do not manifest signs or symptoms that may indicate their high risk of SCD. Since most cases of SCD are due to CAD or underlying structural heart disease, screening for disease in at-risk individuals may reduce the incidence of SCD by identifying patients with predisposing conditions and allowing for adequate therapy before SCD occurs. In general, correcting, or at least improving, cardiac function in those diseases known to cause SCD can reduce its incidence.

Patients with a depressed left ventricular ejection fraction (especially those with underlying CAD) who also have nonsustained VT, have a significantly increased risk of developing SCD. These patients may warrant EPS, and, if VT can be induced at the time of the study, may require ICD placement.

◆ KEY POINTS ◆

1. SCD is a major cause of death in the United States.

2. Coronary artery disease is the leading cause of SCD and accounts for over 80% of cases.

3. SCD is most often the result of ventricular tachyarrhythmias; bradyarrhythmias are a less common cause.

4. The initial evaluation of SCD survivors should include an ECG, electrolyte panel, and echocardiogram.

5. If SCD results from CAD, cardiac catheterization and revascularization are indicated.

6. Treatment depends in large part on the underlying cause and the left ventricular function. Antiarrhythmic agents may be necessary to prevent recurrences, whereas ICD placement is often necessary to treat recurrences.

27

Pacemakers and Implantable Cardioverter Defibrillators

With the major advances in microprocessor technology in the last two decades, patients who have symptomatic bradycardias and malignant tachycardias can be treated effectively with permanent pacemakers and implantable cardioverter defibrillators (ICDs), respectively. This chapter outlines the basic components, function, and indications for implantation of these devices.

PACEMAKERS

A cardiac pacemaker consists of a battery-powered pulse generator connected to a system of electrical leads. With a permanent pacemaker, the pulse generator is implanted subcutaneously in the chest wall, usually below the left clavicle. The leads pass from the pulse generator, through the cephalic or subclavian veins, and are anchored into the right atrium and/or ventricle (Figure 27–1). The device can be programmed to sense intrinsic cardiac electrical activity. If the intrinsic heart rate falls below a predetermined rate, the device delivers an electrical impulse to the myocardium, causing it to depolarize. Temporary pacemakers are also available and can be inserted transvenously or can deliver the electrical impulse through the chest wall (transcutaneously). The electrical impulses from the pacemaker can be seen on an electrocardiogram (ECG) as an elec-

trical spike immediately preceding the P wave or QRS complex (Figure 27–2).

Indications for Pacemaker Implantation

The most common indications for placement of a pacemaker are outlined in Table 27–1. In general, pacemakers are implanted for the therapy of symptomatic bradyarrhythmias (see Chapter 24). Asymptomatic bradyarrhythmias are usually benign, but occasionally require pacemaker placement owing to a high likelihood of progression to symptomatic bradycardia in some settings. Temporary pacemakers are used to treat transient bradyarrhythmias that result from reversible causes, whereas permanent pacemakers are used to treat irreversible disorders.

Pacemaker Modes

Single chamber pacemakers have a lead in the right atrium or ventricle, whereas dual chamber pacemakers have a lead in both chambers. These leads allow the device both to sense the electrical activity in the atrium and/or ventricle, and to pace the chambers at a preset rate.

Pacemakers can be programmed to various modes of activity that are described by a standardized three- or four-letter code. The first letter refers to the chamber

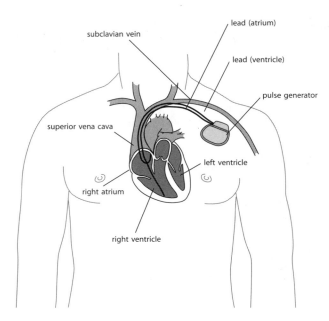

Figure 27–1   Diagram of pacemaker placement. *Illustration by Shawn Girsberger Graphic Design.*

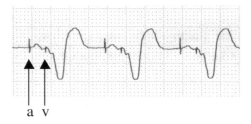

a v

Figure 27–2   Rhythm strip of patient with a dual chamber pacemaker. Note the atrial (a) and ventricular (v) pacemaker spikes that precede the P wave and QRS complex. Also note the wide QRS complex that results from direct activation of the ventricular myocardium.

being paced and the second refers to the chamber being sensed (A = atrium; V = ventricle; D = dual [both atrium and ventricle]; and O = neither). The third letter refers to the response of the pacemaker to a sensed native heart beat. The sensed beat may inhibit (I) the pacemaker from pacing; may trigger (T) the pacemaker to pace; or may have a dual effect (D) whereby it inhibits atrial pacing while triggering subsequent ventricular pacing. The fourth letter refers to special functions of the pace-

TABLE 27–1

Indications for Implantation of a Permanent Pacemaker

Heart Block
Symptomatic 3rd degree AV block
Asystole >3 seconds
Symptomatic 2nd degree HB, regardless of Mobitz type
Asymptomatic 3rd degree HB with escape rate <40 bpm
Mobitz II 2nd degree HB

Sinus node Dysfunction (sick sinus syndrome)
Sick sinus syndrome with symptomatic bradycardia
Symptomatic chronotropic incompetence
Tachycardia-bradycardia syndrome with symptomatic bradycardia

Syncope
Recurrent syncope caused by carotid sinus stimulation
Cardioinhibitory response (asystole >3 seconds) with minimal CSM

HB: heart block; SND: sinus node dysfunction; CSM: carotid sinus massage.

maker. Some pacemakers can sense an increase in a person's activity level and respond by increasing the pacing rate (denoted by R for **rate responsive**).

Choice of Pacemaker Mode

The choice of pacing mode depends mainly on the underlying arrhythmia. For patients with bradycardia but with an underlying sinus rhythm (sick sinus syndrome, heart block, etc.), dual chamber pacing (usually DDD mode) is preferred because it maintains atrioventricular synchrony. For patients with atrial fibrillation and bradycardia, single chamber ventricular pacing is used (usually VVI mode) because the fibrillating atrium cannot be paced. Other pacing modes are used less frequently.

IMPLANTABLE CARDIOVERTER DEFIBRILLATORS

An ICD is a device that is similar to a pacemaker in that it consists of an endocardial lead in the right ventricu-

TABLE 27–2

Indications for Implantation of a Cardioverter-Defibrillator

1. Non-sustained VT with CAD, LV systolic dysfunction and prior MI, with inducible VT on EPS
2. Spontaneous, sustained VT in the absence of a reversible cause
3. Survivors of cardiac arrest resulting from VT or VF, without reversible cause
4. Syncope of undetermined etiology with inducible VT on EPS (when drug therapy is ineffective or not tolerated)

VT: ventricular tachycardia; VF: ventricular fibrillation, EPS: electrophysiologic study.

lar apex connected to a pulse generator that is implanted in the chest wall. However, although ICDs have pacing capability, their primary role is in treating ventricular tachyarrhythmias (tachycardia [VT] or fibrillation [VF]). When the device detects one of these arrhythmias, it attempts to terminate the arrhythmia either by transiently pacing the heart faster than the rate of the arrhythmia (**overdrive pacing**), or by delivering a high-energy shock to the myocardium (**cardioversion/ defibrillation**).

Indications for ICD Implantation

ICDs are highly effective at terminating ventricular tachyarrhythmias and decrease the risk of sudden cardiac death in certain patient populations. The patients who benefit the most from ICDs include those with coronary artery disease, depressed left ventricular systolic function, and documented non-sustained runs of VT; and those who survive an episode of sudden cardiac death. Other patients who are felt to

be at increased risk of sudden cardiac death can be further risk-stratified by electrophysiological study (see Chapter 9). Some of these patients who have inducible VT may benefit from ICD implantation. Table 27–2 outlines the currently accepted indications for ICD placement.

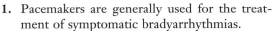

◆ KEY POINTS ◆

1. Pacemakers are generally used for the treatment of symptomatic bradyarrhythmias.
2. Dual chamber pacing maintains atrioventricular synchrony.
3. Implantable cardioverter defibrillators are used for the treatment of ventricular tachyarrhythmias and decrease mortality in certain patient populations.

Part VI
Valvular Heart
Disease

28 Rheumatic Fever

Acute rheumatic fever (RF) is an immune-mediated, inflammatory disease that is the result of untreated group A beta-hemolytic streptococcal pharyngitis. The chronic sequela of this disease is progressive cardiac valvular dysfunction with resulting heart failure.

EPIDEMIOLOGY

Acute RF is an uncommon illness in developed nations. It is rare in infancy, uncommon in adulthood, and is usually seen in the 5–15 year old age group. Males and females are equally affected. Its incidence is directly related to the prevalence of streptococcal pharyngitis in the community. During prior streptococcal pharyngitis epidemics, approximately 3% of those affected developed acute RF. Patients with a prior history of acute RF have a high risk of recurrence (5–50%) with subsequent untreated streptococcal pharyngitis. Most cases in the US are sporadic, although clusters have been reported in dormitories, military barracks, closed institutions, and densely-populated, poor, urban neighborhoods.

ETIOLOGY AND PATHOGENESIS

Several epidemiological and prospective studies have established the association of rheumatic fever with antecedent streptococcal pharyngitis. Group A strepto-cocci with M protein serotypes 1, 3, 5, 6, 18, 19, and 24 are the most rheumatogenic strains. Streptococcal skin infections, even when caused by the above serotypes, are not associated with rheumatic fever. The exact mechanism whereby the disease process is initiated remains uncertain, but likely involves molecular mimicry. Neither streptococci nor streptococcal antigens can be demonstrated in the pathologic lesions of rheumatic fever.

The principal organs involved in RF are the heart, large joints, brain, skin, and subcutaneous tissues. The pathognomonic lesion of rheumatic carditis is the Aschoff body, which consists of interstitial edema, fragmentation of collagen fibers, and mononuclear cell infiltration. Valvulitis, as a result of rheumatic endocarditis, can result in acute valvular regurgitation. More commonly, as the valvulitis heals, scarring, thickening, and adhesion of valve cusps and chordae occur and lead to valvular stenosis and/or regurgitation.

CLINICAL FEATURES

All patients with RF have had preceding strepto-coccal pharyngitis; this may have been asymptomatic in as many as 50% of cases. The symptoms and signs of RF begin several weeks after the incident pharyngitis.

Major Manifestations

Carditis

Acute rheumatic carditis varies in severity, is often asymptomatic, and affects all three layers of the heart. **Endocarditis** most commonly involves the mitral valve, followed by the aortic valve, and rarely the tricuspid and pulmonic valves. Acute valvular regurgitation can occur and may result in heart failure. Most patients with acute rheumatic carditis have a systolic murmur of mitral regurgitation and may have a low-pitched, apical, mid-diastolic murmur (Carey-Coombs murmur) resulting from flow across the inflamed valve. Rheumatic **myocarditis** usually manifests as sinus tachycardia disproportionate to the degree of fever, with or without other symptoms and signs of heart failure. Rheumatic **pericarditis** may result in chest pain, an audible friction rub, and pericardial effusion. Tamponade is a rare sequela.

Arthritis

An asymmetric, nonerosive, migratory polyarthritis with a predilection for large joints of the extremities is the most common symptom of RF. Effusions are common, but there is no residual joint deformity.

Erythema Marginatum

This transient, erythematous, migratory, non-pruritic rash is characteristic of RF, but is seen in only 5% of affected patients. The rash may vary in size with serpiginous, slightly raised margins and a pale center. It is usually localized to the trunk and proximal extremities.

Subcutaneous Nodules

Pea-sized, firm, painless, freely mobile nodules on the extensor surface of the elbows, knees, and wrists, and over the scapulae, vertebrae, and occipital scalp are seen in ~3% of patients with RF (usually in patients with carditis).

Chorea

(Sydenham's chorea, St. Vitus' dance):

Chorea is seen in 20% of RF patients and reflects inflammation of the basal ganglia and caudate nucleus. It is characterized by purposeless, involuntary movements of the face and extremities, nervousness, explosive speech, and emotional lability. Symptoms are absent during sleep and resolve spontaneously in 1–2 weeks. Unlike the other symptoms, chorea appears 3–6 months after the initial pharyngitis.

Minor Manifestations

Fever, arthralgia (without arthritis), epistaxis, abdominal pain, and tachycardia (without other features of carditis) may all be present in acute RF.

Late Manifestations

Approximately 50% of patients who have carditis during an episode of acute RF will eventually develop chronic rheumatic valvular disease. Aortic and mitral regurgitation may occur during the acute phase, or develop years later. Valvular stenosis is a late sequela, usually occurring decades after the acute illness. The mitral valve is most commonly affected, the aortic valve less commonly affected, the tricuspid valve rarely affected, and the pulmonary valve least commonly affected. Combined mitral and aortic valve disease is more common than isolated rheumatic aortic valve disease; tricuspid valve disease is invariably accompanied by mitral valve disease.

DIAGNOSTIC EVALUATION

There is no definitive diagnostic test for acute RF; the Jones Criteria (Table 28–1) is the standard diagnostic modality. The presence of either two major criteria or one major and two minor criteria, with supporting evidence of antecedent streptococcal infection, indicates a high probability of rheumatic fever. The absence of positive cultures or serologic evidence of recent streptococcal infection makes the diagnosis of RF doubtful, except when the presenting symptom is chorea. Diagnostic workup should include a pharyngeal swab, blood cultures, blood tests for acute phase reactants, and serum analysis for anti-streptococcal antibodies. An ECG and echocardiogram should be performed to evaluate for evidence of conduction disturbance and carditis, respectively.

DIFFERENTIAL DIAGNOSIS

Several illnesses can mimic acute RF, including infective endocarditis and various arthritides. However, with infective endocarditis, blood cultures are usually positive, vegetations are seen on echocardiography, and the associated arthritis is non-migratory. Hepatosplenomegaly and lymphadenopathy are prominent features of juvenile rheumatoid arthritis but not of

TABLE 28–1

Clinical Criteria for the Diagnosis of Acute Rheumatic Fever

Modified Duckett Jones Criteria (AHA 1992)

Major Criteria	Minor Criteria
Carditis	Clinical Findings
Polyarthritis	- Fever
Erythema marginatum	- Arthralgia
Subcutaneous nodules	Laboratory Findings
Chorea	- Elevated acute phase reactants (ESR or CRP)
	- Prolonged PR interval

Evidence of antecedent streptococcal infection
- Positive pharyngeal culture or rapid streptococcal antigen test
- Elevated or rising titers of anti-streptococcal antibodies (anti-streptolysin O, anti-DNase B, anti-hyaluronidase, Anti-streptozyme)

ESR: erythrocyte sedimentation rate; CRP: C-reactive protein.

TABLE 28–2

Antibiotic Regimens for the Treatment and Prevention of Acute Rheumatic Fever

Treatment of Streptococcal Pharyngitis	Secondary Prophylaxis after Acute RF
Benzathine PCN G 0.6–1.2 million U IM (as single injection)	Benzathine PCN G 1.2 million U IM every 4 wks
Or	Or
PCN VK 250–500 mg po TID for 10 days	PCN VK 250 mg BID
Or	Or
Erythromycin 20–40 mg/kg/d (divided TID) for 10 days	Sulfadiazine 0.5–1.0 g daily
	Or
	Erythromycin 250 mg BID

RF: rheumatic fever; PCN: penicillin; IM: intramuscular; TID: three times daily; BID: twice daily.

RF. Rheumatoid arthritis is not related to RF and is typically a disease of adults characterized by erosive, non-migratory polyarthritis.

TREATMENT OF ACUTE RF
(see Table 28–2)

Most patients with acute RF should be admitted to the hospital for observation, and those with arthritis and/or carditis should be placed at bed rest until their joint inflammation has subsided and the acute phase reactants have returned to normal. Even if pharyngeal swabs are negative for streptococci, all patients should receive a 10-day course of penicillin VK, 250–500 milligrams four times daily (erythromycin if penicillin allergic), to eradicate residual infection. Arthritis usually responds well to high-dose salicylates (100 mg/kg/day in four to five divided doses); treatment duration depends on the disease severity and clinical response. Patients with significant carditis, and those who do not respond to an adequate dose of aspirin, are treated with steroids (usually prednisone 1–2 mg/kg/day). Most patients require 4–12 weeks of therapy, followed by gradual tapering of the dose. As many as 5% of patients may have attacks that last 6 months or longer. Occasionally, symptoms recur when salicylates or steroids are tapered. Chorea usually responds to benzodiazepines; phenothiazines may also help ameliorate this symptom.

PREVENTION OF RF
(see Table 28–2)

Primary Prevention

Prompt treatment of streptococcal pharyngitis will prevent rheumatic fever. Oral penicillin VK 250–500 milligrams four times daily for 10 days or a single intramuscular injection of benzathine penicillin (0.6–1.2 million units) are acceptable regimens. Erythromycin may be used in penicillin allergic patients. Sulfa drugs are not acceptable because they do not eradicate streptococci.

Secondary Prevention

All patients with an established diagnosis of RF, Sydenham's chorea, or rheumatic heart disease should receive secondary prophylaxis to prevent recurrent acute RF. Intramuscular benzathine penicillin (1.2 million units every 3–4 weeks) or oral penicillin VK (250 milligrams twice daily) are the preferred antibiotic regimens. For those patients allergic to penicillin, oral sulfadiazine (0.5–1 gram once daily) or oral erythromycin (250 milligrams twice daily) are acceptable alternatives. Prophylaxis is recommended for at least 10 years after the most recent episode of acute RF, and generally until age 40. Lifelong prophylaxis is probably advisable for those patients with established rheumatic heart disease, especially if they are living in an endemic area.

◆ **KEY POINTS** ◆

1. Rheumatic fever follows untreated group A beta-hemolytic streptococcal pharyngitis.

2. Carditis, arthritis, erythema marginatum, chorea, and subcutaneous nodules are the cardinal manifestations of acute RF.

3. Carditis can lead to both acute and chronic valvular disease. The mitral valve is most commonly involved, followed by the aortic valve. Tricuspid and pulmonic valve involvement is unusual.

4. Prompt treatment of streptococcal pharyngitis is essential to prevent rheumatic fever.

5. Following an episode of acute RF, all patients should receive long-term antibiotic prophylaxis.

29

Disorders of the Aortic Valve

Valvular heart disease encompasses a wide array of disorders ranging from asymptomatic murmurs to life-threatening disease. In general, diseases of the aortic and mitral valves are far more common and clinically important than diseases of the tricuspid or pulmonic valves. This chapter and the next will, therefore, be limited to a discussion of aortic and mitral valve disorders.

AORTIC STENOSIS (AS)

Etiology

Aortic stenosis may be congenital (bicuspid or unicuspid valve), but is more commonly acquired. Acquired AS is three times more common in men than women and is most often the result of senile degenerative changes ("wear and tear") or rheumatic heart disease.

Pathophysiology

Aortic stenosis is a disease of pressure overload and produces progressive obstruction to left ventricle (LV) outflow. As the obstruction worsens, the pressure required to pump blood across the valve increases and a transvalvular pressure gradient results (Figure 29–1). As compensatory hypertrophy develops, the LV becomes poorly compliant, resulting in elevated ventricular diastolic pressure. This pressure is transmitted to the left atrium (LA) and pulmonary system, resulting in pulmonary congestion and dyspnea. The noncompliant LV is dependent on the "atrial kick" to maintain adequate

filling during diastole; thus, the onset of atrial fibrillation in a patient with AS may precipitate rapid decompensation. Over time, the ventricle weakens and systolic failure occurs.

In congenital AS, the valve leaflets are fused at the commissures, resulting in a reduced effective orifice. In the acquired cases, there is thickening, calcification, fibrosis, and fusion of the leaflets resulting in reduced leaflet excursion. Most patients with rheumatic AS have associated aortic insufficiency and rheumatic mitral valve disease.

Clinical Features

History

The cardinal symptoms of AS are dyspnea (congestive heart failure [CHF]), chest pain (angina), and syncope. CHF may result from systolic or diastolic dysfunction. Angina may reflect concomitant coronary artery disease (CAD), but may also result from myocardial oxygen supply/demand mismatch as a result of increased LV mass and LV diastolic pressure in the face of decreased cardiac output and diminished coronary perfusion pressure. Exertional syncope occurs as a result of peripheral vasodilation and consequent hypotension in the presence of a fixed cardiac output. Syncope at rest is usually secondary to arrhythmias.

Symptoms usually develop in the 3rd to 4th decade of life in patients with bicuspid AS, in the 4th to 5th decade with rheumatic AS, and in the 6th or later decades with degenerative AS. Symptoms are of prognostic impor-

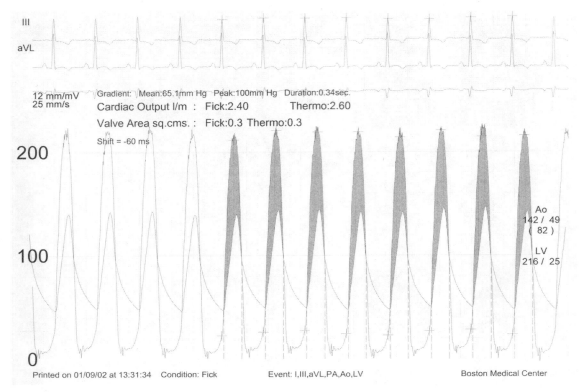

III

aVL

12 mm/mV
25 mm/s

Gradient: Mean:65.1mm Hg   Peak:100mm Hg   Duration:0.34sec.
Cardiac Output l/m : Fick:2.40   Thermo:2.60
Valve Area sq.cms. : Fick:0.3 Thermo:0.3

Shift = -60 ms

200

100

0

Ao
142 / 49
(82)

LV
216 / 25

Printed on 01/09/02 at 13:31:34   Condition: Fick   Event: I,III,aVL,PA,Ao,LV   Boston Medical Center

Figure 29–1   Hemodynamic tracing in a patient with critical aortic stenosis. Note that the left ventricular (LV) pressure exceeds the aortic (Ao) pressure. The shaded area represents the pressure gradient. The aortic valve area was 0.3 cm^2.

tance—once angina, syncope, or heart failure develops, the average survival without surgery is 5, 3, and 1½ years, respectively.

Physical Examination

Characteristic physical findings of AS include:

- **pulsus parvus et tardus** (diminished upstroke and a delayed peak of carotid pulse)

- sustained and LV apical impulse; often bifid as a result of a palpable S_4

- a low pitched, harsh, crescendo-decrescendo, systolic murmur, loudest at the second left intercostal space, and radiating to the carotid arteries (Table 4–2)

- soft or absent aortic valve closure sound (A_2)

- paradoxical splitting of the second heart sound

- a systolic thrill over the upper sternal border

The peak intensity of the murmur helps to estimate the severity of AS. An early-peaking murmur is associated with mild disease, whereas a late-peaking murmur is heard with severe stenosis. The murmur may also radiate to the LV apex (Gallavardin phenomenon). An S_4 is often heard. In patients with bicuspid AS, an aortic ejection sound may be heard immediately after S_1.

Diagnostic Evaluation

The electrocardiogram (ECG) usually demonstrates left ventricular hypertrophy (LVH) if significant AS is present, and chest x-ray may demonstrate aortic valve calcification and LV enlargement. However, the key component of the evaluation is the measurement of the transvalvular pressure gradient and calculation of the valve area. The normal aortic valve area is 3.5 cm^2. An area of 1.5–2.0 cm^2 is considered mild stenosis, 1.0–1.5 cm^2 moderate stenosis, and <1.0 cm^2 (or a mean

gradient of >50 mmHg) severe stenosis. "Critical" stenosis refers to an aortic valve area of <0.75 cm². These values
are usually estimated by echocardiography. Once valve
replacement is felt to be warranted, cardiac catheterization is usually performed to confirm the severity of the
valve disease and to assess for concomitant CAD.

Management

There is no effective medical management for symptomatic AS. In fact, many medications may cause adverse
affects by decreasing preload or afterload and precipitating hemodynamic collapse.

Patients with moderate or severe asymptomatic AS
should be carefully followed with clinical examinations
and serial echocardiograms every 6–12 months. Such
patients should avoid strenuous exertion.

Symptomatic AS, asymptomatic critical AS, and
severe AS with LV dysfunction even if asymptomatic,
are indications for surgical valve replacement. The decision to operate is usually based on symptoms and not on
an absolute valve area or pressure gradient. Percutaneous balloon valvuloplasty is associated with an unac-
ceptably high re-stenosis rate in patients with AS, but
may be attempted in critically ill patients as a bridge to
surgery or in those who are not surgical candidates
owing to significant co-morbid disease.

AORTIC INSUFFICIENCY (AI)

Etiology

Aortic insufficiency may be caused by a variety of
valvular disorders, including:

- rheumatic fever (usually with concomitant AS)
- bicuspid aortic valve
- infective endocarditis
- trauma
- connective tissue disease (systemic lupus erythematosus, rheumatoid arthritis).

It may also result from disorders that primarily cause
dilation of the ascending aorta and aortic root, including Marfan's syndrome, aortic dissection, syphilitic
aortitis, and the seronegative spondylarthropathies.

Epidemiology

Aortic insufficiency is more common in men than in
women. When associated with rheumatic heart disease,

AI is usually accompanied by some degree of AS and
mitral valve disease.

Pathophysiology

Aortic insufficiency is a disease of volume overload, and
may be acute or chronic. In acute AI, the abrupt increase
in blood volume entering the small, non-compliant LV
during diastole results in a sudden rise in LV diastolic
pressure. This is transmitted to the pulmonary system
and results in pulmonary edema and dyspnea.

In chronic AI, the excess volume initially results in
LV hypertrophy. This is followed by ventricular dilation
and increased end-diastolic volume, thereby augmenting contractility by the Frank-Starling mechanism. The
increased stroke volume results in bounding pulses with
an increased systolic pressure. Peripheral vasodilation
and the regurgitation of blood back into the LV results
in a lower diastolic pressure and a widened pulse pressure. Such patients are often well compensated and
asymptomatic. However, with continued enlargement,
the LV systolic function declines and heart failure ensues.

Clinical Features

History

Patients with acute AI often present with pulmonary
edema and hemodynamic instability. The symptoms
of the underlying disease (i.e., aortic dissection, endocarditis) may predominate. Patients with chronic AI
usually present with exertional dyspnea, and may complain of a pounding sensation in their neck resulting
from the increased LV stroke volume. Angina may result
from the combination of increased oxygen demand from
LVH, and low diastolic pressures causing reduced coronary perfusion.

Physical Examination

Chronic AI is associated with a variety of physical findings, all of which relate to the increased stroke volume
and widened pulse pressure (Table 29–1).

Severe AI may be associated with a double peaking
bisferiens pulse. The apical impulse is usually hyperdynamic and displaced downward and laterally signify-
ing LV dilation and hypertrophy. The characteristic
murmur of AI is a high-pitched, decrescendo, diastolic
murmur (see Table 4–2) that is best heard at the second
right or third left intercostal space. The longer the
murmur, the more chronic and severe the AI. A systolic
aortic flow murmur is usually present and is the result
of increased flow across the valve. The first heart sound

TABLE 29–1

Peripheral Signs of Aortic Insufficiency

Sign	Eponym
Systolic head bobbing	DeMusset's sign
Visible pulsations in the nail beds	Quincke's pulses
Rapid-rising and rapid-collapsing carotid pulse	Corrigan's pulse
Pistol shot sounds over the radial or femoral artery	Traube's sign
To-and-fro bruit over the femoral artery	Duroziez's sign
Systolic bobbing of the uvula	Muller's sign
Systolic blood pressure in leg >20 mm Hg higher than in arm	Hill's sign

(S_1) may be soft owing to premature mitral valve closure, and a mitral mid-diastolic murmur (Austin-Flint murmur) may be audible at the apex.

Patients with acute AI frequently have hemodynamic instability and signs of pulmonary edema, but the murmur may be inaudible and peripheral manifestations are frequently absent.

Diagnostic Evaluation

The ECG usually reveals LVH. Echocardiography is the initial test of choice to confirm the diagnosis, assess the severity of AI, and assess LV dimensions and function. Cardiac catheterization and aortography can also assess the severity of AI and identify associated aortic pathology. Magnetic resonance imaging is a useful tool for anatomic assessment of the thoracic aorta, especially in the presence of aneurysms.

Management

Most patients with mild to moderate AI are asymptomatic and require no specific therapy aside from anti-biotic prophylaxis for procedures and close monitoring for the development of symptoms. Many patients with severe AI are also asymptomatic. If such patients have normal LV size and function, surgery can be deferred. They should be closely monitored for symptoms, with exercise testing if necessary, and with periodic echocardiography to assess LV systolic function and dimensions. Chronic administration of nifedipine or angiotensin-converting enzyme (ACE) inhibitors may delay the development of symptoms and the need for surgery in these patients.

Indications for surgery include:

- onset of symptoms attributable to AI
- progressive LV dysfunction (LV ejection fraction <55%)
- progressive LV dilation (end-systolic dimension >55 mm)

Valve replacement is usually necessary for primary valvular disorders. When AI is secondary to a dilated aortic root, root repair alone may be adequate.

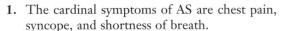

◆ KEY POINTS ◆

1. The cardinal symptoms of AS are chest pain, syncope, and shortness of breath.

2. Patients with symptoms of AS and a valve area <1.0 cm^2 should undergo valve replacement. Valvuloplasty is not an effective long-term therapy for AS.

3. Patients with AI should undergo valve replacement if their LV ejection fraction falls below 55% or their end-systolic LV dimension increases to >55 mm.

30

Disorders of the Mitral Valve

Disorders of the mitral valve are the most common types of valvular heart disease and may occur as either the sequela of a primary valve disorder or the secondary result of other cardiac disease. These disorders may be categorized as those that result in valvular stenosis and those that result in valvular regurgitation.

MITRAL STENOSIS

Etiology

Mitral stenosis (MS) is predominantly a sequela of rheumatic fever (see Chapter 28). Rarely it may be congenital, iatrogenic (following mitral valve repair or replacement), or secondary to rheumatoid arthritis, systemic lupus, or carcinoid heart disease. It is more common in women than in men.

Pathophysiology

The normal mitral valve area (MVA) is 4.0–6.0 cm². The stenosis is considered mild if the MVA is 1.5–2.5 cm², moderate if it is 1.0–1.5 cm², and severe if it is <1.0 cm². With rheumatic MS, fibrosis of the valve occurs producing commissural fusion, and the narrowed orifice takes on the classic "fish-mouth" appearance. As the valve narrows, the pressure gradient across it increases (see Figure 30–1). During tachycardia, there is reduced time available for transmitral flow, and the transvalvar gradient increases even further. The increased pressure gradient then leads to elevated left atrium (LA) pressure,

LA enlargement, pulmonary venous congestion, and pulmonary hypertension. Eventually, right ventricle (RV) dilation, tricuspid regurgitation, and RV failure ensue. In MS, the LV is relatively protected and does not dilate or hypertrophy in the absence of other cardiovascular disease.

Clinical Features

History

The most common symptoms of patients with MS include:

- left heart failure (dyspnea on exertion, paroxysmal nocturnal dyspnea, orthopnea)
- hemoptysis
- embolic events (central nervous system or peripheral)
- chest pain (from pulmonary hypertension)
- right heart failure (fatigue, ascites, edema)
- palpitations (atrial fibrillation)

Patients generally have a gradual onset of symptoms, usually by age 30. Severe enlargement of the left atrium may occasionally compress the left recurrent laryngeal nerve, resulting in hoarseness, or compress the esophagus, causing dysphagia.

Physical Examination

Patients with MS frequently demonstrate signs of chronic left and/or right heart failure and pulmonary hypertension.

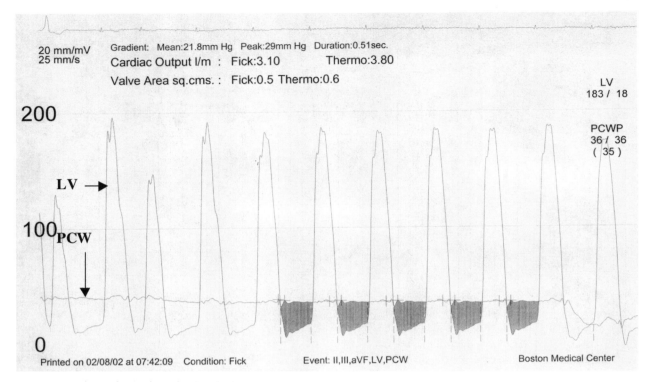

Figure 30–1 Hemodynamic tracing in mitral stenosis. The stenotic mitral valve impairs the flow of blood from the left atrium (measured as pulmonary capillary wedge pressure, PCW) to the left ventricle (LV). Thus, during diastole, there is a continuous pressure gradient (shaded region) between these two chambers.

Classic physical findings of MS include:

- loud S_1
- loud P_2 (pulmonary hypertension)
- opening snap (crisp sound after S_2, heard best with the diaphragm of the stethoscope)
- diastolic "rumble" (with pre-systolic accentuation if in sinus rhythm; see Table 4–2)
- right parasternal heave (right ventricular enlargement)

Diagnostic Evaluation

The electrocardiogram (ECG) often demonstrates sinus tachycardia, left atrial enlargement, and right ventricular hypertrophy. Atrial fibrillation is frequently present. Chest x-ray may reveal straightening of the left heart border (LA and RV dilation), dilated pulmonary arteries, and pulmonary vascular congestion.

Echocardiography is the test of choice by which to confirm the diagnosis of MS and assess its severity (see

Figure 30–2). The size of the MV orifice can be measured, the extent of valvular thickening and calcification assessed, the severity of pulmonary hypertension estimated, and associated valvular abnormalities identified. Cardiac catheterization can also quantify MS severity and measure pulmonary arterial pressure. It is often performed in conjunction with coronary angiography before valve surgery.

Management

Endocarditis prophylaxis is essential for any patient with MS. Asymptomatic patients should be closely monitored for the development of symptoms, atrial arrhythmias, and silent systemic embolism. Serial echocardiograms (every 6 to 12 months depending on valve severity) should be performed to evaluate progression of valvular stenosis.

Symptomatic patients with MS may initially be managed with beta-blockers (calcium channel blockers

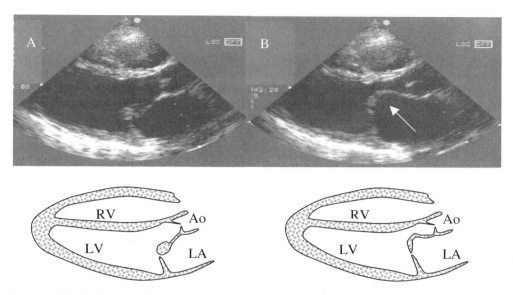

Figure 30–2 Echocardiogram in mitral stenosis. In systole (a) thickening of the mitral leaflets is seen. In diastole (b) the anterior mitral leaflet is seen "doming" into the left ventricular (LV) cavity (arrow).

or digoxin are alternatives) to control the ventricular heart rate, thereby prolonging diastole and minimizing the transvalvar pressure gradient. Diuretics are used to reduce pulmonary congestion. When atrial fibrillation (AF) accompanies MS, it is associated with ~12% per year risk of stroke, compared with ~4–6% in non-valvular related AF. Every effort must be made to maintain sinus rhythm, including electrical cardioversion and administration of antiarrhythmic agents (see Chapter 23). If atrial fibrillation is chronic, patients should be anticoagulated to prevent systemic embolization, and the ventricular rate controlled with beta-blockers, calcium channel blockers, or digoxin.

Patients with symptomatic severe or moderately severe MS, worsening pulmonary hypertension, or recurrent systemic embolization should undergo mitral valvotomy or valve replacement. Valvotomy may be performed percutaneously by balloon dilation, or by surgical commissurotomy. Balloon valvuloplasty is the procedure of choice in young patients with pliable valves, minimal valvular calcification, and no significant associated mitral regurgitation. Patients who undergo valvotomy usually require a second procedure in 5–15 years. Patients with heavily calcified valves and/or associated significant mitral regurgitation require valve replacement.

MITRAL REGURGITATION

Etiology/Epidemiology

Mitral regurgitation (MR) may result from a variety of conditions and may be acute or chronic (Table 30–1). Mitral valve prolapse (MVP) is the most common cause of isolated MR; the posterior leaflet is more frequently involved than the anterior leaflet. MVP affects 2–3% of the population and is slightly more common in women. It is often an isolated condition, but may be associated with congenital heart disease (e.g., atrial septal defect, bicuspid aortic valve), and connective tissue disorders. Rheumatic MR is more common in men than in women, and may occur in isolation or in association with MS.

Pathophysiology

The significance of MR depends in part on its acuity and the compliance of the LA. In acute MR, the LA is normal in size and poorly compliant. The acute regurgitation of blood into the atrium results in marked elevation of left atrial and pulmonary venous pressures, resulting in pulmonary edema. In chronic MR, the regurgitation progresses over time, allowing the LA to dilate gradually and become compliant. In this setting, patients are able to tolerate moderate to severe MR for

TABLE 30–1

Causes of Mitral Regurgitation (MR)

Acute MR	Chronic MR
- Valve leaflet perforation (endocarditis) - Ruptured chord (endocarditis, trauma, myxomatous degeneration) - Papillary muscle dysfunction or rupture (ischemia, blunt chest trauma) - Acute mechanical failure of prosthetic valve (strut fracture, cusp perforation, or degeneration)	- Mitral valve prolapse - Rheumatic heart disease - Annular dilation (cardiomyopathies) - Rheumatologic diseases (SLE, scleroderma) - Disorders of connective tissue (Marfan's, Ehlers-Danlos, pseudoxanthoma elasticum) - Congenital (parachute mitral valve, cleft mitral valve, endocardial cushion defects) - Hypertrophic cardiomyopathy - Mitral annular calcification - Anorexigenic drugs (e.g., Fen-Phen) - Any cause of acute MR

SLE: systemic lupus erythematosus; Fen-Phen: fenfluramine-phentermine.

several years with only a slight increase in left atrial and pulmonary arterial pressures.

Initially with MR, the augmented LV preload results in increased contractility (Starling mechanism) resulting in hyperdynamic LV function. Over time, the LV hypertrophies and dilates, stretching the mitral annulus and worsening the MR severity. Eventually, LV systolic function deteriorates and heart failure ensues.

Clinical Features

History

Patients with acute MR have an abrupt onset of symptoms and often present with acute pulmonary edema. Patients with chronic, severe MR usually have slowly progressive exertional dyspnea. A history of anginal chest pain (ischemic MR), recent dental work (endocarditis), or distant rheumatic fever should be noted. Most patients with MVP are asymptomatic, although many report non-specific symptoms, such as vague chest discomfort, palpitations, presyncope, and fatigue (the MVP syndrome).

Physical Examination

Patients with MR frequently demonstrate signs of chronic left and/or right heart failure and pulmonary hypertension. Patients with acute MR are often hypotensive and tachycardic, and may be in acute respiratory distress.

Classic findings of MR include:

- holosystolic murmur (may be late systolic with MVP)
- apical systolic thrill (with severe MR)
- soft S_1 (incomplete coaptation of the mitral leaflets)
- loud P_2 and RV heave (pulmonary hypertension)
- mid-systolic click (with MVP)

Diagnostic Evaluation

The ECG often demonstrates left atrial enlargement and LVH. Atrial fibrillation is often present. Chest x-ray may reveal straightening of the left heart border (LA dilation), a dilated left ventricle, and pulmonary vascular congestion.

Echocardiography is the test of choice for the assessment of MR. The severity of MR is graded from 1 to 4, based on the volume of regurgitant flow seen by color Doppler. In addition, the atrial and ventricular chamber sizes can be measured, LV systolic function can be quantified, pulmonary hypertension assessed, and associated valvular abnormalities identified. Echocardiographic findings may suggest the etiology of MR by revealing rheumatic changes, MVP, ruptured chordae, vegetations (endocarditis), or LV dilation. Cardiac catheterization has been the gold standard for the quantification of MR, and can also directly measure pulmonary artery pres-

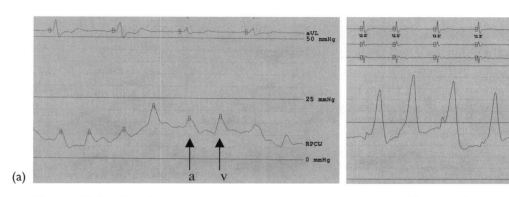

Figure 30–3 Hemodynamic tracing in severe mitral regurgitation. (a) Normal a and v waves in a pulmonary capillary wedge (PCW) pressure tracing. (b) PCW tracing in severe mitral regurgitation. Note the prominent v-wave reflecting direct transmission of the LV pressure to the pulmonary system.

sure. In severe MR, the LV pressure is transmitted to the pulmonary system and produces a prominent v-wave in the pulmonary capillary wedge (PCW) pressure tracing (see Figure 30–3). Cardiac catheterization is usually performed to confirm the severity of MR and to assess for concomitant CAD prior to valve surgery.

Management

Medical management of asymptomatic or minimally symptomatic patients with mild or moderate MR includes afterload reduction (angiotensin-converting enzyme [ACE] inhibitors) and endocarditis prophylaxis. Diuretics should be used if signs of congestion are present. Serial echocardiograms (every 6 to 12 months, depending on valve severity) should be performed to evaluate progression of regurgitation and to assess left ventricular size and systolic function.

Surgery is indicated in patients with severe, symptomatic MR. Valve repair is desirable, if possible, as it avoids the risks of anticoagulation and prosthetic valve dysfunction. If the valve is replaced, the papillary muscles and the chordae are often preserved and help to maintain left ventricular morphology and function.

The ideal timing of surgery for the asymptomatic or mildly symptomatic patient with severe MR remains controversial. Nonetheless, there is general consensus that a decrease in the LVEF to ≤60% and/or an increase

in end-systolic LV dimension to >45 mm are indications for surgery.

Patients with acute, severe MR require urgent therapy. Hypotensive patients should have an intra-aortic balloon pump inserted followed by emergent valve repair or replacement. Patients who are not hypotensive should be managed with diuretics and vasodilators such as nitroprusside or ACE inhibitors while arrangements are being made for surgery.

◆ KEY POINTS ◆

1. Mitral stenosis is predominantly a sequela of rheumatic fever.

2. The most common etiology of mitral regurgitation and most common indication for MVR is mitral valve prolapse.

3. The classic physical findings of MS include a loud S$_1$, an opening snap, and a diastolic rumble. The classic physical finding of MR is a holosystolic murmur that is associated with a mid-systolic click in the presence of MVP.

4. Patients with moderate to severe MS or MR, who have symptoms despite medical therapy, should undergo valve surgery.

31 Infective Endocarditis

Infective endocarditis (IE) is an infection of the endocardial surface of the heart. The structures most commonly affected are the valves; however, valvular chordae and the atrial and ventricular walls may also be involved. IE is associated with significant morbidity and mortality; early diagnosis, appropriate treatment, and prompt recognition of complications are essential for the management of these patients.

EPIDEMIOLOGY

The incidence of IE in the US is 15,000–20,000 new cases per year. Males are affected twice as often as females, and the average age of those affected is 54 years. The mitral valve is the most commonly affected, followed in order by the aortic, tricuspid and pulmonary valves. IE in intravenous drug users has a predilection for the tricuspid valve. IE can be divided into three general categories: native valve endocarditis (NVE), prosthetic valve endocarditis (PVE), and endocarditis in intravenous drug users. The causative organisms, symptoms, treatment, and prognosis differ significantly among these groups.

RISK FACTORS

Predisposing factors for IE include:

- acquired valvular heart disease (rheumatic heart disease [RHD], mitral valve prolapse, degenerative valve disease)
- prosthetic heart valves
- congenital heart disease (ventricular septal defect, bicuspid aortic valve, patent ductus arteriosus)
- hypertrophic cardiomyopathy
- indwelling central venous catheters or temporary pacing catheters
- intravenous drug use
- prior endocarditis

In the past, the most common predisposition for IE was rheumatic heart disease; however, RHD now accounts for less than 25% of cases. Mitral valve prolapse and degenerative valvular disease are now the most common antecedent conditions. In 20–40% of adults with IE, no obvious risk factor is identified.

PATHOGENESIS

The normal cardiac endothelium is resistant to infection. However, endothelial injury may occur as a result of turbulent blood flow across a valve or valvular trauma from intravascular catheters. This results in the deposition of platelets and fibrin on the valve surface (nonbacterial thrombotic endocarditis). During subsequent bacteremia, microorganisms adhere to the fibrinous material, colonize it, and proliferate. This bacteremia may occur during dental, gastrointestinal, genitourinary, or gynecological procedures; dental procedures are associated with the highest incidence. Transient bacteremia also frequently occurs after tooth brushing, eating, and bowel movements. Bacteria that produce dextran and those that have surface receptors for fibronectin are especially likely to adhere to these vegetations. Prosthetic valve endocarditis occurring in the first year after surgery is usually the result of contamination at the time of surgery, whereas that occurring later results from transient bacteremia.

CAUSATIVE ORGANISMS

The microbiology of IE depends upon the underlying predisposing factors (Table 31–1). NVE in nonintravenous drug users is usually caused by streptococci and less commonly by staphylococci. The reverse is true of NVE in intravenous drug users. Prosthetic valve

TABLE 31–1

Microorganisms Causing Endocarditis

Prosthetic valve: <1 year after implant	Native valve endocarditis
Staphylococcus epidermidis	Viridans streptococci
Staphylococcus aureus	Group A streptococci
Gram negative bacilli	Enterococci
Candida	Staphylococcus aureus
Diphtheroids	Staphylococcus epidermidis
Enterococci	HACEK organisms
Streptococci	
Prosthetic valve: <1 year after implant	**Intravenous drug use**
Viridans streptococci	Staphylococcus aureus
Staphylococcus epidermidis	Streptococci
Staphylococcus aureus	Enterocci
Enterococci	Gram negative bacilli
HACEK organisms	Candida

HACEK: *Haemophilus parainfluenzae, Haemophilus aphrophilus, Actinobacillus actinomycetemcomitans, Cardiobacterium hominis, Eikenella corrodens,* and *Kingella kingae*

endocarditis occurring within the first year after surgery is predominantly caused by coagulase-negative staphylococci (*Staphylococcus epidermidis*), whereas that occurring after the first year is usually caused by streptococci. IE caused by enterococci usually follows genitourinary tract procedures; patients with *S. bovis* endocarditis often have colonic neoplasms and should be evaluated with colonoscopy.

CLINICAL MANIFESTATIONS

History

IE may be an indolent disease (subacute bacterial endocarditis, **SBE**) or have a dramatic clinical course (acute bacterial endocarditis, **ABE**). Patients may present with constitutional symptoms resulting from activation of the immune system, or with symptoms of acute valvular dysfunction or embolic events. Common constitutional symptoms include:

- fever (present in 80% of affected individuals)
- rigors
- night sweats
- fatigue, malaise
- anorexia, weight loss
- myalgias, arthralgias

Patients with SBE tend to present with constitutional symptoms whereas patients with ABE tend to present with congestive heart failure from valvular dysfunction. Occasionally the initial symptom is the result of an embolic event and manifests as stroke (central nervous system [CNS] embolism), limb ischemia (vascular embolism), flank pain and hematuria (renal embolism), left upper quadrant or left shoulder pain (splenic embolism), diffuse abdominal pain and hematochezia (mesenteric embolism), or myocardial infarction (coronary artery embolism). Intravenous drug users with tricuspid or pulmonic valve endocarditis may present with cough, hemoptysis, and pleuritic chest pain resulting from septic pulmonary emboli. When obtaining the history from a patient with suspected IE, it is important to ask about predisposing conditions and recent procedures.

Physical Examination

Most patients with IE have a murmur. In those with pre-existing valvular disease, a new or changing murmur may occasionally be noted. A significant proportion of

TABLE 31–2

Cutaneous Manifestations of Infective Endocarditis

Cutaneous Finding	Etiology	Description
Petechiae	Immunologic	Tiny, hemorrhagic lesions in the conjunctiva and oral mucosa
Splinter hemorrhages	Immunologic	Linear hemorrhages in the proximal 2/3 of the nail beds
Osler's nodes	Immunologic	Small, raised, painful lesions in the finger pads
Janeway lesions	Embolic	Erythematous, painless lesions on the palms and soles
Roth spots	Immunologic	Whitish, oval, retinal lesions with surrounding hemorrhage

patients with IE and a new regurgitant murmur will develop signs of congestive heart failure. Cutaneous manifestations may be present and reflect peripheral embolic phenomena and immunologic vascular injury (see Table 31–2). Cutaneous manifestations as well as digital clubbing and splenomegaly are much more common in the subacute forms of endocarditis.

DIFFERENTIAL DIAGNOSIS

The differential diagnosis of IE includes other forms of intravascular infection (septic thromboembolism, infected indwelling vascular catheters). IE may mimic other chronic inflammatory diseases and must be considered in the differential diagnosis of patients with fever of unknown etiology or persistent bacteremia.

DIAGNOSTIC EVALUATION

The diagnosis of IE is usually suspected on the basis of clinical findings and confirmed by blood cultures and echocardiography. When IE is suspected, at least three sets of blood cultures should be drawn over 24 hours from different venipuncture sites, ideally before antibiotics are administered. Blood cultures may be negative in ≤5% of patients with IE, usually as a result of inadequate microbiological techniques, infection with highly fastidious bacteria or nonbacterial microorganisms, or from the administration of antimicrobial agents before blood cultures are drawn. Infection with organisms such as *Coxiella burnetti*, *Bartonella* spp., *Brucella abortus*, and *Chlamydia pneumoniae* may only be identifiable by serological tests or polymerase chain reaction.

Transthoracic echocardiography is the initial test of choice to visualize valvular vegetations and quantitate valvular dysfunction. However, transesophageal echocardiography (TEE) is more sensitive (>80%) for the detection of vegetations (see Figure 31–1), and for assessing local complications such as valve ring or aortic root abscesses and valvular destruction or perforation. A negative TEE does not exclude IE and may occur when the vegetation is very small, the vegetation has embolized, or inadequate images are obtained. When the clinical suspicion of IE is high, a repeat study in 7–10 days may demonstrate previously undetected vegetations.

Laboratory evaluation in patients with IE frequently reveals:

- normocytic anemia (~75% of cases)
- leukocytosis (~30% of cases)
- elevated erythrocyte sedimentation rate (~75% of cases)
- proteinuria (~50% of cases)
- microscopic hematuria (~50% of cases)

A positive rheumatoid factor, and false-positive VDRL and Lyme titers may also be noted.

The chest x-ray (CXR) may show consolidation or evidence of parenchymal abscesses as a result of septic emboli from right-sided endocarditis. The electrocardiogram (ECG) is of limited diagnostic value, but may show conduction abnormalities (progressive atrioventricular [AV] block) when a perivalvular abscess burrows into the conduction system.

The diagnosis of IE is relatively easy in patients with the classic features of bacteremia, vegetations, and

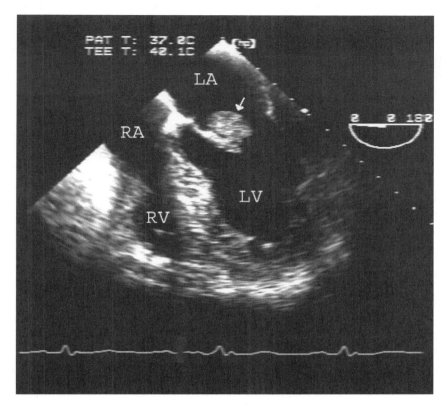

Figure 31–1 Transesophageal echocardiogram in a patient with mitral valve endocarditis. There is a large, rounded vegetation (arrow) on the atrial surface of the anterior mitral valve leaflet. LA: left atrium; LV: left ventricle; RA: right atrium; RV: right ventricle.

TABLE 31–3

Clinical Criteria for Diagnosing Infective Endocarditis (IE)

The clinical diagnosis of IE can be made if a patient has:
  2 major criteria, OR
  1 major and 3 minor criteria, OR
  5 minor criteria

Major criteria
- Positive blood culture (≥2 positive cultures drawn >12 hours apart OR all 3 cultures positive if drawn at least one hour apart OR a majority positive if 4 or more cultures are drawn)
- Echocardiographic evidence of endocardial involvement

Minor criteria
- Predisposing cardiac condition or intravenous drug use
- Fever (temperature ≥38.0°C)
- Vascular phenomena: major arterial emboli, septic pulmonary infarcts, mycotic aneurysm, intracranial hemorrhage, conjunctival hemorrhages, and Janeway lesions
- Immunologic phenomena: glomerulonephritis, Osler's nodes, Roth spots, and elevated rheumatoid factor
- Microbiological evidence: positive blood culture but does not meet a major criterion as noted above
- Echocardiographic findings: consistent with IE but do not meet a major criterion as noted above

TABLE 31-4

Antibiotic Therapy for Infective Endocarditis

Situation	*Antibiotic*
NVE with PCN G-susceptible *S. viridans* or *S. bovis*	PCN G 12–18 million U every 24 hours for 4 weeks, OR Ceftriaxone 2 g once daily IV/IM for 4 weeks, OR PCN G 12–18 million U every 24 hours with gentamicin 1 mg/kg IM/IV every 8 hours for 2 weeks. If PCN allergic: vancomycin 1 g IV twice daily for 4 weeks
NVE with relatively PCN-resistant *S. viridans* or *S. bovis*	PCN G 12–18 million U every 24 hours for 4 weeks with gentamicin 1 mg/kg IM/IV every 8 hours for 2 weeks. If PCN allergic: vancomycin 1 g IV twice daily for 4 weeks
IE due to enterococci	PCN G 12–18 million U every 24 hours with gentamicin 1 mg/kg IM/IV every 8 hours for 4–6 weeks, OR Ampicillin 12 g every 24 hours with gentamicin 1 mg/kg IM/IV every 8 hours for 4–6 weeks.
NVE due to MRSA	Nafcillin sodium or oxacillin sodium 2 g IV every 4 hours for 4–6 weeks with optional addition of gentamicin 1 mg/kg IM/IV every 8 hours for 3–5 days. If PCN allergic: vancomycin 1 g IV twice daily for 4–6 weeks
PVE due to Staphylococcus	Nafcillin sodium or oxacillin sodium 2 g IV every 4 hours with rifampin 300 mg every 8 hours for at least 6 weeks, with gentamicin 1.0 mg/kg IM/IV every 8 hours for 2 weeks. If MRSA or PCN allergic: vancomycin 1 g IV twice daily with rifampin 300 mg every 8 hours for at least 6 weeks, with gentamicin 1.0 mg/kg IM/IV every 8 hours for 2 weeks.
IE due to HACEK microorganisms	Ceftriaxone 2 g once daily IV/IM for 4 weeks OR Ampicillin 12 g every 24 hours IV either continuously or in six equally divided doses with gentamicin sulfate 1 mg/kg IM/IV every 8 hours for 4 weeks

NVE: native valve endocarditis; PVE: prosthetic valve endocarditis; PCN G: aqueous penicillin G; IM: intramuscular; IV: intravenous; MRSA: methicillin-resistant *Staphylococcus aureus*; HACEK: *Haemophilus parainfluenzae, Haemophilus aphrophilus, Actinobacillus actinomycetemcomitans, Cardiobacterium hominis, Eikenella corrodens,* and *Kingella kingae.*

embolic phenomena. In those without such features, the Duke criteria may aid in the diagnosis (see Table 31–3).

TREATMENT (see Table 31–4)

Once IE is suspected, empiric antibiotic therapy should be started until the diagnosis is confirmed and an orga-

nism identified. It is important that bactericidal antibiotics be used in order to effectively eradicate the infection. High dose penicillin G (12 million units daily) is the usual initial regimen; vancomycin may be substituted in penicillin-allergic patients. The addition of an aminoglycoside during the first week of therapy has been shown to hasten sterilization of the blood, but does not improve the cure rate. Once the infecting organism

TABLE 31–5

Indications for Surgery in Infective Endocarditis (IE)

Native Valve Endocarditis	Prosthetic Valve Endocarditis
Acute AI or MR with heart failure	Early IE (within 2 months of surgery)
Fungal endocarditis	Heart failure with valve dysfunction
Annular or aortic abscess or aneurysm	Fungal endocarditis
Persistent infection with valve dysfunction	Evidence of significant paravalvular regurgitation
Recurrent emboli despite therapy	Annular or aortic abscess or aneurysm
IE with Gram-negative organisms, or organisms with poor response to antibiotics	IE with Gram-negative organisms, or organisms with poor response to antibiotics
Large mobile vegetations	Persistent bacteremia despite 7–10 days of antibiotic therapy
	Recurrent emboli despite therapy

AI: aortic insufficiency; MR: mitral regurgitation.

TABLE 31–6

Cardiac Conditions Associated with Infective Endocarditis (IE)

IE Prophylaxis Recommended		IE Prophylaxis Not Recommended
High risk category	**Moderate risk category**	**Low or negligible risk category**
Prosthetic heart valves	Most other congenital cardiac malformations	Isolated secundum ASD
Previous IE	Acquired valvular dysfunction (e.g., senile degenerative valve disease, RHD)	Successfully repaired ASD, VSD, or ductus
Congenital cyanotic heart disease	Hypertrophic cardiomyopathy	Previous CABG
Surgically constructed systemic pulmonary shunts or conduits	MVP with regurgitation and/or thickened leaflets	MVP without regurgitation
		Previous rheumatic fever without valve dysfunction
		Cardiac pacemakers, ICD

MVP: mitral valve prolapse; RHD: rheumatic heart disease; ASD: atrial septal defect; VSD: ventricular septal defect; CABG: coronary artery bypass surgery; ICD: implantable cardioverter-defibrillator.

has been identified, antibiotic treatment should be guided by sensitivity studies. Most patients will become afebrile within one week of starting antibiotic therapy. In general, however, 4 to 6 weeks of intravenous antibiotic therapy is required to treat IE adequately.

Patients should be closely observed for response to treatment and the development of complications, including:

- emboli to major organs resulting in ischemia, infarction, or abscess

- congestive heart failure from valvular destruction

- perivalvular abscess formation

- intracranial hemorrhage from ruptured mycotic aneurysms

- immune-complex mediated glomerulonephritis resulting in renal insufficiency

Patients at a higher risk of complications include those with prosthetic heart valves, cyanotic congenital heart disease, systemic to pulmonary shunts, left-sided IE, *S. aureus* or fungal IE, recurrent IE, symptoms of >3 months duration, and poor response to antimicrobial therapy. Serial clinical exam in association with echocardiography will identify most mechanical complications. Recurrence of fever may indicate treatment failure, but may also result from hypersensitivity reactions to antibiotics. "Surveillance" blood cultures are recommended during antibiotic therapy, especially in staphylococcal IE, in order to detect persistent bacteremia. Cultures should also be drawn in the first 8 weeks following completion of treatment to diagnose relapses.

Despite appropriate antibiotic therapy, many patients with IE will require surgery to replace or repair an infected valve. Table 31–5 summarizes the currently accepted indications for surgery in the setting of IE.

PROGNOSIS

The overall mortality rate in NVE is ~15%. Markers of increased mortality include advanced age (>65 years old), aortic valve infection, congestive heart failure, and central nervous system involvement. The overall mortality rate for PVE is 20–25%.

PREVENTION OF INFECTIOUS ENDOCARDITIS

In those patients at risk for IE (see Table 31–6) who are undergoing dental, genitourinary, or gastrointestinal procedures, antibiotic prophylaxis is essential to minimize the risk. In general, amoxicillin, 2 grams, or clindamycin, 600 mg (if penicillin-allergic) given one hour before the procedure is the recommended prophylactic regimen. In high risk patients undergoing genitourinary or gastrointestinal procedures, the addition of gentamicin (1.5 mg/kg IV) is suggested.

◆ KEY POINTS ◆

1. Risk factors for infective endocarditis include acquired valvular heart disease, congenital heart disease, prosthetic heart valves, intravenous drug abuse, indwelling central venous catheters, and prior endocarditis.

2. Mitral valve prolapse and degenerative valvular disease are the most common antecedent conditions.

3. NVE in non-intravenous drug users is usually caused by streptococci and less commonly by staphylococci. The reverse is true of NVE in intravenous drug users.

4. Prosthetic valve endocarditis occurring within the first year after surgery is predominantly caused by coagulase-negative staphylococci (*Staphylococcus epidermidis*), whereas that occurring after the first year is usually caused by streptococci.

5. Over 80% of patients with IE present with a fever; the vast majority also have a murmur.

6. When IE is suspected, at least three sets of blood cultures should be drawn over 24 hours from different venipuncture sites.

7. Four to six weeks of intravenous antibiotic therapy is required to adequately treat IE, although most patients will become afebrile within one week of starting treatment.

8. Antibiotic prophylaxis is essential in patients at risk for developing IE.

32

Prosthetic Heart Valves

Valve replacement surgery is the treatment of choice for severe valvular heart disease. A variety of prosthetic valves exist; each has its own benefits and drawbacks. These valves are quite effective at correcting a variety of valvular disorders. Unfortunately, they are also prone to a variety of complications, including infection, thrombosis, and degeneration.

TYPES OF PROSTHETIC VALVES
(see Figure 32–1)

Prosthetic valves may be classified as mechanical prosthetic valves (MPVs) or tissue valves (bioprosthetic valves [BPVs]). Mechanical valves are usually composed of metal or carbon alloys, and are available in three main types:

- ball-in-cage (Starr-Edwards)
- single tilting disk (Björk-Shiley, Medtronic-Hall, or Omniscience)
- bileaflet tilting disk (St. Jude, Medtronic-Hall)

Mechanical prostheses are very durable, lasting at least 20 years; however, they are thrombogenic and require lifelong anticoagulation. Ball-in-cage valves are the most thrombogenic, followed by single-tilting-disk valves; bileaflet-tilting-disk valves are the least thrombogenic. The thrombotic potential of these valves is also dependent, in part, on the position in which they are placed—mitral valve prostheses have a higher risk of thrombosis than do aortic valve prostheses.

Tissue valves may also be of several different types:

- **heterograft (xenograft)**: either an explanted animal valve (usually porcine, i.e., Carpentier-Edwards, Hancock) or a valve created from bovine or porcine pericardial tissue (Edwards)

- **homograft**: aortic valves that are harvested from human cadavers

- **autografts**: the patient's own pulmonary valve is harvested and placed in the aortic position; a prosthetic valve is then placed in the pulmonary position (see below)

The main advantage of BPVs is that they are less thrombogenic than MPVs and require only short-term anticoagulation (~3 months) after implantation; however, with the exception of the pulmonary autograft, they are not as durable and often need to be replaced 10–15 years after implantation.

CLINICAL EVALUATION

Heterografts may produce mildly accentuated heart sounds, and, when placed in the aortic or pulmonary position, may produce a short ejection systolic murmur. Frequently, however, tissue valves may be indistinguish-

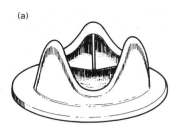
(a)

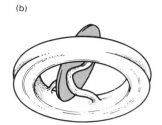
(b)

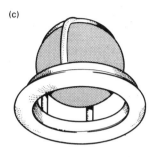
(c)

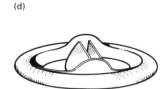
(d)

Figure 32–1 Diagram of various prosthetic valves. (a) Carpenter—Edwards porcine xenograft. (b) Björk-Shiley tilting disc valve. (c) Starr-Edwards ball-in-cage valve. (d) St.-Jude Medical bileaflet valve. (Used with permission from Swanton, RH. Pocket Consultant: Cardiology. Oxford: Blackwell Science, 1998: 108.)

able from native valves by auscultation. Mechanical prostheses produce crisp, metallic opening and closing sounds; in some cases these may be audible without a stethoscope. Mechanical prostheses also result in short flow murmurs—systolic in the aortic and pulmonary positions and mid-diastolic in the mitral and tricuspid positions. All mechanical valves have mild transvalvar regurgitation, which is rarely audible. In general, audible prosthetic valve regurgitation should trigger an evaluation for valve dysfunction.

DIAGNOSTIC EVALUATION

A baseline electrocardiogram (ECG) and an echocardiogram should be obtained postoperatively in all patients who have undergone valve replacement. In the absence of specific concerns, patients with bioprosthetic valves should have an annual transthoracic echocardiogram for the first five years and then biannually thereafter to evaluate valve function and identify early valvular dysfunction. Signs and symptoms of heart failure, new murmurs, significant changes in the intensity of the prosthetic valve sounds, embolic events, per-

sistent fevers, and bacteremia should also prompt evaluation with a transthoracic echocardiogram. Frequently, a transesophageal echocardiogram (TEE) is also required to evaluate suspected prosthetic valve endocarditis and/or valvular dysfunction. Mechanical valve leaflet mobility and integrity can also be evaluated with fluoroscopy.

FACTORS AFFECTING THE CHOICE OF PROSTHETIC VALVE TYPE
(see Table 32–1)

The major advantage of an MPV is its durability, whereas the major advantage of a BPV is the avoidance of anticoagulation. Factors to consider when selecting a valve for a particular patient include:

- patient's age
- risk of bleeding
- other indications for anticoagulation (e.g., atrial fibrillation)
- potential for pregnancy

TABLE 32-1

Preferred Type of Prosthetic Valve in Specific Clinical Scenarios

Clinical Scenario	Preferred Valve	Reasons for Choice
Age >70	BPV	- Slow valve deterioration in this age group - Patient less likely to outlive valve
Patient with bleeding risk	BPV	- Avoids need for anticoagulation
Medication noncompliance	BPV	- Avoids subtherapeutic anticoagulation of mechanical valve
Women desiring pregnancy	BPV	- Avoids need for anticoagulation due to bleeding risk and teratogenicity
Other indication for anticoagulation	MPV	- Need for anticoagulation negates advantage of tissue valve
Most patients age <70	MPV	- Greater durability; patients likely to outlive tissue valve
Children; adults age <35	MPV	- Rapid deterioration of tissue valve in this age group - Greater durability
Chronic renal failure	MPV	- Rapid deterioration of tissue valve in this group
Young patients (<40) with aortic valve disease	Pulmonary autograft	- Avoids long-term anticoagulation risk - Excellent durability of autograft in this group

BPV: bioprosthetic valve. MPV: mechanical prosthetic valve.

- medication compliance
- surgical considerations (size of the aortic root)

The surgeon has a central role in valve selection and must consider such factors as the patient's size, the size of the valvular annulus into which the prosthesis will be sewn, and the hemodynamic profile of the specific valve (bileaflet tilting discs or bioprosthetic valves offer a slightly larger orifice than other prosthetic valves).

The pulmonary autograft (the Ross procedure) may be the valve replacement procedure of choice in young patients with aortic valve disease. In this procedure, the patient's own pulmonary valve is used to replace the diseased aortic valve and a tissue valve (usually a homograft) is placed in the pulmonary position. This is a technically challenging operation, but the autograft provides excellent durability, grows with the adolescent or child, and obviates the need for anticoagulation.

PROBLEMS ASSOCIATED WITH PROSTHETIC VALVES

Although valve replacement surgery can be lifesaving and provides significant symptom relief in patients with severe disease, prosthetic valves themselves are associated with several potential problems that carry substantial risks of morbidity and mortality.

Valve Thrombosis and Thromboembolism

With mechanical valves, the risk of valve thrombosis is related to valve type, valve position, and the number of prosthetic valves present. Ball-in-cage valves, older tilting disk valves (Bjork-Shiley, Omniscience), tricuspid and mitral valve positions, and multiple valve prostheses are associated with higher thrombotic risk. Other predisposing factors include left ventricle (LV) dysfunction, inadequate anticoagulation, and a prior history of thromboembolism. Valve thrombosis can present as embolic episodes or valve dysfunction, the latter frequently precipitating heart failure. Despite anticoagulation of mechanical valves, there is at least a 1–2%-per-year risk of thromboembolism, which is associated with a 0.2% rate mortality. Tissue valves do not require long-term anticoagulation, and have a slightly lower thromboembolic complication rate.

Hemorrhagic Complications

Anticoagulation with warfarin carries a 0.2%-per-year risk of fatal intracranial bleeding and 2%-per-year risk of non-fatal but significant bleeding. Predisposing factors include advanced age, gait instability, alcoholism, and the use of medications that potentiate the effect of warfarin.

Valve Degeneration

Valve degeneration is the main complication limiting the use of tissue valves. Degeneration, fibrosis, perforation, and calcification can affect the valve cusps as early as the fifth postoperative year, and may result in hemodynamically significant stenosis and/or regurgitation. Usually, the deterioration is insidious; rarely it is acute with resultant catastrophic heart failure. As many as 60% of bioprosthetic valves may need to be replaced within 15 years; re-operation carries a 5–15% mortality risk. Valvular degeneration may be particularly rapid in the young, and in those with chronic renal failure or hyperparathyroidism.

Hemodynamic Issues

Prosthetic valves generally have a smaller orifice area than the normal, native valve and are intrinsically mildly stenotic. In patients with a small aortic annulus, this degree of obstruction may be hemodynamically significant.

Infective Endocarditis (see also Chapter 31)

With the exception of the pulmonary autograft, all prosthetic valves are prone to endocarditis. This complication occurs in 3–6% of patients with prosthetic valves. Early endocarditis (<60 days after surgery) principally results from perioperative seeding of bacteria, and is most commonly caused by staphylococcal organisms. It is associated with a mortality of 30–80%. Late prosthetic valve endocarditis (>60 days post-op) is usually caused by streptococci, and is associated with a mortal-

ity of 20–40%. Meticulous attention to dental hygiene, appropriate antibiotic prophylaxis for invasive procedures, and early aggressive treatment of infections elsewhere are essential for the prevention of prosthetic valve endocarditis.

Hemolysis

Mechanical valves usually result in mild intravascular hemolysis owing to traumatic destruction of red blood cells. Perivalvular regurgitation from endocarditis or suture dehiscence may also cause clinically significant hemolysis.

Pregnancy-related Problems

Anticoagulation during pregnancy increases the risk of fetal loss and the risk of peripartum hemorrhage. Pregnancy also increases the risk of thromboembolic complications. In addition, warfarin is teratogenic, and first trimester fetal exposure results in a 4–10% risk of an embryopathy characterized by telecanthus, small nasal bones, choanal hypoplasia, and long bone epiphyseal dysplasia.

◆ KEY POINTS ◆

1. Prosthetic heart valve recipients require close lifelong follow-up.

2. Mechanical valves are durable for the lifetime of the patient, but carry a risk of thromboembolism and require lifelong anticoagulation.

3. Tissue valves do not require chronic anticoagulation, but are not as durable.

4. Factors to consider when deciding which type of valve should be used in a particular patient includes his or her age, risk of bleeding, presence of other indications for anticoagulation, and pregnancy potential.

5. Fatal intracranial hemorrhage, endocarditis, hemolysis, and warfarin-induced teratogenicity are other potential complications.

6. TEE is useful when valvular dysfunction is present or subacute bacterial endocarditis suspected.

Part VII
Pericardial Diseases

33 Pericarditis

Acute pericarditis is a syndrome caused by inflammation of the pericardium and is characterized by chest pain, distinctive electrocardiographic changes, and a pericardial friction rub on physical examination.

EPIDEMIOLOGY

The incidence of pericardial inflammation noted at autopsy ranges from 2–6%; however, pericarditis is diagnosed in only 1 in 1000 hospital admissions, suggesting that this process is often clinically inapparent. Pericarditis is generally more common in men than women and is fairly uncommon in children.

PATHOPHYSIOLOGY

The normal pericardium is a smooth, double-layered structure. The visceral pericardium constitutes the epicardial surface of the heart and is separated from the parietal pericardium by the pericardial space. This space usually contains less than 50 mL of fluid, which lubricates the pericardium and prevents friction between the layers during cardiac contraction. Pericarditis is marked by infiltration of the pericardium by polymorphonuclear leukocytes with eventual deposition of fibrin in the pericardial space. The inflamed pericardial layers rub against each other during each cardiac contraction, often resulting in pain and an audible friction rub.

Inflammatory fluid may collect in the pericardium, producing a pericardial effusion; large effusions may result in pericardial tamponade (see Chapter 34). Chronically, the inflammatory process may produce pericardial thickening and reduced pericardial compliance, resulting in pericardial constriction (see Chapter 35).

ETIOLOGY

The most common causes of acute pericarditis are viral infections and idiopathic, the latter of which is usually presumed to be viral. A variety of other causes have been identified, including other infections and systemic diseases (Table 33–1).

CLINICAL MANIFESTATIONS

History

The clinical history may provide clues to the cause of pericarditis. For example, a preceding upper respiratory tract infection suggests viral pericarditis, whereas a prior history of systemic lupus erythematosus or rheumatoid arthritis suggests autoimmune pericarditis. Regardless of the cause, most patients with acute pericarditis complain of chest pain. This pain is usually sudden in onset, retrosternal in location, variable in intensity, and may be confused with angina. Several characteristic features of pericardial pain include:

TABLE 33–1

Selected Causes of Pericarditis

Category	Examples
Idiopathic	Unknown, by definition
Viral	Coxsackie A and B virus, HIV, adenovirus, EBV
Autoimmune	SLE, scleroderma, rheumatoid arthritis, Wegener's granulomatosis
Radiation	Mantle radiation for chest malignancies
Bacterial	Pneumococcus, streptococcus, *Neisseria* spp., tuberculosis
Myocardial infarction	Dressler syndrome, acute regional pericarditis
Medications	Procainamide, hydralazine
Trauma	Cardiac surgery (post-pericardiotomy syndrome), cardiac contusion
Renal	Uremia, hemodialysis associated
Neoplastic	Lung and breast cancer, lymphoma, melanoma
Miscellaneous	Amyloidosis, sarcoidosis

EBV: Epstein-Barr virus; HIV: human immunodeficiency virus; SLE: systemic lupus erythematosus.

- **pleuritic** in nature, exacerbated by deep breathing or coughing
- alleviated by sitting upright and leaning forward, aggravated in the supine position
- may radiate to the trapezius ridge and neck
- may be worse with swallowing

Patients with pericarditis will often complain of systemic symptoms, including fevers, myalgias, and generalized fatigue.

Physical Examination

The classic physical examination finding for acute pericarditis is a **pericardial friction rub**. This is a scratching, high-pitched, superficial sound noted on cardiac auscultation, and may be localized over the left lower sternal border or heard across the precordium. A rub is

TABLE 33–2

Electrocardiographic Stages of Pericarditis

Stage	ST Segment	PR Interval	T waves
I	Elevated	Depressed or normal	Upright
II	Normal	Depressed or normal	Upright
III	Normal	Normal	Inverted
IV	Normal	Normal	Upright

best appreciated with the **diaphragm** of the stethoscope, with the patient leaning forward or in the left lateral decubitus position. Classically, the rub consists of three components corresponding to atrial systole, ventricular systole, and ventricular diastole. In many instances, only one or two components may be heard and are often mistaken for murmurs. A rub may be intermittent; its presence is diagnostic for acute pericarditis but its absence does not exclude the diagnosis. The clinician should always examine the patient for any signs of underlying disorders that may cause pericarditis.

DIAGNOSTIC EVALUATION

Electrocardiographic abnormalities during acute pericarditis reflect inflammation of the myocardium underlying the visceral pericardium. They may develop within hours of the onset of chest pain, and may persist for days. The typical electrocardiogram (ECG) abnormalities include (see Figure 33–1):

- diffuse ST segment elevation
- PR segment depression

Over a period of days, a typical evolution of ECG abnormalities occurs (see Table 33–2). Once pericarditis has been diagnosed, a search for the underlying cause is warranted. Serum markers of inflammation (e.g., erythrocyte sedimentation rate) are invariably elevated. Specific testing for human immunodeficiency virus (HIV) or other viral antigens, blood cultures, ASO (anti streptolysin O) titer, autoimmune antibodies, and tuberculin skin testing should be considered. An echocardiogram is not necessary in uncomplicated cases of pericarditis, but can be useful if associated myocardi-

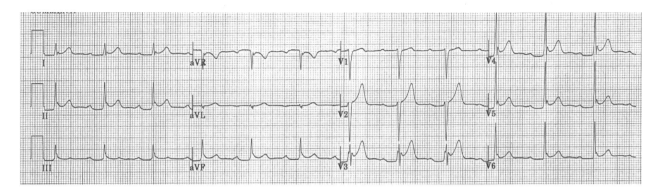

Figure 33–1 ECG of Stage I pericarditis. Note the diffuse ST segment elevation, and the PR depression in lead II. A first degree AV block is also present (unrelated).

tis is suspected, and to assess for associated pericardial effusion.

THERAPY

The cornerstone of acute pericarditis therapy involves treating the underlying disorder. The inflammatory process and the associated pericardial pain usually respond to treatment with nonsteroidal anti-inflammatory agents (e.g., indomethacin); systemic steroids may be required for severe, unremitting pain. Anticoagulant drugs should be avoided in the early stages of pericarditis owing to the risk of intrapericardial hemorrhage. Viral pericarditis is usually self-limited and resolves spontaneously over a period of days without significant sequelae. Occasionally, recurrent pericarditis may develop weeks or months later. Acute bacterial pericarditis is a life-threatening disease and requires emergent drainage of purulent pericardial fluid and administration of intravenous antibiotics. Some forms of pericarditis (especially malignancy-associated) may result in cardiac tamponade and require emergent percutaneous or surgical drainage. Chronically, pericarditis can result in pericardial scarring and constriction.

◆ **KEY POINTS** ◆

1. Pericarditis is an inflammatory disease of the pericardium.
2. The most common causes of pericarditis are viral and idiopathic.
3. The classic features of pericarditis include pleuritic chest pain, a pericardial friction rub, and diffuse ST segment elevation and PR segment depression on ECG.
4. Treatment involves treating the underlying cause and administration of anti-inflammatory agents.

34

Cardiac Tamponade

Cardiac tamponade is a characteristic hemodynamic syndrome resulting from the accumulation of fluid in the pericardial space with resultant compression of the cardiac chambers.

ETIOLOGY

Cardiac tamponade may result from any disease process that can produce pericarditis or a pericardial effusion (see Table 33–1). The most common causes of cardiac tamponade include:

- neoplasm (50% of cases)
- idiopathic/viral pericarditis (15% of cases)
- uremia (10% of cases)

Other causes include bacterial and tuberculous pericarditis, blunt or penetrating chest trauma, myxedema, systemic lupus erythematosus, aortic dissection with rupture into the pericardial space, and myocardial infarction with left ventricular free wall rupture.

PATHOPHYSIOLOGY

Normally, the pericardial space contains approximately 50 mL of fluid and the intrapericardial pressure is similar to intrathoracic pressure (i.e., lower than right and left ventricular diastolic pressures). When addi-

tional fluid enters the pericardial space, intrapericardial pressure rises. If the fluid accumulation is rapid, intrapericardial pressure will rise significantly after only 80–100 mL. If the fluid accumulates gradually, the pericardium may be able to accommodate several liters of fluid with only a small rise in pressure.

During diastole, the increased intrapericardial pressure is transmitted to the heart resulting in the simultaneous elevation of diastolic pressure in all cardiac chambers (**equilibration of pressures**). The increased ventricular diastolic pressures impair ventricular filling and result in decreased cardiac output and elevated jugular venous pressure (JVP). Tachycardia and peripheral vasoconstriction occur as a compensatory mechanism. Once the intrapericardial pressure exceeds intracardiac pressure, cardiac compression occurs, cardiac output falls precipitously, and hypotension ensues.

CLINICAL MANIFESTATIONS

History

Patients with tamponade often present with shortness of breath, lightheadedness, presyncope, or hemodynamic collapse. Palpitations or chest pain may also be present, as may symptoms of poor peripheral perfusion such as confusion and agitation. Patients with slowly developing tamponade may present with symptoms of progressive right heart failure (edema, fatigue).

Physical Examination

The classic features of cardiac tamponade are described by Beck's triad:

- elevated jugular venous pressure
- systemic hypotension
- "quiet" heart sounds (blunted transmission of sound across the precordium as a result of pericardial fluid)

Other physical findings include:

- **pulsus paradoxus**
- tachypnea
- tachycardia
- pericardial friction rub (often absent or evanescent)

The jugular venous pulsations in tamponade classically demonstrate a rapid x-descent (rapid atrial filling after atrial contraction) and an absent y-descent (no passive filling of the ventricle owing to increased ventricular diastolic pressure) (see Figure 4–1). **Pulsus paradoxus** is the inspiratory fall in systolic arterial blood pressure. Normally during inspiration the increased venous return causes the right heart to expand, pushing the intraventricular septum slightly to the left. This impairs left ventricular stroke volume, and accounts for the normal pulsus paradoxus of <10 mmHg. In tamponade, the pericardial effusion limits the total volume capacity of the heart and the augmented right ventricular (RV) filling occurs at the expense of left ventricular (LV) filling, resulting in a marked fall in LV stroke volume and a pulsus paradoxus of >10 mmHg. Other causes of an increased pulsus paradoxus include severe chronic obstructive pulmonary disease (COPD) and constrictive pericarditis.

- electrocardiogram (ECG)—usually demonstrates tachycardia; low QRS amplitude may be present with large effusions; electrical alternans may occur as the heart swings back and forth within the pericardial fluid (Figure 34–2)
- right cardiac catheterization—demonstrates elevated pressure and equalization of diastolic pressures

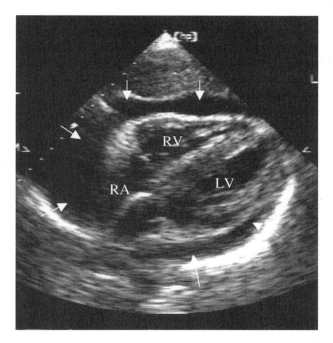

Figure 34–1 Echocardiogram demonstrating a large circumferential pericardial effusion (arrows) in a patient with pericardial tamponade. The right atrium is compressed by the fluid and is poorly visualized.

DIAGNOSIS

The diagnosis of cardiac tamponade is made on the basis of historical features and physical findings. Ancillary testing should be used to confirm the clinically suspected diagnosis. Helpful diagnostic modalities include:

- echocardiogram—demonstrates pericardial fluid, compression of cardiac chambers, and impaired ventricular diastolic filling (Figure 34–1)
- chest x-ray—cardiac silhouette may appear as a "water bottle" due to a large pericardial effusion

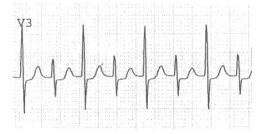

Figure 34–2 ECG demonstrating electrical alternans. The QRS axis alternates with each beat as the heart swings within a large effusion.

THERAPY

Cardiac tamponade is a medical emergency requiring rapid diagnosis and treatment. The cornerstone of therapy is immediate drainage of the pericardial fluid. This may be performed percutaneously via a hollow bore needle inserted into the pericardium from the subxiphoid region (pericardiocentesis). Hemodynamically unstable patients should be supported with volume expansion and vasopressors (i.e., dopamine) while preparing for pericardiocentesis. Following pericardial drainage, rapid recovery of blood pressure and normalization of heart rate is the rule. The pericardial fluid should be sent for chemical analysis, culture, and cytology. Often, a catheter is left in the pericardial space for 1–2 days after pericardiocentesis to allow continued drainage. In patients in whom percutaneous drainage is unsuccessful or rapid reaccumulation of the fluid occurs, surgical resection of a portion of the pericardium (pericardiectomy or "pericardial window") can be performed. This allows for chronic drainage of the fluid from the pericardial space into the left thorax, thereby preventing recurrent tamponade.

◆ KEY POINTS ◆

1. Cardiac tamponade is caused by the accumulation of excessive pericardial fluid.

2. The most common causes of pericardial tamponade include malignancies, viral pericarditis, and uremia.

3. The hemodynamic hallmarks of tamponade include increased intrapericardial pressure, elevated and equilibrated intracardiac diastolic pressures, reduced diastolic filling of the ventricles, and reduced cardiac output.

4. Classic features of tamponade include hypotension, elevated JVP, and muffled heart sounds (Beck's triad).

5. Other physical findings characteristic of tamponade include tachycardia, prominent x-descent and absent y-descent in the jugular venous waveform, and elevated pulsus paradoxus.

6. Definitive therapy for tamponade is emergent pericardiocentesis (acutely) and surgical pericardiotomy (for recurrent effusions).

35 Constrictive Pericarditis

Constrictive pericarditis, one of the sequelae of acute pericarditis, is characterized by a thickened, noncompliant pericardium that impairs filling of the cardiac chambers, and, thereby, results in heart failure.

ETIOLOGY

Most cases of constrictive pericarditis evolve following an initial episode of acute pericarditis; therefore, the etiologies are similar (Table 35–1). Worldwide, tuberculosis is the leading cause of constrictive pericarditis; however, in developed countries, idiopathic constrictive pericarditis predominates.

PATHOPHYSIOLOGY

The hallmark of constrictive pericarditis is impairment of diastole without impairment of systole. Normally, the pericardium is compliant and allows the ventricles to fill freely during diastole. After an episode of acute pericarditis, fibrosis may develop and can severely reduce pericardial elasticity. When this occurs, intracardiac pressures begin to rise. Early in diastole, the ventricles fill rapidly owing to unimpeded ventricular relaxation and increased atrial pressure. However, once the cardiac volume has reached the limits of the constrictive pericardium, further diastolic filling is severely reduced.

Throughout diastole, as a result of equivalent effects of the constrictive pericardium on the right and left ventricles, the ventricular pressures are elevated and equal (Figure 35–1). This is to be distinguished from the hemodynamic pattern of restrictive cardiac disease, which predominantly affects the left ventricle resulting in elevated, but unequal, right and left ventricular pressures during diastole (see Figure 21–3). The elevated diastolic pressures produce many of the clinical features of this syndrome. Systolic cardiac function, however, remains intact.

CLINICAL FEATURES

History
Elevated right and left ventricular end-diastolic pressure may manifest as right and left heart failure, respectively. However, in most patients with pericardial constriction, right-sided symptoms predominate and include:

- Peripheral edema
- Abdominal fullness, nausea (resulting from intestinal edema and ascites)
- Right upper quadrant tenderness (owing to liver congestion)
- Fullness in the neck (resulting from elevated jugular venous pressure [JVP])

TABLE 35–1

Common Causes of Constrictive Pericarditis

Category	Examples
Infectious	Tuberculosis, viral, bacterial
Connective tissue disorders	Systemic lupus erythematosus, rheumatoid arthritis
Neoplasms	Lung and breast cancer, mesothelioma, lymphoma, melanoma
Radiation-induced	Following mantle radiation
Trauma	Post-cardiac surgery
Idiopathic	Nonspecific

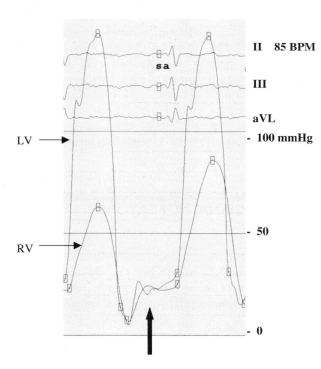

Figure 35–1 Intraventricular pressure tracings in a patient with pericardial constriction. The ventricular diastolic pressures are equal, elevated, and demonstrate the "square-root sign" (block arrow) characteristic of this condition.

Physical Examination

The *sine qua non* of constrictive physiology is elevated JVP. Classically, the JVP will exhibit a prominent y-descent reflecting rapid, initial atrial emptying after the opening of the tricuspid valve (Figure 4–1e). This occurs as a result of elevated atrial pressure and unimpeded early ventricular diastolic filling. Often, the x-descent is also prominent. This is to be distinguished from cardiac tamponade in which the x-descent is prominent but the y-descent is blunted or absent, owing to the compressive effects of the pericardial fluid throughout the cardiac cycle. Detecting these signs may be difficult, especially during tachycardia.

As a result of pericardial constriction, the normal inspiratory decrease in intrathoracic pressure is not transmitted to the cardiac chambers and right ventricular volume therefore does not increase. The increased venous return instead results in a paradoxical increase in the JVP with inspiration (**Kussmaul's sign**). This pattern is not seen with tamponade. **Pulsus paradoxus**, an exaggerated drop in the systemic blood pressure with inspiration, is usually absent in constriction, whereas it is characteristically present during cardiac tamponade (see Table 35–2 and Chapter 34).

Cardiac auscultation may demonstrate an early, relatively high-pitched, 3rd heart sound known as a **pericardial knock**. This sound occurs early in diastole as a result of the rapid cessation of ventricular filling as the pericardium is stretched to its limit. Other signs of right heart failure may be present such as hepatic congestion, peripheral edema, and ascites. Left heart failure is less common, but may be present.

DIAGNOSTIC EVALUATION

The clinician should suspect this syndrome in any patient who presents with new-onset heart failure and a recent history of pericarditis. There are several diagnostic modalities that may aid in diagnosing this condition (Table 35–3). A chest x-ray may reveal pericardial calcification in tuberculous pericarditis or other forms of long-standing pericardial constriction; however, computed tomography (CT) scanning is a more accurate method of assessing pericardial thickness. An echocardiogram will reveal an abnormal diastolic filling pattern with diminished late diastolic ventricular filling. Cardiac catheterization remains the gold standard for diagnosis and will reveal:

TABLE 35–2

Comparative Features of Pericardial Constriction, Pericardial Tamponade, and Restrictive Cardiomyopathy

	Pericardial Constriction	Pericardial Tamponade	Restrictive Cardiomyopathy
Pulsus paradoxus	Usually absent	Present	Absent
Jugular venous pressure waveform	Prominent x- and y-descents	Prominent x-descent, absent y-descent	Prominent x- and y-descents
Kussmaul's sign	Usually present	Absent	May be present
Hemodynamic pattern	LV and RV diastolic pressure equal and have "dip and plateau" pattern	Equalization of all cardiac diastolic pressures	LV diastolic pressure >5 mmHg higher than RV, both have "dip and plateau" pattern

LV: left ventricle; RV: right ventricle.

TABLE 35–3

Some Typical Findings of Constrictive Pericarditis Using Various Diagnostic Modalities

Modality	Typical Findings
Chest x-ray	Normal cardiac size, calcification of the pericardium
CT scan	Thickened pericardium, dilated superior and inferior venae cavae
ECG	Low voltage of QRS complexes; commonly, atrial fibrillation
Echocardiogram	Dilated IVC, augmented early diastolic transmitral flow, diastolic posterior wall flattening, thickened pericardium
Cardiac catheterization	Elevated right and left heart diastolic pressures, elevated right atrial mean pressure, rapid y-descent, equal LV and RV end-diastolic pressures, "dip and plateau" or "square root" sign, normal cardiac output

ECG: electrocardiogram; IVC: inferior vena cava; LV: left ventricle; RV: right ventricle.

- elevated diastolic pressure in all cardiac chambers
- rapid x- and y-descents on the right atrial and pulmonary capillary wedge pressures
- rapid early diastolic fall in ventricular pressure followed by a sustained elevation in pressure ("dip and plateau pattern"; see Figure 35–1)

The "dip" in the ventricular pressure tracing is the result of rapid, unimpeded, early diastolic ventricular relaxation, whereas the "plateau" reflects constant ventricular pressure once the ventricle expands to the limits of the constrictive pericardium. Occasionally, pericardial biopsy is required to confirm the diagnosis.

TREATMENT

Patients with limited symptoms of heart failure can usually be treated effectively with sodium restriction and diuretics. However, despite maximal medical therapy, many patients develop progressive symptomatic right and left heart failure, and subsequently require surgical resection of the pericardium (pericardiectomy, or **pericardial stripping**). The operative mortality of pericardiectomy may be as high as 10%; however, over 90% of patients who survive surgery will improve significantly. The proper timing of surgery is controversial; however, it should be performed before severe right heart failure develops.

◆ KEY POINTS ◆

1. Constrictive pericarditis is usually a sequela of acute pericarditis.
2. Classic physical findings of pericardial constriction include rapid x- and y-descents in the jugular venous waveform and a pericardial knock.
3. The thickened pericardium is best visualized by CT scanning.
4. The gold standard for diagnosis of constrictive pericarditis is invasive measurement of intracardiac pressures (Swan-Ganz catheter).
5. Medical treatment of pericardial constriction consists of diuretics and salt restriction; surgical pericardiectomy may be required to alleviate the hemodynamic disturbance.

Part VIII
Vascular Diseases

36 Hypertension

Although no true physiological threshold exists by which to define hypertension, it has somewhat arbitrarily been defined as a systolic blood pressure >140 mmHg or a diastolic blood pressure >90 mmHg based on the average of two or more measurements on two or more occasions. The severity of hypertension can be further classified according to the degree of systolic or diastolic pressure elevation (see Table 36–1).

EPIDEMIOLOGY

The estimated prevalence of hypertension in the United States is 20–30%. It is more common in men than in women (up to the age of 55 years) and in African Americans than Caucasians, and increases in incidence with advancing age. Among patients with hypertension, approximately 30% are unaware that they have elevated blood pressure and only 25–30% of patients with hypertension are optimally controlled (<140/90 mmHg) on their present medical regimen.

ETIOLOGY

In the vast majority of patients, no cause for hypertension can be determined (**primary** or **essential** hypertension). Nonetheless, several risk factors for the development of essential hypertension have been identified, including:

- genetic predisposition (family history)
- male gender
- excessive alcohol consumption
- obesity
- inactivity
- increased sodium intake
- African American race

Secondary hypertension is defined as hypertension due to an identifiable cause and accounts for only 5–10% of cases. Etiologies include:

- renovascular disease (renal artery stenosis, fibromuscular dysplasia)
- renal parenchymal disease (glomerulonephritis, polycystic kidney disease)
- endocrine disorders (primary hyperaldosteronism, Cushing's syndrome, hyper- or hypothyroidism, hyperparathyriodism, pheochromocytoma)
- carcinoid syndrome
- alcohol and drug use
- coarctation of the aorta

TABLE 36–1

Classification of Blood Pressure

Classification*	Systolic (mmHg)		Diastolic (mmHg)
Optimal	<120	**AND**	<80
Normal	<130	**AND**	<85
High-normal	130–139	**OR**	85–89
Stage 1 hypertension	140–159	**OR**	90–99
Stage 2 hypertension	160–179	**OR**	100–109
Stage 3 hypertension	>180	**OR**	>110

*For adults who are not taking antihypertensive medications and are not acutely ill.

TABLE 36–2

Target Organ Damage

Target Organ	Disease Manifestations
Heart	Left ventricular hypertrophy, congestive heart failure, cardiomyopathy, coronary artery disease (angina, myocardial infarction)
Brain	Hemorrhagic stroke, encephalopathy
Kidney	Proteinuria, renal failure, acute glomerulonephritis
Eye	Retinopathy, papilledema
Peripheral arteries	Aortic dissection, transient ischemic attacks, claudication

- obstructive sleep apnea
- oral contraceptive use

CLINICAL MANIFESTATIONS

The goals of the clinical evaluation of a person with hypertension are to determine the presence and extent of target organ damage (see Table 36–2); to identify secondary causes of hypertension and precipitating or exacerbating factors; and to identify concomitant cardiovascular disease risk factors.

History

In general, hypertension is a silent disease until complications develop, at which time the patient may report symptoms of cardiovascular, cerebrovascular, or peripheral vascular disease. Nonetheless, the elevated pressure itself may cause headaches, chest pain, shortness of breath, or palpitations. Other important historical points that should be addressed include the following:

- duration and degree of hypertension
- family history of hypertension, coronary artery disease (CAD), stroke, diabetes, renal disease, or dyslipidemia
- history of tobacco, alcohol, or illicit drug use (including androgen steroids), herbal preparations (including sympathomimetics such as ephedrine)

- level of physical activity
- dietary intake of sodium, caffeine, and saturated fat
- symptoms of target organ damage
- presence of other CAD risk factors (see Chapter 11)

A secondary cause of hypertension should be suspected in patients with the following historical features:

- new-onset hypertension in a patient <20 years old or >50 years old
- severe or refractory hypertension despite maximal treatment with three or more antihypertensive agents
- an acute rise in blood pressure over a previously stable baseline
- moderate-to-severe hypertension precipitating flash pulmonary edema
- negative family history of hypertension

Physical Examination

The physical examination should also be directed toward identifying signs of end-organ damage, including:

- retinopathy (arteriolar narrowing, arteriovenous nicking, hemorrhages, exudates, papilledema)
- vascular disease (arterial bruits, diminished peripheral pulses)

- cardiac disease (displaced left ventricular apex, S_3, S_4, pulmonary rales, elevated jugular venous pressure)
- neurological disease (motor or sensory deficits)

Several physical findings suggest specific secondary causes of hypertension, including thyromegaly, cutaneous striae (Cushing's syndrome), abdominal bruits (renovascular disease), and arm-leg pressure discrepancy (aortic coarctation).

DIAGNOSTIC EVALUATION

Routine testing in the initial evaluation of hypertension should include a complete blood count, electrolytes, urinalysis, fasting glucose, lipid profile, and electrocardiography. Additional testing should be directed at establishing a secondary cause or identifying specific target organ damage, as directed by the history and physical examination.

TREATMENT

General Approach

The need for and intensity of antihypertensive therapy can be determined by considering the absolute level of blood pressure elevation as well as a patient's cardiovascular risk factors and target organ damage. Patients who have clinical evidence of cardiovascular disease or have diabetes are considered to be in the same high-risk group as patients who have target organ damage. General guidelines with regard to risk classification and treatment options are summarized in Table 36–3.

The goal of hypertension therapy is to reduce blood pressure to a level at which target organ damage will be prevented or limited. The recommended goal blood pressure levels are as follows:

- for uncomplicated hypertension: BP <140/90 mmHg
- for patients with diabetes, renal failure, or heart failure: BP <130/85 mmHg
- for patients with proteinuria: BP <125/75 mmHg

Non-Pharmacological Therapy

Antihypertensive treatment generally begins with non-pharmacological therapy and lifestyle modifications, including weight loss in obese patients, reduction of dietary sodium intake to <2–3 grams/day, regular exercise, and avoidance of excess alcohol intake. All patients, regardless of their blood pressure, should be counseled with regard to smoking cessation. In general, lifestyle changes can decrease systolic pressure by 2–4 mmHg and diastolic pressure by 1–2 mmHg.

TABLE 36–3

Treatment Recommendations in Hypertension

Risk	High Normal BP (130–139/85–89)	Stage 1 (140–159/90–99)	Stage 2 or 3 (>160/>100)
No RF	Lifestyle modifications	Lifestyle modifications (for up to 1 yr)	Drug therapy + lifestyle modifications
>1 RF, excluding DM	Lifestyle modifications (for up to 1 yr)	Lifestyle modifications (for up to 6 mo)	Drug therapy + lifestyle modifications
CHD, TOD, DM	Drug therapy if HF, DM, renal failure; otherwise, lifestyle modifications	Drug therapy + lifestyle modifications	Drug therapy + lifestyle modifications

RF: risk factor; DM: diabetes mellitus; CHD: coronary heart disease; HF: heart failure; TOD: target organ damage. Modified from The Sixth Report of the Joint National Committee on the Prevention, Detection, Evaluation, and Treatment of High Blood Pressure (JNC VI).

Pharmacological Therapy

Several classes of antihypertensive agents exist including:

- diuretics (e.g., hydrochlorothiazide, furosemide, spironolactone)
- beta-blockers (e.g., metoprolol, atenolol, propranolol)
- calcium channel blockers (e.g., verapamil, diltiazem, nifedipine, amlodipine)
- angiotensin converting enzyme (ACE) inhibitors (e.g., captopril, enalapril, lisinopril)
- angiotensin receptor blockers (e.g., losartan, valsartan)
- alpha-blockers (e.g., clonidine, prazosin)
- mixed alpha- and beta-blockers (e.g., carvedilol, labetolol)
- direct vasodilators (e.g., hydralazine, minoxidil)

Almost all agents are reasonable choices for initial drug therapy. Most antihypertensive agents will result in an adequate blood pressure response in 40–60% of patients; however, much variability exists in individual responses to different agents. Patients who do not respond to one antihypertensive drug have a 50% chance of responding to a different agent.

The general recommendations for initial therapy of uncomplicated hypertension consist of monotherapy with either a thiazide diuretic or beta-blocker. However, in certain situations there are compelling indications for use of a specific agent (see Table 36–4). Several points regarding antihypertensive therapy are worth noting:

1. Medications should be started at lower doses and up-titrated every 1–2 weeks until the optimal effect is achieved.
2. If a person has no response to a particular agent after 2–3 weeks of therapy, a different agent should be substituted.
3. If a person responds to one agent but the blood pressure is still not optimally controlled, a second agent of a different class should be added.
4. If combination therapy is required, the dose of the first agent should be maximized before initiating a second drug.

Aggressive pharmacological therapy results in optimal blood pressure control in 75–80% of patients; however, on average at least three agents are required to achieve this result.

HYPERTENSIVE CRISIS

The term hypertensive crisis encompasses a variety syndromes associated with marked elevation of blood pressure (systolic BP >230mmHg, diastolic BP >130 mmHg), including:

- hypertensive urgency: markedly elevated BP **without** acute target organ damage
- hypertensive emergency: markedly elevated BP **with** acute target organ damage
- accelerated hypertension: markedly elevated BP with associated retinal hemorrhages or exudates
- malignant hypertension: markedly elevated BP with associated papilledema

Such profound hypertension requires aggressive blood pressure reduction. In the absence of symptoms or acute target organ damage, blood pressure should be decreased within hours to days. In the presence of symptoms or target organ damage, immediate blood pressure reduction is indicated. Hypertensive crises should be managed with intravenous agents to achieve an initial goal of not more than a 25% reduction in the mean arterial pressure in the first two hours (Table 36–5). Blood pressure should be further reduced toward 160/100 mmHg over the next several hours. More rapid reductions in blood pressure may precipitate cerebral hypoperfusion as a result of altered autoregulation of cerebral blood flow.

TABLE 36–4

Indications for Specific Drug Therapy

Disease State	Agents of Choice
Diabetes mellitus	ACE inhibitor
Heart failure/ cardiomyopathy	ACE inhibitor, beta-blocker, diuretic
Coronary heart disease	Beta-blocker, ACE inhibitor
Isolated systolic hypertension	Diuretic, calcium channel blocker

ACE: angiotensin-converting enzyme.

TABLE 36–5

Medications Used in the Treatment of Hypertensive Crises

Drug	Initial Dose	Onset of Action	Duration of Action	Special Indications
Sodium nitroprusside	5–10 µg/kg/min	Immediate	1–2 min	Most hypertensive emergencies; use with caution in elevated ICP
Nitroglycerin	5–100 µg/min	2–5 min	3–5 min	Myocardial ischemia
Labetolol	20–80 mg every 10 min OR 0.5–2 mg/min infusion	5–10 min	3–6 hr	Most hypertensive emergencies with exception of acute HF
Nicardipine	5–15 mg/hr	5–10 min	1–4 hr	Most hypertensive emergencies with exception of acute HF; use with caution in coronary ischemia
Phentolamine	5–15 mg	1–2 min	3–10 min	Catecholamine excess (pheochromocytoma, MAO interaction)
Hydralazine	10–20 mg	10–20 min	3–8 hr	Eclampsia
Esmolol	250–500 µg/kg/min for 1 min, then 50–100 µg/kg/min for 4 min	1–2 min	10–20 min	Aortic dissection, perioperative
Enalaprilat	1.25–5 mg every 6 hr	15–30 min	6 hr	Acute heart failure

ICP: intracranial pressure.

◆ KEY POINTS ◆

1. Hypertension is defined as a systolic blood pressure >140 mm Hg or a diastolic blood pressure >90 mm Hg based upon the average of two or more measurements on two or more occasions.
2. Hypertension is categorized as essential or secondary.
3. Treatment generally begins with lifestyle modifications unless the patient has multiple CAD risk factors or Stage 2 (Table 36–1) or greater hypertension.
4. Drug therapy should be aimed at maximal blood pressure reduction while minimizing side effects and ensuring compliance.
5. Hypertensive crises are potentially life-threatening conditions that require immediate reduction in blood pressure.

37 Peripheral Arterial Disorders

The peripheral arteries can be affected by a variety of disorders, including atherosclerosis, thromboembolic disease, and vasoconstrictive disorders. These conditions result in impaired blood flow to the brain or extremities and account for significant morbidity and mortality.

PERIPHERAL ARTERIAL DISEASE

Pathogenesis

Peripheral arterial disease (PAD) is most often a manifestation of atherosclerosis (see Chapter 11). In the peripheral vasculature, atheromatous lesions tend to develop at arterial branch points. The increased turbulence and shear stress in these areas result in intimal injury and stimulate plaque formation. The disease tends to be diffuse, affecting multiple arteries, the most frequent of which include:

- femoral and popliteal arteries (80–90% of affected patients)
- tibial, peroneal, and more distal arteries (40–50% of affected patients)
- abdominal aorta and iliac arteries (30% of affected patients)

Risk Factors

The risk factors for PAD are the same as for coronary artery disease (CAD), and include:

- advanced age
- hypertension
- diabetes mellitus
- dyslipidemia
- male gender
- cigarette smoking

Atherosclerotic peripheral arterial disease is frequently associated with coronary and carotid atherosclerotic disease. Therefore, one should always look for evidence of CAD in patients presenting with PAD, and vice versa.

Clinical Manifestations

History

The principal symptom of PAD is intermittent claudication, a manifestation of skeletal muscle ischemia resulting from inadequate peripheral blood flow. The symptoms occur distal to the obstructing lesion and are usually described as a dull ache, cramp, or limb fatigue that occurs with exertion and resolves after a few minutes of rest. Symptoms may be limited to the calf in the case of femoral-popliteal disease, or may extend to the buttock, hip, and thigh in the presence of aortoiliac disease. This latter manifestation may be associated with impotence (**Leriche's syndrome**). In severe, occlusive PAD, the arterial blood supply may become inadequate to support resting metabolic demands and patients may develop claudication at rest.

A thorough history includes a search for cardiac risk factors and symptoms of CAD, as these two disorders frequently coexist.

Physical Examination

Physical findings of PAD include:

- diminished peripheral pulses with cool, pale extremities
- vascular bruits
- shiny, smooth, hairless skin (atrophic changes)
- **dependent rubor** (reactive hyperemia of legs in dependent position)

Differential Diagnosis

True claudication must be distinguished from **pseudoclaudication** ("neurogenic claudication"). True claudication results from vascular compromise, is precipitated by walking, and resolves after standing still. Pseudoclaudication, a symptom of lumbar spinal stenosis, may mimic true claudication by causing exertional leg pain; however, pseudoclaudication resolves only after sitting down or changing position.

Diagnostic Evaluation

The diagnosis of peripheral arterial disease can usually be established by a thorough history and physical examination. Diagnostic testing is reserved for assessing the severity of the disease. The most commonly used test to assess PAD is the ankle-brachial index (ABI). Normally, the systolic blood pressure in the legs is higher than that in the arms and the ABI is greater than 1.0. Values less than 0.9 predict peripheral arterial disease with 95% sensitivity; values less than 0.5 are consistent with severe ischemia. Duplex ultrasonography can be useful in localizing the level of the disease and assessing its severity. Magnetic resonance angiography (MRA) and contrast angiography are rarely necessary to diagnose PAD; however, they are essential tests in patients being considered for surgical revascularization.

Treatment

The treatment of peripheral arterial disease consists of nonpharmacological, pharmacological, and surgical therapies. Nonpharmacological therapies should always be employed, and include:

- exercise therapy
- risk factor modification (smoking cessation, lipid-lowering therapy, aggressive blood sugar control, antihypertensive therapy)
- meticulous foot care to avoid injury and infection

Exercise rehabilitation programs dramatically reduce symptoms and improve walking distance, likely through improved endothelial function and collateral vessel formation.

Antiplatelet agents (i.e., aspirin, dipyridamole, clopidogrel) have been the mainstay of medical therapy for PAD and may improve symptoms as well as decrease the need for surgical revascularization. Pentoxifylline (400 mg three times daily), a xanthine derivative with hemorheologic properties, appears to offer no advantage over exercise rehabilitation alone. Cilostazol (100 mg twice daily), a phosphodiesterase inhibitor that inhibits platelet aggregation and causes direct vasodilation, reduces claudication time by 30–60% compared with placebo and appears to be more effective than pentoxifylline. Several novel pharmacotherapies are under investigation, including serotonin, L-arginine, carnitine derivatives, and parenteral angiogenic growth factors (vascular endothelial growth factor, basic fibroblast growth factor).

Revascularization of peripheral arteries is indicated for patients with:

- incapacitating claudication
- rest pain
- evidence of tissue necrosis

Revascularization may be performed percutaneously or through an open surgical procedure. The success and patency rates associated with percutaneous transluminal angioplasty (PTA) with stent implantation vary with the location of the vascular lesion. PTA and stent of the iliac arteries is associated with a greater than 90% acute success rate, and good long-term patency (80% remain patent after 1 year; 60% after 5 years). Less favorable outcomes are associated with femoral and popliteal interventions (65% 1-year and 40% 5-year patency rates).

Surgical revascularization procedures can be classified as aortoiliac or infrainguinal. Aortoiliac reconstruction is typically performed with placement of an aorto-bifemoral prosthetic bypass graft. Infrainguinal bypass procedures utilize saphenous vein grafts for the reconstruction. Long-term patency varies with location and type of graft utilized, and ranges from 70–85% patency at 5 years.

ACUTE ARTERIAL OCCLUSION

Acute arterial occlusion is a medical emergency. It results in acute limb ischemia and requires emergent therapy to prevent limb loss.

Pathogenesis

Acute arterial occlusion can occur as a result of embolic disease, thrombotic disease, dissection or trauma. Most arterial emboli originate in the heart, usually as a result of atrial fibrillation or mural thrombi in the left ventricle. Less commonly, peripheral emboli may originate from thrombi associated with prosthetic heart valves, from valvular vegetations (endocarditis), or from atrial myxomas. *In situ* thrombosis of a peripheral artery may occur in patients with PAD, infrainguinal bypass grafts, and peripheral aneurysms, especially in patients with concomitant hypercoagulable states.

Clinical Manifestations

History & Physical Examination

The history and physical examination of the patient with acute arterial occlusion are characterized by the "6 P's" in the affected extremity:

- pulselessness
- pallor
- pain
- paresthesias
- paralysis
- poikilothermia

A thorough history may disclose prior symptoms of a preexisting condition (e.g., atrial fibrillation, PAD, etc.). Additional physical findings may include muscle stiffness, absent deep tendon reflexes, cyanosis, and cutaneous mottling.

Diagnostic Evaluation

The clinical presentation should strongly suggest this diagnosis. Contrast angiography is typically used to confirm the diagnosis. Following definitive therapy for the acute occlusion, transesophageal echocardiography should be performed in patients with a presumed cardiac source of the embolism.

Treatment

The initial management of acute arterial occlusion consists of analgesia and anticoagulation with unfractionated heparin. Intra-arterial thrombolytic therapy has been used successfully to treat acute thrombotic occlusion and decreases the need for surgical thrombectomy by approximately 50%. In cases in which limb viability is threatened, expedient surgical thromboembolectomy or arterial bypass surgery is indicated. Following a thromboembolic vascular event, long-term anticoagulation with warfarin is usually warranted.

RAYNAUD'S PHENOMENON

Clinical Manifestations

Raynaud's phenomenon is a symptom or physical finding that is characterized by the sequential development of clearly demarcated digital blanching, cyanosis, and rubor (white-blue-red) upon cold exposure. This episodic digital ischemia is attributed to arterial vasospasm. Raynaud's disease, i.e., idiopathic or primary Raynaud's phenomenon, most commonly occurs in young women (20–40 years old), is bilateral, may involve the feet, and follows a benign course. Secondary Raynaud's phenomena occur in association with a variety of systemic disorders, including collagen vascular diseases (e.g., systemic lupus erythematosus, progressive systemic sclerosis), vasculitis, pulmonary hypertension, neurological disorders, and blood dyscrasias. This form of Raynaud's syndrome is more common in older men, is frequently unilateral, is usually limited to the hands, and may be associated with digital necrosis.

Treatment

Most patients with Raynaud's phenomenon can be managed with reassurance and avoidance of unnecessary cold exposure. Pharmacotherapy should be instituted in severe cases. Calcium channel blockers (e.g., nifedipine 10–30 mg three times daily, diltiazem 30–90 mg three times daily) have been shown to decrease the frequency and severity of attacks.

THROMBOANGIITIS OBLITERANS

Thromboangiitis obliterans (TAO), also known as **Buerger's disease**, is a vasculitis of the small- and medium-sized arteries and veins of the upper and lower extremities. Cerebral, visceral, and coronary vessels may also be involved. Young men (<45 years of age) are most commonly affected. The etiology of TAO is unknown, but there appears to be a definite relationship to cigarette smoking (in virtually all patients) and an increased incidence of HLA-B5 and HLA-A9 antigens in affected individuals.

Clinical Manifestations

Patients with TAO frequently present with the triad of claudication, Raynaud's phenomenon, and migratory superficial thrombophlebitis. Physical examination typically reveals reduced or absent distal pulses (radial, ulnar, dorsalis pedis, posterior tibial). Trophic nail changes, digital ulcerations, and gangrene may develop in severe cases.

Diagnostic Evaluation

The diagnosis is suggested by the disorder's characteristic appearance on arteriography. Smooth tapering segmental lesions of the distal vessels with surrounding collateral vessels at the site of occlusion are the hallmark of TAO. Definitive confirmation is obtained by excisional biopsy.

Treatment

No specific therapy exists for TAO. Smoking cessation appears moderately effective at halting disease progression. Surgical reconstruction is of limited applicability owing to the distal nature of the disease. In severe cases, amputation may be required.

◆ KEY POINTS ◆

1. PAD is frequently associated with coronary and cerebral vascular disease.

2. True claudication is a symptom of PAD and must be distinguished from pseudoclaudication, a symptom of lumbosacral spine disease.

3. Acute arterial occlusion is heralded by the 6 P's: pain, pulselessness, pallor, paresthesias, paralysis, and poikilothermia.

4. Raynaud's phenomenon is the result of vasospasm and produces sequential white, blue, then red discoloration of the digits upon exposure to the cold.

5. Thromboangiitis obliterans is almost universally a disease of young, male smokers.

38

Diseases of the Aorta

The aorta, like other vascular structures, is subject to a variety of disorders, including atherosclerosis, aneurysm formation, dissection, inflammation, and collagen vascular diseases. Disease of this vessel may impair blood flow to one or more vital organs, thus producing a variety of symptoms depending on the particular vascular territory affected.

AORTIC ANEURYSMS

An aneurysm is a focal (saccular) or diffuse (fusiform) area of vascular dilation. A true aneurysm is at least 50% greater than the normal vessel diameter and involves all three layers of the vessel wall. This is in contrast to a false aneurysm (**pseudoaneurysm**), which is, essentially, a contained vascular rupture. The walls of a pseudoaneurysm do not include any of the normal vascular layers; rather, the pseudoaneurysm is contained by perivascular tissue. Aneurysms may arise at any point in the aorta; involvement of the abdominal aorta is the most common.

Epidemiology

The prevalence of abdominal aortic aneurysms in the US is approximately 50 per 100,000 men and 10 per 100,000 women. The incidence increases significantly with age; more than 3% of people over the age of 55 years have abdominal aortic aneurysms. Thoracic aortic aneurysms are less common. In the US alone, aortic aneurysms account for nearly 70,000 hospitalizations, 40,000 operations, and 20,000 deaths annually.

Risk Factors

Factors associated with a higher incidence of aortic aneurysms include:

- smoking
- male gender
- advanced age
- hypertension

Other cardiac risk factors (e.g., diabetes mellitus, hyperlipidemia) may contribute by accelerating the development of atherosclerosis. Genetic factors also play a role; over one-third of affected patients have a family history of aneurysmal disease.

Etiology

Several diseases are associated with the development of aortic aneurysms (Table 38–1). Atherosclerosis is the most common predisposing factor for the development of abdominal and descending thoracic aortic aneurysms. Cystic medial necrosis, as occurs with hypertension and connective tissue disorders, is the most common cause of ascending aortic aneurysms.

Pathogenesis

Atherosclerosis clearly plays a large part in the formation of aortic aneurysms. These aneurysms have a

TABLE 38–1

Diseases Associated with Aortic Aneurysms

Disease Category	Examples
Atherosclerosis	—
Cystic medial necrosis	Hypertension, Marfan's syndrome, Ehlers-Danlos disease, Turner's syndrome, osteogenesis imperfecta
Congenital abnormalities	Bicuspid or unicuspid aortic valve, aortic coarctation
Infection	Syphilis, tuberculosis
Spondyloarthropathy	Reiter's syndrome, ankylosing spondylitis, rheumatoid arthritis
Vasculitis	Takayasu's arteritis, giant cell arteritis
Trauma	Blunt chest trauma, iatrogenic

predilection for the infrarenal abdominal aorta, owing in part to the absence of vasa vasorum in the media of this region of the aorta. Altered synthesis and expression of types I and III procollagen, destruction of elastin and collagen in the vascular media by cytokine-induced metalloproteinases, and medial neovascularization also contribute to the pathogenesis. These changes weaken the aortic wall allowing it to expand. As the aorta enlarges, wall tension increases (LaPlace's law), and progressive dilation ensues.

Clinical Manifestations

History

The majority of abdominal aortic aneurysms and almost half of thoracic aortic aneurysms are asymptomatic at the time of diagnosis. When symptoms are present, they relate to the size and location of the aneurysm.

Thoracic aneurysms may cause:

- chest or back pain (compression of adjacent thoracic structures)
- dyspnea (compression of phrenic nerve or tracheobronchial tree; aortic insufficiency)
- dysphagia (esophageal compression)
- hoarseness (compression of the left recurrent laryngeal nerve)
- cough, wheezing, hemoptysis (compression of tracheobronchial tree)
- superior vena cava syndrome

- symptoms of coronary, cerebral, renal, mesenteric, lower extremity, or spinal ischemia (rarely)

Abdominal aneurysms may cause:

- abdominal, back, leg, groin, or flank pain
- anorexia, nausea, vomiting (compression of gastrointestinal tract)
- unilateral leg swelling (compression of left iliac vein)

The pain of an aortic aneurysm is usually a steady, gnawing pain that is unaffected by exertion. An acute increase in the pain usually heralds aneurysm expansion or rupture. Thrombus may form within an aneurysm and subsequently embolize, resulting in acute vascular occlusion (see below).

Physical Examination

Physical findings of aortic aneurysms vary with the location of the aneurysm. Ascending aortic aneurysms may be associated with:

- a diastolic murmur of aortic regurgitation due to distortion of the aortic annulus
- a pulsatile mass in the sternal notch

Abdominal aortic aneurysms may be associated with:

- a pulsatile abdominal mass
- an abdominal bruit

Carotid and femoral bruits as well as diminished peripheral pulses are frequently present in patients with aortic aneurysms, and are caused by coexistent peripheral vascular disease (see Chapter 37).

Diagnostic Evaluation

Asymptomatic thoracic aneurysms may be detected by routine chest x-ray because they result in widening of the mediastinum, enlargement of the aortic knob, or displacement of the trachea. Abdominal aneurysms may also be an incidental finding noted by calcification of a dilated aorta on abdominal radiographs. In patients with suspected thoracic aortic aneurysms, computed tomography (CT) with intravenous contrast and magnetic resonance angiography (MRA) are both accurate methods of assessing aneurysm size and determining its location with regard to branch vessels. Ultrasound is the usual initial imaging modality for the diagnosis of abdominal aortic aneurysms (sensitivity approaches 100%), and it can be used as a screening tool in high-risk patients. Angiography remains the preferred modality for imaging aortic aneurysms before corrective surgery.

Approximately 25% of patients with thoracic aortic aneurysms have coexistent abdominal aneurysms, and more than 10% of patients with aortic aneurysms have peripheral vascular aneurysms. Therefore, a full vascular evaluation is warranted when an aortic aneurysm is identified.

Natural History

The major risks associated with aortic aneurysms are dissection (see below) and vascular rupture. The risk of rupture is directly related to:

- the size of the aneurysm (risk is very low for aneurysms <4 cm in diameter. Risk is high for abdominal aneurysms >5 cm in diameter [two-year risk >20%] or thoracic aneurysms >6 cm in diameter [risk of rupture ~30%])
- the rate of expansion of the aneurysm (risk increased if expansion >0.5 cm/yr)
- the presence of symptoms

Treatment

Surgical correction is the definitive therapy for aortic aneurysms. Indications for surgery include:

- the presence of symptoms attributable to the aneurysm
- abdominal aortic aneurysms >5 cm

- thoracic aortic aneurysms >6 cm (>5.5 cm in Marfan's syndrome)
- rapidly expanding aneurysms (>0.5 cm/yr)
- thrombotic or embolic complications

Endoluminal stent grafting is a novel, less invasive alternative for the repair of aortic aneurysms. Successful repair is achieved in 80–90% of cases with a mortality rate of 9–10%. This technique is currently applied to abdominal aneurysms in limited cases, and remains investigational in thoracic aneurysm repair.

Smaller, asymptomatic aneurysms may be managed medically with aggressive blood pressure control and beta-blocker therapy. Beta-blockers decrease shear stress in the aorta and may decrease the rate of aneurysm expansion and risk of rupture. Reduction of other cardiovascular risk factors is also essential (see Chapter 11). In patients managed medically, serial imaging every 6 months (usually with CT scanning for thoracic aneurysms, or ultrasound for abdominal aneurysms) is required to assess for aneurysm expansion.

Prognosis

Sixty percent of patients who suffer a ruptured aortic aneurysm die before reaching the hospital and 50% of the remainder die perioperatively. Elective thoracic aneurysm repair is associated with a 30-day mortality that approaches 10% and a significant risk of morbidity, namely stroke and renal failure. The mortality of abdominal aortic aneurysm repair is somewhat less (2–5%).

AORTIC DISSECTION

An aortic dissection is a tear of the intimal lining of the aorta that allows intraluminal blood to enter the vascular wall and then propagate down a dissection plane between the intima and media of the vessel. More than 2,000 cases occur in the US each year.

Classification

Aortic dissections are classified according to their anatomic location (see Figure 38–1) and their duration. Sixty-five percent of aortic dissections begin in the ascending aorta, 20% in the descending thoracic aorta (distal to the left subclavian artery at the ligamentum arteriosum), and 10% in the aortic arch. Only 5% originate in the abdominal aorta. Dissections that have

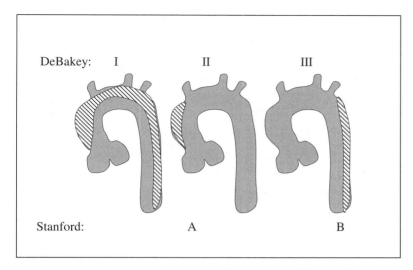

Figure 38–1 Anatomic classifications of aortic dissections. DeBakey classes I and II and Stanford class A involve the ascending aorta. DeBakey class III and Stanford class B involve only the descending aorta. Hatched areas represent the false lumen.

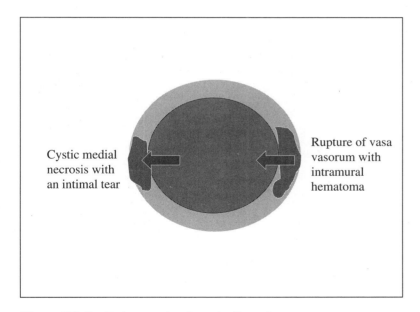

Figure 38–2 Pathogenesis of aortic dissection.

been present for less than two weeks are classified as acute, while dissections of greater than two weeks' duration are termed chronic. Both prognosis and management vary with the different types of aortic dissections (see below).

Pathogenesis

The intimal tear may occur following rupture of an atherosclerotic plaque or as a result of stretching of an aortic aneurysm. It may also follow rupture of the vasa vasorum within the aortic media (see Figure 38–2). This later mechanism results in hemorrhage within the vascular media (an intramural hematoma) that may then rupture into the vascular lumen creating an intimal tear. Once the dissection plane is established, it may propagate proximally or distally, thereby creating a false channel. This channel may subsequently thrombose, or may rupture back into the vascular space, allowing continued flow in both the true and false lumen.

Several conditions predispose to aortic dissection, including:

- aortic aneurysms (mainly atherosclerotic)
- connective tissue diseases (Marfan's syndrome, Ehlers-Danlos syndrome)
- trauma

Clinical Manifestations

History

More than 90% of patients with acute aortic dissection present with the abrupt onset of severe pain that is localized to the chest or back and described as sharp, "ripping," or "tearing." The pain often radiates to the neck, jaw, flanks, or legs. Less common symptoms include:

- syncope
- congestive heart failure (acute aortic valve insufficiency)
- stroke (carotid artery dissection or impaired cerebral blood flow)
- paraplegia (spinal artery occlusion)
- myocardial infarction (coronary artery occlusion)
- sudden cardiac death (pericardial tamponade, aortic rupture)

Physical Examination

Hypertension is the most common finding in patients with distal dissections, whereas those with proximal dissections frequently present with hypotension as a result of acute aortic insufficiency or pericardial tamponade. Other physical findings may include:

- pulse deficits, asymmetric extremity blood pressures (>30 mmHg difference), or acute limb ischemia (occlusion of limb vessel by dissection flap)
- diastolic murmur of aortic insufficiency
- left pleural effusion (hemothorax from rupture of aneurysm into the pleural space)

- paraparesis, paraplegia, focal neurological deficits
- cardiac tamponade (rupture into pericardial space)

Rarely, patients with dissection of the aorta may present with hoarseness, hemoptysis, pulsating neck mass, Horner's syndrome, hematemesis, or upper airway obstruction.

Diagnostic Evaluation

Chest x-ray often provides the first clues to the diagnosis of aortic dissections by revealing:

- widening of the mediastinum (Figure 38–3)
- "calcium sign" (separation of intimal calcification from outer aortic soft tissue border)
- pleural effusion
- tracheal deviation

Routine blood tests are typically nondiagnostic, although a novel immunoassay for smooth muscle myosin heavy chain has been recently introduced and

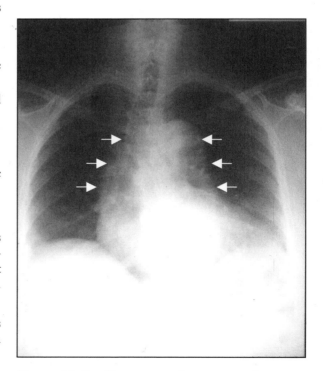

Figure 38–3 Chest x-ray of a patient with an acute aortic dissection. Note the marked widening of the mediastinal shadow (arrows).

appears to be a promising diagnostic technique in acute dissections.

Several imaging modalities, including CT, MRI, and echocardiography, have been employed to aid in the rapid diagnosis of this disorder (see Table 38–2). Selection of a diagnostic test requires knowledge of the testing and expertise available at the institution as well as consideration of the patient's clinical status. In critically ill, hemodynamically unstable patients, transesophageal echocardiography is the test of choice because it is rapid, portable, and highly sensitive for identifying thoracic aortic dissections (Figure 38–4). In more stable patients, and patients with suspected abdominal aortic dissections, CT or MRI is invaluable (Figure 38–5).

Treatment

Prompt, aggressive medical therapy aimed at lowering blood pressure and decreasing left ventricular contractility is crucial to the management of aortic dissections (see Table 38–3). All patients should be treated with beta-blockers to decrease the rate of pressure development (dP/dT) within the aorta, even if they are normotensive. The overall mortality of an untreated aortic dissection is ~1% per hour for the first 48 hours, and

TABLE 38–2

Diagnostic Tests in the Evaluation of Aortic Dissection

Test	Advantages	Limitations	Sens/Spec
Transesophageal echocardiogram (TEE)	Performed at bedside; rapid; readily available; can assess LV function, valvular function, and pericardial disease; no contrast required; reasonable cost	Distal dissections may be missed; specificity dependent on strictness of diagnostic criteria	Sensitivity: 98% Specificity: 77–97%
Contrast enhanced computed tomography (I + CT)	Rapid; readily available; can assess entire aorta; noninvasive; reasonable cost	Intimal flap often not identified; site of entry rarely seen; requires intravenous contrast; no information about aortic regurgitation	Sensitivity: 85–95% Specificity: 87–100%
Magnetic resonance angiography (MRA)	Fairly rapid; noninvasive; no contrast required; can assess entire aorta and its branches; can assess LV function and aortic regurgitation	Not ideal for very unstable patients as patients are inaccessible during study; metal objects cannot be in vicinity of scanner; moderate cost	Sensitivity: 98% Specificity: 98%
Aortography	Fairly rapid; can assess entire aorta and its branches; can assess LV function and aortic regurgitation	False negative results occur with simultaneous opacification of true and false lumens; invasive; requires intravenous contrast; high cost	Sensitivity: 85–90% Specificity: 94%

LV: left ventricle.

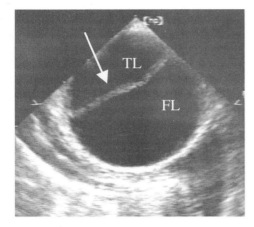

Figure 38–4   Transesophageal echocardiogram in a patient with a dissection of the descending thoracic aorta. An intimal flap (arrow) separates the true lumen (TL) from the false lumen (FL).

65–75% in the first two weeks. Mortality of ascending aortic dissections is significantly improved with emergent surgical repair (~25% with surgery versus ~60% with medical therapy). Conversely, descending aortic dissections are better managed without surgery unless vascular compromise is present (mortality ~10% with medical management versus ~30% with surgery).

Surgical therapy includes resection of the damaged aortic segment, decompression of the false channel, and, often, resuspension of the aortic valve. Indications for surgery include:

- acute ascending aortic dissection
- any aortic dissection in patients with Marfan's syndrome
- acute distal dissections complicated by vascular compromise, aneurysm formation, rupture or impending

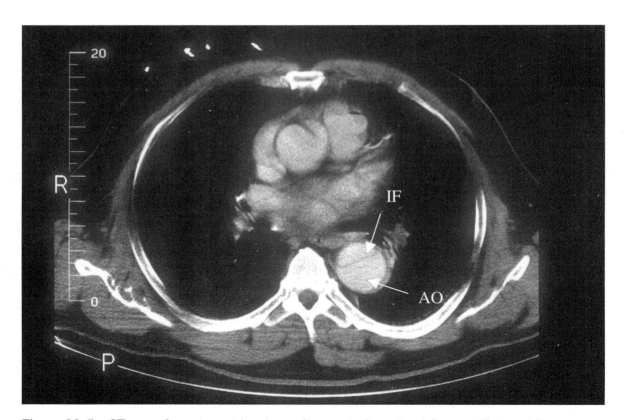

Figure 38–5   CT scan of a patient with a descending aortic dissection. AO: aorta; IF: intimal flap.

TABLE 38–3

Medications Used in the Acute Management of Aortic Dissection Complicated by Hypertension

Drug	Dose
Propanolol	5 mg IV load; 1 mg IV every 5 min (maximum dose 10 mg)
Labetolol	5–10 mg IV every 2 min; then 40–120 mg/hr
Metoprolol	5 mg IV every 2 min up to 15 mg; then 50 mg PO every 6 hr
Esmolol	30 mg IV load; 3–12 mg/min infusion
Sodium nitroprusside*	20 μg/min, titrate up to control BP (maximum 800 μg/min)
Enalaprilat	0.625 mg IV; 0.625–5.0 mg every 6 hr

*It is recommended that therapy with sodium nitroprusside be preceded by the administration of beta-blockers, because the vasodilation associated with nitroprusside can result in reflex activation of the sympathetic nervous system with enhanced contractility and increased shear stress.

IV: intravenous; PO: by mouth; BP: blood pressure.

rupture, or retrograde propagation to the ascending aorta.

As in the elective repair of aortic aneurysms, the use of endovascular stents in the treatment of acute aortic dissection is under investigation.

AORTITIS

Takayasu's arteritis and giant cell arteritis are the principal inflammatory diseases of the aorta. Aortitis can also occur in diseases such as systemic lupus erythematosus, syphilis, Wegener's granulomatosis, Behçet's disease, and Cogan syndrome, and as a complication of Kawasaki's disease. Systemic manifestations including fevers, malaise, fatigue, and weight loss are common. The aortic inflammation may narrow the aorta or its major branches and result in limb or organ ischemia. Treatment usually includes glucocorticoid therapy; however, recurrences may occur.

◆ **KEY POINTS** ◆

1. Leaking/ruptured aortic aneurysms and acute ascending aortic dissections require emergent surgical treatment.

2. Ascending aortic aneurysms are usually the result of cystic medial necrosis, whereas descending aortic aneurysms are usually atherosclerotic.

3. Asymptomatic thoracic aortic aneurysms should undergo surgical repair if they are >6 cm, whereas asymptomatic abdominal aortic aneurysms should undergo surgical repair if they are >5 cm.

4. Ascending aortic dissections require surgical repair, whereas descending aortic dissections are usually managed medically.

5. Takayasu's arteritis and giant cell arteritis are the principal inflammatory diseases of the aorta.

39 Carotid Arterial Disease

Cerebrovascular disease (CVD) is the third leading cause of death in the United States. A cerebrovascular accident (CVA) (i.e., stroke) carries an acute mortality of 20%, has a five-year mortality of 50%, and produces substantial morbidity in survivors. Carotid artery disease represents a major cause of CVD. This chapter discusses the evaluation and management of carotid arterial disease, but does not discuss the management of the neurological syndromes that result.

PATHOPHYSIOLOGY

The pathophysiology of carotid disease is that of atherosclerosis (see Chapter 11). The most common site of atheromatous lesion formation in the cerebral circulation is within 2 cm of the origin of the internal carotid arteries. These lesions impair cerebral blood flow and result in cerebral ischemia, that produces neurological symptoms. The ischemia may result from either a severe flow-limiting carotid stenosis with inadequate collateral circulation, or from embolic phenomena originating from the site of the stenosis.

A carotid stenosis causes local acceleration of blood flow that can be heard as a **bruit** over the involved vessel. Among patients with carotid bruits, only 35–40% have hemodynamically significant carotid artery disease. Moreover, the absence of a carotid bruit does not exclude the presence of significant carotid artery disease. Patients with carotid bruits have an increased risk of

transient ischemic attack (TIA) or CVA; however, these events are not always in the vascular territory supplied by the affected artery.

CLINICAL MANIFESTATIONS

History

The vast majority of patients with carotid artery disease are asymptomatic. Symptoms, when present, occur as a result of cerebral ischemia and reflect the specific cerebral territory involved. Common presenting symptoms include:

- arm and/or leg weakness
- change in vision
- difficulty speaking
- difficulty walking
- unilateral facial droop

Less common symptoms include headache, confusion, and seizure. Loss of consciousness is a distinctly uncommon presentation of carotid disease owing to the fact that it requires either bilateral cortical ischemia or brainstem ischemia, neither of which should occur in the setting of unilateral carotid disease. Many patients do not recognize their own neurological deficits, and are instead brought to medical attention at the insistence of others.

The clinical syndromes resulting from carotid arterial disease may be classified on the basis of the duration of the associated neurological deficit.

- A **transient ischemic attack** is an ischemic neurological symptom lasting less than 24 hours.
- A **reversible ischemic neurologic deficit (RIND)** is an ischemic event of 24 hours to 72 hours in duration.
- A permanent neurological deficit is termed a **cerebrovascular accident** or **stroke**.

Physical Examination

In the absence of a cerebral ischemic event, the physical examination may be completely normal, although a carotid bruit may be noted. The specific neurological abnormalities present during a TIA or following a CVA vary depending on the location and extent of cerebral ischemia/infarction present. Common findings include:

- contralateral homonymous hemianopsia
- hemiparesis
- hemisensory loss
- aphasia (dominant hemisphere ischemia)
- hemineglect (nondominant hemisphere ischemia)
- transient monocular blindness (**amuarosis fugax**)

- constructional apraxia (nondominant hemisphere ischemia)

Careful physical examination may also disclose evidence of coronary or peripheral vascular disease, as these conditions often coexist.

Diagnostic Evaluation

Imaging of the carotid arteries is warranted both in patients with asymptomatic carotid bruits and in patients who have suffered a transient or permanent cerebral ischemic event. Carotid duplex ultrasound is the usual initial test following a TIA/CVA and can be used as a screening test in patients with suspected carotid disease. Although reasonably accurate (sensitivity: 91–94%; specificity 95–99%), it can only visualize the cervical portion or the carotid artery. Magnetic resonance angiography (MRA) and computed tomography (CT) are more sensitive studies and can image the intracranial as well as the carotid vessels. However, these studies are more expensive and less readily available. Additionally, MRA cannot be performed in patients with pacemakers or other metal implants, and CT angiography is invasive and requires the use of intravenous contrast. Cerebral angiography remains the gold standard for imaging the carotid arteries; however, it is usually reserved for patients who are undergoing carotid endarterectomy (see below).

TABLE 39–1

Recommendations Regarding Carotid Endarterectomy (CEA) in Patients with Carotid Artery Disease, Based on Stenosis Severity and the Presence or Absence of Symptoms

	CEA Not Indicated	CEA Acceptable but of No Proven Benefit	CEA Beneficial
Symptomatic	<30% stenosis (NNT* 67)	30–69% stenosis (NNT 20)	70–99% stenosis[a] (NNT 8)
Asymptomatic	<60% stenosis (NNT 83)		60–99% stenosis[b] (NNT 48)

*NNT signifies the number needed to treat to prevent one ischemic stroke.
[a] Provided surgical risk <6%.
[b] Provided surgical risk <3%.

Treatment

The treatment of carotid artery disease depends upon the presence or absence of symptoms and the severity of the stenosis. Nonpharmacological therapy is applied to all patient groups with carotid artery disease and consists of aggressive risk factor modification (blood pressure control, blood sugar control, smoking cessation, and lipid-lowering therapy).

Antiplatelet therapy is the mainstay of medical management for carotid artery disease. Aspirin has been shown clearly to decrease the risk of subsequent stroke in patients who have suffered a TIA or CVA. The appropriate dose is not yet clear, but low doses (81 mg/day) appear to be as effective as higher doses (≥325 mg/day). The efficacy of stroke prevention with clopidogrel (75 mg/day) is at least equal to, and may exceed that of, aspirin. The utility of either of these agents in patients with asymptomatic carotid disease is not clear. Warfarin is not routinely indicated in the therapy of carotid artery disease (in the absence of stroke), but it is often used in patients with very severe stenoses awaiting surgery, and in patients who have recurrent ischemic events despite antiplatelet therapy.

Surgical therapy for carotid artery stenosis consists of resection of the carotid plaque, i.e., carotid endarterectomy (CEA). Long-term antiplatelet therapy is an obligatory adjunct to this surgery. CEA clearly reduces the long-term risk of CVA in patients with symptomatic carotid disease. The data is less clear for patients with asymptomatic carotid stenoses, although patients with moderate to severe carotid artery stenoses (>60%) likely benefit. Table 39–1 summarizes the currently accepted criteria for CEA in symptomatic and asymptomatic carotid disease. Percutaneous transluminal carotid angioplasty and carotid stent placement hold promise for the treatment of carotid disease; however, they currently remain experimental procedures in the US.

◆ KEY POINTS ◆

1. Carotid artery disease is predominantly the result of atherosclerosis.

2. Significant stenosis of the carotid artery may occur in the absence of symptoms.

3. Neurological symptoms resulting from carotid artery disease may be transient (TIA, RIND) or permanent (CVA).

4. All patients with symptomatic carotid disease should receive antiplatelet therapy.

5. Carotid endarterectomy is indicated in patients with symptomatic, moderate to severe carotid artery stenoses (>70%), and should be considered in asymptomatic patients with >60% carotid artery stenosis.

40 Deep Venous Thrombosis and Pulmonary Embolic Disease

VENOUS THROMBOEMBOLIC DISEASE

Venous thromboembolic (VTE) disease accounts for significant morbidity and mortality. Over 300,000 cases of pulmonary embolism (PE) occur in the United States annually, accounting for 50,000 to 150,000 deaths each year. The mortality rate of untreated PE is approximately 30%. Despite advances in diagnostic modalities and therapeutic strategies, it is estimated that the majority of patients with PE remain undiagnosed.

PATHOPHYSIOLOGY OF VENOUS THROMBOSIS AND PULMONARY EMBOLI

Venous thrombosis most commonly involves the deep veins of the lower extremities, although the superficial veins, veins of the upper extremity, and pelvic and renal veins may also be involved. Predisposing factors involve **stasis**, **vascular injury**, and **hypercoagulability** (Virchow's triad). Both hereditary and acquired factors contribute (see Table 40–1). Venous thrombosis is usually associated with inflammation of the vessel wall (**thrombophlebitis**). The thrombi may detach, embolize through the venous system, and lodge in the pulmonary arteries. Large thrombi may lodge in the main pulmonary artery bifurcation causing hemodynamic instability (**saddle embolus**), whereas smaller emboli lodge in distal pulmonary arterial branches and may be clinically silent.

Occlusion of small pulmonary arteries results in increased pulmonary vascular resistance (both directly, and indirectly via release of vasoactive substances from the thrombus), pulmonary hypertension, right ventricular hypertrophy, and, eventually, right ventricular failure. The PE also impairs gas exchange in the affected lung regions resulting in hypoxemia and an increased alveolar-arterial oxygen gradient (**A-a gradient**). Pulmonary infarction occurs infrequently (<10% of pulmonary emboli).

CLINICAL MANIFESTATIONS

History

The most common presenting complaint associated with a DVT is calf pain. Additionally, patients may note unilateral leg swelling, erythema or warmth, and may have low-grade fevers. When obtaining a history from a patient with DVT, it is important to note the following:

- history of trauma or other injury
- history of recent prolonged immobility

TABLE 40–1

Causes of Venous Thromboembolic Disease

Hereditary Hypercoagulable States	Acquired Conditions
Factor V Leiden mutation	Stasis:
Activated Protein C resistance	- Immobilization (stroke, spinal
Protein C deficiency	cord injury, prolonged travel)
Protein S deficiency	- Obesity
Antithrombin III deficiency	- Pregnancy
Prothrombin G20210A mutation	- Advanced age
Hyperhomocyst(e)inemia	- Heart failure
Antiphospholipid antibody	Vascular injury:
syndrome	- Trauma
Plasminogen deficiency	- Surgery
Dysfibrinogenemia	- Indwelling venous catheters
Factor XII deficiency	- Prior deep venous thrombosis
Inherited thrombophilia	Hypercoagulability:
Elevated factor VIII coagulant	- Surgery
activity	- Malignancy
	- Oral contraceptives
	- Smoking
	- Pregnancy
	- Nephrotic syndrome

- use of prescription medications, recreational drugs, or tobacco
- prior history of thrombosis or abnormal bleeding
- history of malignancy
- family history of thrombosis

Patients with recurrent DVTs frequently have a hypercoagulable state. Patients with underlying carcinoma (especially adenocarcinomas) may have a migratory superficial thrombophlebitis (Trousseau's syndrome).

The most common presenting symptom of PE is sudden dyspnea, which occurs in approximately 80% of patients. Additional symptoms include:

- pleuritic chest pain (66%)
- cough (35–40%)
- hemoptysis (10–15%)
- syncope (10%)

Physical Examination

Physical findings associated with DVTs may include the following:

- calf asymmetry, erythema, warmth, and/or tenderness
- pedal edema
- **Homans' sign** (calf pain with resisted dorsiflexion of the foot)
- venous engorgement
- palpable thrombosed vein (a **cord**) in the posterior calf
- **phlegmasia cerulea dolens** (cyanotic hue due to deoxygenated hemoglobin in stagnant veins)
- **phlegmasia alba dolens** (pallor associated with massive edema)

The physical examination of patients with PE may be normal but often demonstrates signs of pulmonary hypertension or right heart failure including:

- tachypnea (70%)
- tachycardia (40%)
- elevated jugular venous pressure with prominent V waves
- right-sided S_3 or S_4
- murmur of tricuspid regurgitation
- accentuated pulmonic component of S_2 (P_2)
- right ventricular heave

The lung fields are usually clear, although a pulmonary rub may be heard over the involved area of lung when pulmonary infarction has occurred.

DIFFERENTIAL DIAGNOSIS

The differential diagnosis of DVT includes cellulitis, venous insufficiency, ruptured Baker's cyst, lymphedema, and muscular injury. The differential diagno-

sis of PE includes pneumonia, pleurisy, pneumothorax, myocardial infarction, pericarditis, congestive heart failure, and anxiety.

DIAGNOSTIC EVALUATION
(see Figure 40–1)

Duplex venous ultrasonography is the most common test used to confirm the diagnosis of DVT and has a sensitivity and specificity of >95%. Other noninvasive tests (e.g., impedance plethysmography) are used less frequently. Contrast venography remains the gold standard for the diagnosis of deep venous thrombosis (DVT) (sensitivity and specificity 100%) but is typically reserved for cases in which noninvasive testing is equivocal.

In patients with PE, arterial blood gas analysis typically demonstrates a respiratory alkalosis, hypocapnea, and hypoxemia. Additionally, the A-a gradient is

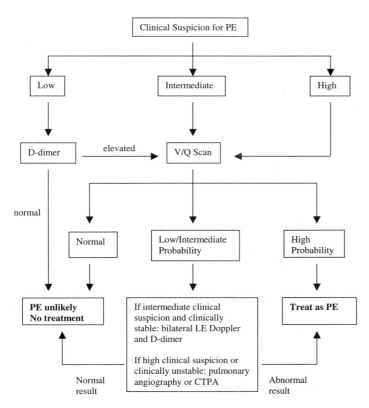

Figure 40–1   Diagnostic algorithm for patients with suspected pulmonary embolism.

increased (>10 mmHg). The A-a gradient can be calculated by the following formula:

$$\text{A-a gradient} = [(P_{atm} - P_{H20})(FIO_2) - (PCO_2/0.8)] - PaO_2$$

Where P_{atm} is atmospheric pressure (760 mmHg), P_{H20} is the partial pressure of water in the atmosphere (47 mmHg), FIO_2 is the percent oxygen in the inspired air (21% in room air), PCO_2 is the partial pressure of carbon dioxide in the blood, and PaO_2 is the partial pressure of oxygen in the blood.

The electrocardiogram (ECG) is abnormal in the majority of patients with an acute PE and may show a deep S wave in lead I and a deep Q wave and T wave inversion in lead III (*S1-Q3-T3*). Other frequent patterns include sinus tachycardia, an incomplete right bundle branch block, or a pseudo-infarction pattern in the inferior leads (II, III, aVF).

Chest radiography is frequently normal in patients with PE but may reveal decreased vascular markings in the affected lung regions (**Westermark's sign**), a wedge-shaped peripheral infiltrate (**Hampton's hump**), or an enlarged right descending pulmonary artery (**Palla's sign**). Ventilation/perfusion (V/Q) lung scan is the usual initial diagnostic test for PE. Normal and near-normal tests virtually exclude the diagnosis, while a high-probability result is confirmatory. However, in patients with a high clinical suspicion of PE, a low or intermediate probability scan is unhelpful, as at least 40% of these patients have a PE.

CT of the pulmonary arteries with intravenous contrast (CTPA) and magnetic resonance angiography (MRA) with gadolinium enhancement can confirm or exclude the diagnosis if the V/Q scan is equivocal, but may miss small peripheral emboli. Pulmonary angiography remains the gold standard for diagnosis of PE.

Other tests that may be helpful in the evaluation of PE include:

- echocardiography—demonstrates signs of pulmonary hypertension and/or right ventricular dysfunction
- lower extremity duplex ultrasonography—a negative result does not exclude the diagnosis of PE as up to 50% of patients with PE have no evidence of DVT
- D-dimer (a fibrin degradation product)—a normal value, if obtained by ELISA technique, essentially excludes PE with a negative predictive value of

~90%. The negative predictive value is even higher when combined with a normal lower extremity duplex.

TREATMENT

In patients with suspected DVT or PE, anticoagulant therapy should be started immediately. It is imperative that therapeutic anticoagulation (1.5–2.0 times the control PTT value if unfractionated heparin is used) be achieved in the first 24 hours to decrease the risk of recurrent DVT/PE and postphlebitic syndrome. Unfractionated heparin may be used initially, although low-molecular-weight heparin (LMWH) may be more effective. Advantages of LMWH include its greater bioavailability, ease of administration (subcutaneous injection), reliable anticoagulant effect, lack of need for laboratory monitoring, and lower incidence of heparin-induced thrombocytopenia.

Oral anticoagulation with warfarin may be begun concurrently with heparin; but should overlap with heparin therapy for 4 to 5 days to avoid the transient hypercoagulability that may occur after warfarin initiation. Heparin may be discontinued once the international normalized ratio (INR) is therapeutic (2.0–3.0). Anticoagulation should be continued for 3–6 months in patients presenting with their first DVT and for 6 months in patients with PE. Prolonged therapy may be required in patients with recurrent DVT/PE, underlying malignancy, or primary hypercoagulable states. Patients with recurrent DVT despite

---

TABLE 40–2

Indications for Inferior Vena Cava Filter Placement

Recurrent pulmonary embolism on therapeutic anticoagulation
Contraindications to anticoagulation
Active bleeding that is life threatening
Post-surgical (relative)
Thrombocytopenia (spontaneous or heparin-induced)
Prophylaxis in high risk patients
Extensive venous thrombosis
Severe pulmonary hypertension, cor pulmonale

therapeutic anticoagulation and patients with contraindications to anticoagulation may benefit from placement of an inferior vena cava (IVC) filter (see Table 40–2).

Patients presenting with massive PE associated with hemodynamic instability should be treated with thrombolytic therapy. If thrombolytic therapy is contraindicated or unsuccessful, percutaneous or open-surgical thrombectomy should be considered.

The treatment of DVTs that are limited to the calf is controversial. These thrombi have a much lower risk of embolism, although 10–15% will progress to the thigh. Conservative therapy with anti-inflammatory agents is the usual course of therapy, coupled with serial noninvasive studies (weekly for 2–3 weeks) to identify thrombi that propagate proximally and, therefore, warrant anticoagulation.

DEEP VENOUS THROMBOSIS PROPHYLAXIS

Prophylaxis against DVT is critical for reducing the morbidity and mortality of this disease and should be considered in high risk clinical situations (hospitalization, postoperative states, prolonged immobility, etc.).

Prophylactic therapy may consist of external pneumatic compression, or low dose subcutaneous administration of unfractionated heparin (5000 U twice daily) or LMWH (e.g., enoxaparin 30 mg twice daily).

◆ KEY POINTS ◆

1. Predisposing factors for DVT include stasis, vascular injury, and hypercoagulability.

2. Only 80% of patients with PE present with dyspnea.

3. The initial diagnostic test of choice for DVT is duplex ultrasonography, whereas V/Q scan is the test of choice for PE.

4. Once DVT or PE is suspected, heparin therapy should be started immediately, and therapeutic anticoagulation established within 24 hours.

5. Thrombolytic therapy or surgical thrombectomy should be considered for patients with hemodynamically significant pulmonary emboli.

41 Pulmonary Hypertension

Pulmonary hypertension is a disorder defined by a mean pulmonary artery (PA) pressure (PA mean = 1/3 PA systolic pressure +2/3 PA diastolic pressure) greater than 25 mmHg at rest or greater than 30 mmHg with exercise. A variety of disorders can result in pulmonary hypertension (**secondary pulmonary hypertension [SPH]**) by producing alterations in pulmonary blood flow, pulmonary vascular tone, pulmonary venous pressure, or the size of the pulmonary vascular bed. When pulmonary hypertension occurs in the absence of an identifiable cause, it is referred to as **primary pulmonary hypertension** (PPH).

EPIDEMIOLOGY AND PATHOGENESIS

The incidence of PPH is estimated at 1–2 cases per million people per year. PPH classically afflicts young and middle-aged women. Its etiology is unknown, but a familial component has been described, suggesting a genetic susceptibility. Current theories implicate the interaction between endothelial and smooth muscle cells, in addition to an imbalance of vasoactive amines, in the pathogenesis of PPH. The classic histopathological finding in PPH consists of intimal proliferation, in-situ thrombosis, and plexogenic arteriopathy.

Secondary pulmonary hypertension may result from:

1. **Increased pulmonary blood flow** associated with:
   - intracardiac shunts (atrial septal defect [ASD], ventricular septal defect [VSD])
   - patent ductus arteriosus

2. **Hypoxic vasoconstriction** associated with:
   - emphysema
   - obstructive sleep apnea and other hypoventilation syndromes
   - high altitude

3. **Pulmonary venous hypertension** associated with:
   - mitral valve disease (stenosis or regurgitation)
   - left ventricular failure
   - pulmonary venous thrombosis
   - constrictive pericarditis
   - congenital anomalies (e.g., cor triatriatum)

4. **A decrease in the size of the pulmonary vascular bed** associated with:
   - chronic obstructive pulmonary diseases
   - connective tissue disorders
   - vasculitis (e.g., systemic lupus erythematosus [SLE], systemic sclerosis)
   - HIV infection
   - pulmonary embolic disease

- toxic injury (e.g., crack cocaine, L-tryptophan, fenfluramine, rapeseed oil)
- liver dysfunction (hepatopulmonary syndrome)

CLINICAL MANIFESTATIONS

History

Patients with pulmonary hypertension commonly present with advanced disease because of the insidious progression of their symptoms. Symptoms generally include:

- dyspnea at resting and/or with exertion (occurs in >95% of patients)
- fatigue, lethargy
- exertional syncope (due to an inability to augment cardiac output)
- chest pain (due to pulmonary artery "stretch" or right ventricular ischemia)
- cough, hemoptysis
- hoarseness (due to left recurrent laryngeal nerve compression by the dilated pulmonary artery)
- anorexia, right upper quadrant pain (from liver congestion)
- peripheral edema (due to right heart failure)

In evaluating a patient with suspected pulmonary hypertension, a detailed history needs to be obtained and should include questions about the following: appetite suppressant or intravenous drug use, smoking, HIV risk factors, symptoms of liver disease, connective tissue disorders, venous thrombotic disease, and lung disease.

Physical Examination

The physical findings in pulmonary hypertension occur as a result of either right ventricular (RV) strain or RV failure (cor pulmonale) secondary to chronically elevated pulmonary artery (PA) pressure. Hypoxia (either ambulatory or nocturnal) is a uniform finding. Other physical findings include:

- tachypnea
- elevated jugular venous pressure
- loud pulmonic component of the second heart sound (P_2)
- palpable P_2

- tricuspid regurgitation
- right ventricular S_3 and/or S_4
- left parasternal (right ventricular) lift
- hepatomegaly, ascites
- pulsatile liver (with severe tricuspid regurgitation)
- peripheral edema

DIFFERENTIAL DIAGNOSIS

The differential diagnosis of pulmonary hypertension is similar to the differential diagnosis of dyspnea (see Chapter 2), and includes cardiac (myocardial and valvular diseases), pulmonary (pulmonary parenchymal and vascular diseases), and systemic (anemia, physical deconditioning) disorders.

DIAGNOSTIC EVALUATION

Several diagnostic studies provide indirect evidence of pulmonary hypertension. The electrocardiogram may reveal right axis deviation, RV hypertrophy or strain, right atrial enlargement, or right bundle branch block (see Figure 41–1). Chest radiography may demonstrate enlargement of the central pulmonary arteries or right ventricle, and pruning of the peripheral pulmonary vessels. Signs of chronic RV pressure overload apparent by echocardiography include RV hypertrophy and dilation, right atrial enlargement, abnormal interventricular septal flattening, and tricuspid regurgitation. The PA pressure can be estimated during Doppler echocardiography by measuring the velocity of the tricuspid regurgitation jet and converting this velocity into a pressure using the equation $P = 4V^2$ (97% correlation with pulmonary artery catheter). Direct measurement of the PA pressure can be obtained using a pulmonary artery catheter (Swan-Ganz catheter), and is the gold standard for the diagnosis of pulmonary hypertension.

In the case of SPH, additional laboratory studies should be undertaken in an attempt to identify the underlying process. These studies may include arterial blood gases, liver function tests, HIV antibody assays, connective tissue serology, pulmonary function testing, sleep studies, ventilation-perfusion (V/Q) lung scanning, or pulmonary angiography. There is no specific test available to diagnose PPH; this is a diagnosis of exclusion.

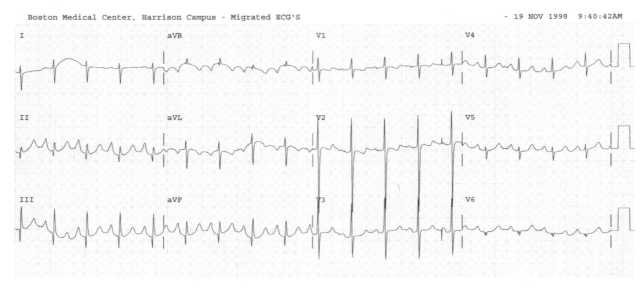

Figure 41–1   ECG of a patient with pulmonary hypertension. Characteristic features include right axis deviation (QRS axis is +130°), right atrial enlargement (P wave in lead II > 2.5 mV), and right ventricular hypertrophy (R > S in V_1, S > R in V_6).

TREATMENT

Primary pulmonary hypertension is an incurable disease with a poor prognosis (median survival of 2–3 years from the time of diagnosis). It is only in the last 15 years that advances in medical and surgical therapies have been able to alter the natural history of this disease.

Vasoconstriction is thought to play an important role in the pathogenesis of PPH. Accordingly, treatment with vasodilators has received a great deal of attention, although not all patients exhibit a uniform response to vasodilator therapy. The oral vasodilators of choice are calcium channel blocking agents such as nifedipine or diltiazem. These agents result in sustained clinical improvement in approximately 25–30% of patients.

Epoprostenol, a potent vasodilator that acts by increasing intracellular levels of cyclic AMP, has been found to produce both acute and sustained hemodynamic improvement in patients with PPH. It can be administered as a continuous infusion or by aerosol inhalation, and has been shown to improve exercise tolerance and prolong survival in these patients. Continuous epoprostenol therapy is currently used either as primary treatment or as a bridge to lung transplant in patients with PPH, depending on the degree of observed hemodynamic improvement.

Retrospective analysis of small, nonrandomized studies suggests that chronic anticoagulation in patients with PPH improves survival. As such, the general consensus is to treat these patients with warfarin to achieve an international normalized ratio (INR) of 1.5–2.5. Single lung and combined heart-lung transplantation remain the only definitive therapies for PPH. One-year survival following lung transplantation approaches 65–70%.

The mainstay of treatment of SPH is treatment of the underlying disease. Accepted general treatment modalities include supplemental oxygen for patients with hypoxemia, diuretics for symptomatic relief of ascites and hepatic congestion, and anticoagulation for patients at high risk for thromboembolic events. Specific therapies aimed at treating or correcting the underlying disorder (e.g., valve replacement for mitral disease, surgical correction of intracardiac shunts, maximization of medical therapy for left heart failure, etc.) may lead to normalization of pulmonary pressures and marked improvement in symptoms. Other treatment options of less clear benefit in SPH include calcium channel blockers and other vasodilators. Patients with certain forms of SPH that have histopathological findings in common with PPH (connective tissue disorders, HIV, hepatopulmonary syndrome) have shown improvement in hemodynamics, exercise tolerance, and survival on epoprostenol therapy.

◆ KEY POINTS ◆

1. Pulmonary hypertension is defined as a mean pulmonary pressure greater than 25 mmHg at rest or greater than 30 mmHg with exercise.

2. Primary pulmonary hypertension is a diagnosis of exclusion and is most commonly seen in young and middle-aged women.

3. Secondary pulmonary hypertension may result from a variety of cardiovascular, pulmonary, and systemic disorders.

4. Swan-Ganz or pulmonary artery catheterization is the gold standard for the diagnosis of PH, but elevated pulmonary pressures can often be identified by noninvasive techniques (echocardiography).

5. Primary pulmonary hypertension is an incurable disease. Vasodilators (calcium channel blocking agents or epoprostenol) are the mainstay of therapy; transplantation is the definitive treatment.

6. The treatment of SPH relies primarily on treatment of the underlying condition.

Part IX
Congenital
Heart Disease

42 Congenital Cardiac Shunts

In the normal setting, the output of the right heart flows to the pulmonary circulation and the output of the left heart flows to the systemic circulation. These two systems are anatomically distinct, being divided by the atrial septum, ventricular septum, and vasculature. Occasionally, a communication between these systems exists and allows for the shunting of blood from the right heart to the left heart and vice versa. This communication may occur at the level of the atrial septum, ventricular septum, or the vasculature.

PATHOPHYSIOLOGY

Prior to birth, the pulmonary and systemic circulation do communicate. Blood entering the right atrium is directed across the **foramen ovale** into the left atrium, and blood entering the pulmonary artery flows through the **ductus arteriosus** into the aorta. These communications help to limit blood flow to the pulmonary system since the lungs are nonfunctional prior to birth. Shortly after birth, these anatomic connections usually seal off.

Occasionally, the formation of the interatrial septum is incomplete, resulting in a defect (atrial septal defect or ASD) that allows for interatrial shunting of blood (Figure 42–1). The defect may be of three general types based on location:

- sinus venosus defect (at the superior aspect of the septum near the vena cava)

- ostium secundum defect (at the site of the **fossa ovalis**)
- ostium primum defect (at the inferior aspect of the interatrial septum near the atrioventricular plane)

Identification of the particular type of ASD is important because each is associated with specific concomitant congenital abnormalities (see Table 42–1).

In approximately 25% of patients, the interatrial septum forms completely but the foramen ovale fails to seal off following birth. This does not lead to shunting of blood in the resting state but can lead to shunt flow if the right atrial pressure exceeds the left atrial pressure (patent foramen ovale).

The interventricular septum may also fail to form correctly resulting in a ventricular septal defect (VSD). These are of two main types:

- membranous VSD (located high in the septum)
- muscular VSD (located in the mid- to distal septum)

Lastly, in some infants, the ductus arteriosus fails to constrict after birth and remains patent (a patent ductus arteriosus or PDA).

ASDs, VSDs, and PDAs allow for the abnormal flow of blood between the right and left circulation. Because the pressure in the left side of the heart is higher than that in the right, the shunt flow is usually from left to right and results in increased flow in the pulmonary circulation (Qp) compared with that in the systemic circulation (Qs). The ratio of these flows (Qp : Qs) is a

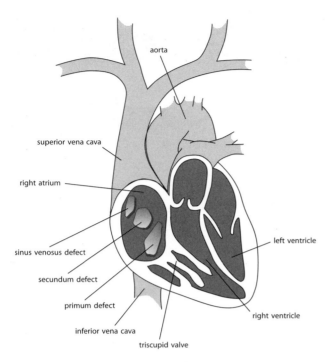

aorta

superior vena cava

right atrium

sinus venosus defect

secundum defect

primum defect

inferior vena cava

triscupid valve

left ventricle

right ventricle

Figure 42–1   Diagram of the various atrial septal defect types. *Illustration by Shawn Girsberger Graphic Design.*

method of quantifying shunt severity. Over time, the increased pulmonary flow results in pulmonary hypertension and right heart failure. Rarely, the right heart pressure may then exceed the left heart pressure resulting in right to left shunting of blood (Eisenmenger's syndrome). The deoxygenated blood thus entering the systemic circulation results in cyanosis and hypoxemia.

INCIDENCE

Intracardiac shunts are the second most common congenital heart defects; only bicuspid aortic valves are more common. VSDs account for 30% of all congenital heart disease and are common findings in infants and children. Fifty to 70% of VSDs close spontaneously during childhood; thus, it is rare that they are first diagnosed in adults. ASDs and PDAs each account for 10% of congenital heart disease. ASDs are the most common congenital heart diseases diagnosed in adulthood but are infrequently diagnosed in infancy.

CLINICAL MANIFESTATIONS

History

Infants and children with ASDs are usually asymptomatic but may occasionally present with signs of congestive heart failure. Large VSDs tend to produce heart failure at a young age. Adults with an ASD, PDA, or small VSD usually present with either arrhythmias (e.g., atrial fibrillation) or symptoms of progressive right heart failure and pulmonary hypertension, including:

- dyspnea with exertion
- peripheral edema
- fatigue
- chest pain

Patients with intracardiac shunts may occasionally present with a stroke caused by a thromboembolism that enters the systemic circulation through the defect (paradoxical embolus).

Physical Examination

Physical examination of patients with cardiac shunts may reveal signs of right heart failure. The characteristic findings on cardiac examination are outlined in Table 42–2.

DIAGNOSTIC EVALUATION

Chest x-ray may demonstrate increased pulmonary vascular markings (shunt vascularity), right and/or left atrial enlargement, and right ventricular enlargement. Patients with suspected cardiac shunts should undergo echocardiography to locate the defect (transesophageal echocardiography may be required to visualize small defects). The extent of shunt flow should be quantified by measurement of Qp:Qs. If echocardiography yields borderline or equivocal findings, cardiac catheterization and measurement of intracardiac oxygen saturations can be performed.

TREATMENT OF CARDIAC SHUNTS IN THE ADULT

Patients with small shunts may tolerate them well, have no long-term ill effects, and require no specific therapy

---

TABLE 42–1

Types of Atrial Septal Defects (ASD) and Associated Abnormalities

Type of ASD	Relative Prevalence	Associated Abnormalities	Classic ECG Findings
Ostium primum	20%	Cleft mitral valve, Down syndrome	Incomplete RBBB, left axis deviation, first degree AV block
Ostium secundum	70%	Mitral valve prolapse	rSr' in V1
Sinus venosus	10%	Anomalous pulmonary venous return	None

RBBB: right bundle branch block; AV: atrioventricular.

TABLE 42–2

Some Physical Characteristics of ASD, VSD, and PDA

Defect	Physical Exam Findings	Useful Diagnostic Modalities
ASD	1. Fixed split S_2 2. Midsystolic pulmonary ejection murmur 3. Prominent RV impulse 4. Cyanosis (if element of R-to-L shunt) 5. Tricuspid diastolic flow murmur	1. Echocardiography 2. ECG (rSr' in V1, RV strain pattern) 3. Cardiac catheterization 4. Chest x-ray
VSD	1. Loud holosystolic murmur at LSB 2. Thrill over precordium 3. Prominent RV impulse	1. Echocardiography 2. Cardiac catheterization 3. Chest x-ray
PDA	1. Wide pulse pressure 2. Continuous (systolic and diastolic) murmur at 2nd left ICS	1. Echocardiography 2. Cardiac catheterization 3. MRA

ASD: atrial septal defect; VSD: ventricular septal defect; PDA: patent ductus arteriosus; RV = right ventricle; LSB = left sternal border; ICS = intercostal space; MRA = magnetic resonance angiography.

---

aside from endocarditis prophylaxis (not necessary for patients with ASDs). Patients with larger shunts may develop progressive pulmonary hypertension and subsequent right heart failure. In these patients, closure of the defect should be considered before irreversible right heart failure occurs.

In patients with ASDs, the defect should be closed if the pulmonary blood flow exceeds the systemic blood flow by at least 50% (i.e., the Qp:Qs is >1.5:1.0), if echocardiography reveals right heart dilation or dysfunction, or if the patient has suffered a paradoxical embolism. Available closure techniques include:

- percutaneous closure with catheter-based devices (usually for ASDs <2 cm in diameter)
- primary surgical closure without a patch (small defects)
- surgical closure with a patch (larger defects)

Management of a VSD is similar with closure recommended when the Qp:Qs exceeds 1.5–2.0:1. Surgical closure of a VSD is the standard therapy.

In the absence of severe pulmonary hypertension and right heart failure, a patent ductus arteriosus in a full-term infant is an indication for closure. Surgical ligation is the usual technique; percutaneous methods are still investigational. In some infants, constriction of the PDA may be stimulated by use of prostaglandin inhibitors (e.g., indomethacin). Patients with large, uncorrected PDAs rarely survive into adulthood.

◆ KEY POINTS ◆

1. ASD, VSD, and PDA allow for left to right shunting of blood and may present as pulmonary hypertension, right heart failure, or an asymptomatic murmur. These defects do not cause cyanosis unless marked pulmonary hypertension develops resulting in reversal of the shunt direction (Eisenmenger's syndrome).

2. The three types of ASD include ostium primum, ostium secundum, and sinus venosus. The most common type is ostium secundum.

3. VSDs may occur in the membranous or the muscular regions of the interventricular septum.

4. ASDs are usually asymptomatic in childhood, but can present late in adulthood with symptoms of right heart failure. ASDs should be closed if the Qp:Qs is >1.5:1.

5. Large VSDs require surgery during infancy whereas small VSDs may require no specific therapy and may close spontaneously before adulthood.

6. PDAs produce a continuous "machinery" murmur and should be surgically closed unless severe pulmonary hypertension and right heart failure are present.

43

Cyanotic Congenital Heart Disease

Although many forms of congenital cyanotic heart disease are fatal in childhood, several disorders (including Eisenmenger's syndrome, tetralogy of Fallot, and corrected transposition) are compatible with survival to adulthood. Affected patients may be minimally limited during childhood but become progressively cyanotic with advancing age.

EISENMENGER'S SYNDROME

Patients who are born with a large VSD or PDA (rarely with a large secundum ASD) initially have a substantial left-to-right shunt. The resultant marked increase in pulmonary flow produces irreversible pulmonary hypertension. As right heart pressure rises, it may exceed left heart pressure, as a result of which the shunt reverses (i.e., right-to-left) This directional change shunts deoxygenated blood to the systemic circulation, leading to cyanosis.

Physical Examination

Prominent cyanosis and digital clubbing are usually present. A right ventricular heave and loud P_2 (pulmonary hypertension) are typical.

Diagnostic Evaluation

Electrocardiogram (ECG) demonstrates right ventricular hypertrophy. Chest radiography reveals prominent central pulmonary arteries with peripheral arterial pruning, and right ventricular enlargement. Echocardiography confirms the diagnosis and demonstrates right-to-left shunt flow, pulmonary hypertension, and right ventricular hypertrophy.

Treatment

Surgical repair of the shunt is not possible after irreversible pulmonary hypertension develops. Vasodilator therapy should be avoided as this will exacerbate the shunting. The only effective therapy is heart-lung transplantation or single-lung transplant and closure of the defect.

Prognosis

Patients may survive into the sixth decade but usually develop right ventricular failure in their 40's. Hypoxia and ventricular arrhythmias are the common causes of death.

TETRALOGY OF FALLOT (TOF)

Tetralogy of Fallot is characterized by:

- ventricular septal defect
- overriding aorta
- obstruction to right ventricular outflow
- right ventricular hypertrophy (RVH)

Incidence

Tetralogy of Fallot accounts for 10% of all congenital cardiac abnormalities, but is the most common congenital abnormality causing cyanosis after 1 year of age. Most patients with uncorrected TOF do not survive to adulthood; only 6% survive to age 30.

Physiology

Tetralogy of Fallot results from anterior displacement of the ventricular septum with an associated membranous VSD. The aorta thus straddles the septum (overriding aorta), allowing flow from both ventricles to enter the systemic circulation (Figure 43–1). In addition, there is a varying degree of RV outflow tract obstruction that results in right ventricular hypertrophy. These abnormalities impair blood flow through the pulmonary system and allows flow of deoxygenated blood from the right ventricle to the aorta, resulting in systemic hypoxemia and cyanosis.

The degree of cyanosis directly depends on two factors:

* severity of right ventricular outflow obstruction
* systemic vascular resistance (SVR)

More severe RV outflow obstruction and low SVR favor flow of deoxygenated blood from the RV to the aorta, increasing cyanosis. However, if SVR is increased, right ventricular blood flows preferentially to the pulmonary artery, and oxygenation improves.

Clinical Presentation

History

Most children with tetralogy of Fallot are cyanotic at birth. They usually develop dyspnea with exertion, and often learn to squat after exercise, thereby increasing their SVR, increasing pulmonary blood flow, and reducing fatigue and cyanosis. Episodic, sudden increases in the shunt may occur resulting in worsened cyanosis and tachypnea. These episodes may progress to syncope, seizure, or death.

Physical Examination

Physical examination reveals a systolic ejection murmur caused by stenosis of the RV outflow tract. A precordial thrill may be present. The second heart sound is single as P_2 is absent. A prominent RV heave may be present, as may digital clubbing, the latter resulting from chronic hypoxemia.

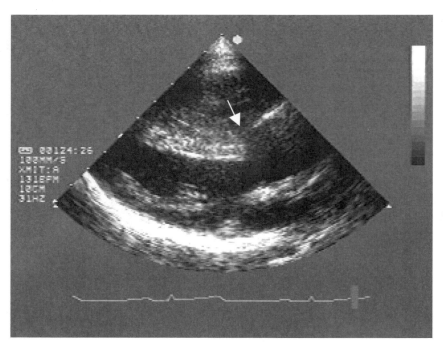
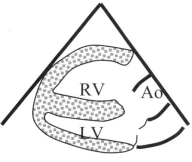

Figure 43–1 Echocardiogram of a patient with tetralogy of Fallot. The right ventricle (RV) is dilated and hypertrophied. The ventricular septal defect (arrow) is obvious, and the aorta (Ao) straddles the interventricular septum, allowing blood from both ventricles to enter the systemic circulation.

Diagnostic Evaluation

ECG may reveal evidence of right atrial enlargement and right ventricular hypertrophy. Chest x-ray usually demonstrates right heart enlargement, resulting in a characteristic "boot-shaped" cardiac silhouette. Echocardiography will demonstrate the classic anatomic abnormalities, which can be confirmed by cardiac catheterization.

Therapy

Surgical correction early in infancy is the treatment of choice. The feasibility of surgery depends on the size of the right ventricular outflow tract and the pulmonary arteries. A severely hypoplastic RV outflow tract or pulmonary artery atresia may not allow for complete surgical repair. In these patients, palliative surgical therapy can be performed to create a systemic-pulmonary artery anastomosis (Blalock-Taussig shunt, Watterson shunt, or Pott's shunt) to allow increased pulmonary blood flow and improve oxygenation.

CORRECTED TRANSPOSITIONS

Complete transposition of the great arteries (aorta arises from the RV; pulmonary artery arises from the LV) is a universally fatal syndrome if not surgically corrected at birth. In congenitally corrected transposition, there is atrioventricular and ventriculoarterial discordance (essentially the ventricles have switched position). Blood flows through the circulation in the appropriate direction; however, the morphologic RV (in the anatomic LV position) pumps blood to the systemic circulation and the morphologic LV pumps blood to the pulmonary circulation. There is frequently an associated VSD, pulmonary stenosis, and complete heart block.

Clinical Presentation

Patients with congenitally corrected transposition without associated anomalies may survive into the 6th decade but often develop left-sided heart failure as the morphologic RV is unable to maintain systemic pressures. Patients with associated VSD have varying degrees of cyanosis.

Treatment

Surgical repair of the VSD and pulmonary stenosis, when present, is the treatment of choice. The left atrioventricular valve frequently becomes regurgitant and requires replacement.

◆ KEY POINTS ◆

1. Eisenmenger's syndrome consists of pulmonary hypertension and right-to-left shunting through an ASD, VSD, or patent ductus arteriosus.

2. Tetralogy of Fallot is the most common cause of cyanotic congenital heart disease after 1 year of age and consists of RVH, VSD, overriding aorta, and pulmonic outflow obstruction.

3. The degree of cyanosis in TOF is dependent on the severity of the pulmonic outflow obstruction and the systemic vascular resistance.

4. Surgical correction early in infancy and childhood is the cornerstone of therapy for TOF.

Part X
Other

44

Pregnancy and Cardiovascular Disease

Significant circulatory changes occur during pregnancy and the peripartum period and can precipitate clinical deterioration in the presence of pre-existing cardiovascular disease. In addition, pregnancy itself may be an etiological factor in the development of certain cardiovascular disorders, including hypertension and dilated cardiomyopathy. An understanding of this altered cardiovascular physiology is essential to the management of the pregnant cardiac patient.

CARDIOVASCULAR PHYSIOLOGY DURING PREGNANCY

Blood volume, heart rate, stroke volume, and cardiac output increase substantially during pregnancy. On average, blood volume increases by 40%, accounting, in part, for an increase in cardiac output of 30–50%. Blood pressure tends to decline during the first trimester, reaching a nadir during the second trimester before returning to normal toward the end of the pregnancy. These hemodynamic changes are summarized in Table 44–1.

Despite the increase in blood volume, venous return is reduced during late pregnancy as a result of compression of the inferior vena cava by the gravid uterus. This compression is relieved after delivery, and, when combined with the shifting of blood from the contracting uterus into the systemic circulation, results in an acute rise in preload, stroke volume, and cardiac output. These volume shifts may result in heart failure in the immediate postpartum period, especially in patients with depressed left ventricular function.

CLINICAL MANIFESTATIONS

The normal hemodynamic changes of pregnancy may result in signs and symptoms that mimic or obscure cardiac disease, including:

- fatigue, decreased exercise capacity
- dyspnea (due to hormonal changes and diaphragmatic elevation)
- orthopnea (due to diaphragmatic elevation)
- lightheadedness, presyncope (due to compression of the vena cava with decreased venous return)
- palpitations (due to sinus tachycardia)
- elevated jugular venous pressure (JVP), edema (due to fluid retention)
- displaced point of maximal impulse (PMI)
- third and/or fourth heart sounds
- systolic flow murmurs (due to increased stroke volume)

Physical findings seen almost exclusively in pregnancy include:

- cervical venous hum (continuous murmur in the right supraclavicular fossa)
- mammary souffle (continuous murmur over the breast)

TABLE 44–1

Hemodynamic Changes During Normal Pregnancy

	1st Trimester	2nd Trimester	3rd Trimester
Blood volume	↑	↑↑	↑↑↑
Stroke volume	↑	↑↑↑	↑, ↔, or ↓
Heart rate	↑	↑↑	↑↑ to ↑↑↑
Cardiac output	↑	↑↑ to ↑↑	↑↑ to ↑↑↑
Systolic BP	↔	↓	↔
Diastolic BP	↓	↓↓	↓
Pulse pressure	↑	↑↑	↔
Systemic vascular resistance	↓	↓↓↓	↓↓

Diastolic murmurs and systolic murmurs that are greater than II/VI in intensity are rarely related solely to pregnancy and warrant further evaluation.

DIAGNOSTIC CARDIAC TESTING IN PREGNANCY

Electrocardiographic changes in normal pregnancy include sinus tachycardia, QRS axis shift, and premature atrial and ventricular complexes. ST-T changes are not routinely seen as part of normal pregnancy and warrant further evaluation.

Echocardiography is safe in pregnancy and frequently reveals atrial and/or ventricular chamber dilation; a small pericardial effusion; and mild mitral, tricuspid, and pulmonic valve regurgitation.

Chest radiography is generally avoided during pregnancy, but when performed may reveal cardiomegaly, increased pulmonary markings, and small pleural effusions.

PRE-EXISTING CARDIAC DISEASE AND PREGNANCY

Congenital Heart Disease (CHD)

Maternal prognosis is influenced by the type of CHD, previous surgical repair, severity of cyanosis, pulmonary vascular resistance, and functional capacity. In general,

a good maternal outcome can be expected in most patients with:

- non-cyanotic CHD
- surgically corrected CHD
- uncorrected atrial (ASD) *or* ventricular (VSD) septal defects
- patent ductus arteriosus (PDA),
- pulmonic stenosis (PS),
- uncomplicated coarctation of the aorta

Patients with uncorrected or partially corrected tetralogy of Fallot do not tolerate pregnancy very well. The increase in blood volume and venous return to the right atrium, combined with a drop in systemic vascular resistance (SVR), can produce or exacerbate right-to-left shunting and cyanosis in these patients. Eisenmenger's syndrome continues to be associated with high maternal morbidity and mortality; pregnancy should be avoided, and abortion should be considered for patients with this disorder who are already pregnant.

Valvular Heart Disease

Mitral and aortic regurgitation is usually well tolerated during pregnancy owing to the reduction in SVR. Symptomatic patients can be treated with diuretics, digoxin, and/or hydralazine. Mild aortic stenosis (valve area > 1.0 cm^2) and mild mitral stenosis (valve area

TABLE 44–2

Antihypertensive Agents in Pregnancy

Medication	? Safe	Comment
Alpha-blocker (methyldopa)	Yes	Safety and efficacy supported in randomized trials
Beta-blockers (metoprolol and atenolol)	Yes, in late pregnancy	Fetal growth retardation noted when used in early- or mid-gestation
Alpha- and beta-blocker (Labetalol)	?	Lack of data; concern for maternal hepatotoxicity
Vasodilator (hydralazine)	Yes	Rare cases of neonatal thrombocytopenia
Angiotensin-converting enzyme inhibitors	No	Fetal death or renal failure in newborns
Diuretics	Yes and no	May continue if prescribed before gestation; thiazides may result in low birth weight, hypoglycemia and bone marrow suppression in fetus

> 1.5 cm^2) are generally well tolerated during pregnancy; more severe valvular stenosis is often problematic. Patients with stenotic valvular disease who develop severe symptoms despite medical therapy may require surgical valve repair or percutaneous balloon valvuloplasty. Those managed medically often require invasive hemodynamic monitoring with a PA catheter in the peripartum period. Termination of the pregnancy is occasionally required.

Hypertension

Women with chronic hypertension have a higher risk of peripartum complications including fetal growth retardation, placental abruption, premature delivery, acute renal failure, and hypertensive crisis. Drug therapy for hypertension during pregnancy is recommended for diastolic BP >100 mmHg, or >90 mmHg in patients with renal disease or evidence of end organ involvement (refer to Table 44–2).

PREGNANCY-RELATED CARDIOVASCULAR DISORDERS

Pre-eclampsia is characterized by hypertension associated with proteinuria, edema, or both. Hypertension in pre-eclampsia is defined as either: (1) an increase in systolic blood pressure (SBP) of >30 mmHg or (2) an increase in diastolic blood pressure (DBP) >15 mmHg over baseline values obtained prior to 20 weeks' gestation. If blood pressures prior to the 20th week of gestation are not known, a blood pressure of >140/90 mmHg is diagnostic. Drug therapy and hospitalization are recommended for pre-eclamptic patients.

Peripartum Cardiomyopathy

Peripartum cardiomyopathy is a form of dilated cardiomyopathy that usually becomes apparent by the third trimester. The reported incidence in the US is 1 in 10,000 pregnancies. Its etiology is unknown. Treatment of resultant heart failure includes use of diuretics, digoxin, and vasodilators (such as hydralazine). Patients should also receive anticoagulant therapy post partum because of an increased incidence of thromboembolic events. Varying degrees of recovery of LV function may occur after delivery. Subsequent pregnancies are associated with a high risk of relapse, in addition to maternal morbidity and mortality. Further pregnancies should be discouraged in patients with persistent LV dysfunction, while patients with recovered LV function should be counseled regarding their increased risk of relapse.

◆ KEY POINTS ◆

1. Substantial hemodynamic changes occur during pregnancy, including increased heart rate, increased stroke volume, increased cardiac output, and decreased systemic vascular resistance.

2. Symptoms and signs of normal pregnancy may mimic or obscure cardiac disease.

3. Pre-existing cardiac conditions, especially heart failure, may be exacerbated by the altered physiology of pregnancy. Regurgitant valvular disease is usually tolerated well while stenotic valvular disease may be problematic and result in heart failure during the pregnancy.

4. Hypertension, pre-eclampsia, and peripartum cardiomyopathy may complicate gestation.

45

Traumatic Heart Disease

Cardiac trauma is one of the leading causes of death among individuals sustaining violent injuries, such as motor vehicle accidents and gunshot or stab wounds. Iatrogenic cardiac trauma can also occur, caused by the use of intravascular and intracardiac catheters, or from the performance of closed chest compressions during cardiopulmonary resuscitation (CPR). Cardiac injuries can be separated into two major types: **non-penetrating** and **penetrating**.

NON-PENETRATING CARDIAC INJURY

Non-penetrating injuries most commonly result from:

- impact during a motor vehicle accident with resultant compression of the chest from the steering wheel
- blows to the chest by any kind of blunt object or missile (e.g., a clenched fist or sporting equipment)
- external chest compression during CPR

Blunt trauma can lead to injuries to the myocardium, pericardium, endocardial structures, coronary arteries, and the aorta (see Table 45–1).

Clinical Manifestations

Cardiac injury should be suspected in patients with an appropriate mechanism of injury, even in the absence of other overt chest trauma. Traumatic **cardiac rupture** usually results in exsanguination or cardiac tamponade, and is almost always fatal. Cardiac rupture can either occur immediately upon injury (acute laceration) or be delayed (e.g., contusion leading to hemorrhage, necrosis, and subsequent rupture), and can affect any cardiac chamber. Rupture of the papillary muscles, chordae tendineae, or any of the valve leaflets results in acute valvular insufficiency with heart failure, hemodynamic instability, and a new murmur. Rupture of the interventricular septum may present similarly, but may be relatively well tolerated. Rupture of the pericardium can present as circulatory collapse owing to cardiac herniation through the pericardial sac.

Less severe blunt injuries may lead to **myocardial contusion**, the presentation of which varies depending on the location and extent of injury. The right ventricle (RV) is most frequently involved owing to its anterior location (see Figure 45–1); the interventricular septum and LV apex are less frequently affected. The most common symptom of cardiac contusion is precordial pain similar to that of a myocardial infarction. Patients with extensive contusion may present with shock resulting from RV and/or LV failure.

Diagnosis

The electrocardiogram (ECG) may be helpful in suspected cases of cardiac contusion. Initially, it may demonstrate non-specific ST-T wave abnormalities or findings of pericarditis. Subsequently, ECG

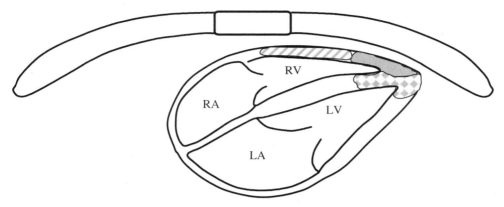

Figure 45–1   Spectrum of myocardial contusion. Myocardial contusion involving the left ventricle (LV) tends to be limited to the LV apex (spotted region). Involvement of the right ventricle (RV) may be limited to the RV apex (shaded region), or involve the RV free wall as well (hatched region). RA: right atrium; LA: left atrium.

<table>

TABLE 45–1

Types of Cardiac Injury Resulting from Blunt Trauma

Myocardium	1. Contusion
	2. Rupture
	3. Septal perforation (ventricular septal defect)
	4. Ventricular aneurysm or pseudoaneurysm
	5. Hemopericardium or tamponade
Pericardium	1. Pericarditis
	2. Post-pericardiotomy syndrome
	3. Constrictive pericarditis
	4. Pericardial laceration
	5. Cardiac herniation
Endocardial structures	1. Papillary muscle rupture
	2. Rupture of chordae tendinae
	3. Valvular leaflet rupture
Coronary artery	1. Thrombosis and myocardial infarction
	2. Laceration
	3. Fistula

</table>

myocardial injury (creatine kinase-MB fraction and cardiac troponins) will be elevated in myocardial contusion.

Two-dimensional echocardiography is very helpful in evaluating cardiac injuries. This study can identify pericardial effusions and determine their hemodynamic significance, identify structural injuries (myocardial or valvular rupture, intracardiac shunts), and demonstrate poorly functioning myocardium in the region of a cardiac contusion.

Treatment

Patients with ventricular free wall rupture or valvular rupture require emergent surgery, whereas patients with rupture of the interventricular septum can often initially be managed conservatively; the ventricular septal defects (VSDs) are often small and may close spontaneously. The treatment of patients with myocardial contusion is similar to that of patients with myocardial infarction excepting that anticoagulation is contraindicated in the setting of contusion. These patients should receive supportive care and observation, including close monitoring for arrhythmias and potential late complications.

findings similar to those of a myocardial infarction may evolve. A variety of supraventricular or ventricular arrhythmias may occur, and transient of persistent right bundle branch block may develop. Markers of

PENETRATING CARDIAC INJURY

The majority of **penetrating cardiac injuries** are caused by sharp objects (such as knives or ice picks) and missiles (mostly bullets). As in myocardial contusion, the chamber most commonly involved is the RV owing to its anterior location. In contrast to blunt trauma, penetrating cardiac wounds generally involve concomitant laceration of both the pericardium and myocardium. Gunshot wounds tend to cause extensive tissue destruction and bleeding along the path of the projectile, whereas stab wounds may seal quickly before disastrous complications occur.

Clinical Manifestations

The clinical presentation depends on the type, location, and extent of injury. Pericardial laceration is common, and the nature of this wound (open or closed) determines whether intrapericardial blood drains freely into the chest, resulting in extensive hemorrhage and hemothorax, or collects in the pericardial space resulting in cardiac tamponade. Although severe penetrating injuries to the heart generally result in immediate death or shock, one must maintain a high index of suspicion in hemodynamically stable patients with penetrating injuries to the chest that involve the lungs and other organs. Delayed clinical manifestations of cardiac injury include infection, retained foreign bodies, and arrhythmias.

Diagnosis

Two-dimensional echocardiography is the diagnostic test of choice for the evaluation of penetrating cardiac trauma and can be invaluable in recognizing pericardial effusion, intracardiac shunts (ASD or VSD), foreign bodies, and valvular disruption. However, echocardiography is not always available in the emergency setting; therefore, emergent thoracotomy is often performed that will allow for the direct visualization of cardiac injury.

Treatment

The definitive therapy for severe hemorrhage accompanying cardiac injuries is immediate thoracotomy and cardiorrhaphy. The heart and its surrounding structures are inspected carefully, and repaired accordingly prior to chest closure. Treatment for retained foreign bodies is more controversial, as one has to balance the risk of the operation against the risk of future embolization or infection. ASD, VSD, and valvular regurgitation, when diagnosed as late complications, are corrected only if symptoms warrant operative repair.

◆ KEY POINTS ◆

1. The most common cause of non-penetrating cardiac injuries is motor vehicle accidents.

2. Blunt chest trauma can lead to cardiac rupture, valvular disruption, pericardial effusion, and myocardial contusion.

3. Myocardial contusion may mimic myocardial infarction in both symptoms and associated complications. The treatment of contusion is similar to the medical treatment of infarction excepting that anticoagulation is contraindicated in the setting of contusion.

4. Penetrating cardiac injuries usually result from knife and gunshot wounds, and lead to immediate death or shock if severe. Survivors usually require emergent thoracotomy and cardiorrhaphy.

46 Cardiac Tumors

Primary tumors of the heart are rare, with an incidence of less than 0.3% by autopsy, and may be **benign** or **malignant** (see Table 46–1). Of the primary cardiac tumors, myxomas are the most common. Other benign tumors include papillary fibroelastomas, lipomas, and rhabdomyomas. Angiosarcomas, rhadomyosarcomas, mesotheliomas, and fibrosarcomas account for the majority of malignant primary cardiac tumors in adults. Metastatic tumors to the heart are far more common, and may involve the myocardium, pericardium, or endocardial surface. The most common primary source of metastatic cardiac tumors is the lung, followed by breast and kidney. Cardiac involvement may also occur with melanomas and lymphomas.

CLINICAL MANIFESTATIONS

History

The specific signs and symptoms of cardiac tumors are more dependent on their anatomical location rather than their histological type. One notable exception is cardiac myxomas, which are frequently associated with nonspecific systemic symptoms such as fever, malaise, weight loss, arthralgias, and rash.

Tumors arising on the endocardial surface of the heart commonly present with symptoms of pulmonary emboli (right-sided tumors), or systemic or cerebral emboli (left-sided tumors). These result from emboliza-tion of tumor fragments or of thrombi from the surface of the tumor.

Left atrial tumors (predominantly myxomas) often mimic mitral valve disease. These tumors may prolapse into the mitral valve orifice during diastole, thereby impairing left ventricular filling, mimicking mitral stenosis, and resulting in symptoms of congestive heart failure. Patients who have such tumors may report symptoms that occur in relation to body position. **Right atrial tumors** are frequently asymptomatic but may produce symptoms of right heart failure if they are large. Myxomas occur more frequently in the left atrium, and sarcomas are more commonly found in the right atrium.

Left ventricular tumors are often asymptomatic, unless significant obstruction of the left ventricular outflow tract or impairment of myocardial function causing left heart failure is present. Systemic embolization may also occur. **Right ventricular tumors** often present with right heart failure. If right ventricular outflow tract obstruction is present, patients may present more dramatically with syncope or sudden death.

Intramyocardial tumors most commonly result in rhythm or conduction disturbances and may produce palpitations or syncope. They can occasionally present as sudden cardiac death due to cardiac rupture. **Pericardial tumors** result in the accumulation of blood or exudative fluid in the pericardial space and may produce symptoms of pericarditis or pericardial tamponade (see Chapters 33 and 34).

TABLE 46–1

Primary Cardiac Tumors

Benign	Malignant
1. Myxoma	1. Angiosarcoma
2. Lipoma	2. Rhabdomyosarcoma
3. Papillary fibroelastoma	3. Mesothelioma
4. Rhabdomyoma	4. Fibrosarcoma
5. Fibroma	5. Malignant lymphoma
6. Hemangioma	6. Osteosarcoma
7. Teratoma (in childhood)	7. Thymoma
8. Mesothelioma of the atrioventricular node	8. Neurogenic sarcoma
9. Granular cell tumor	9. Malignant teratoma (in childhood)

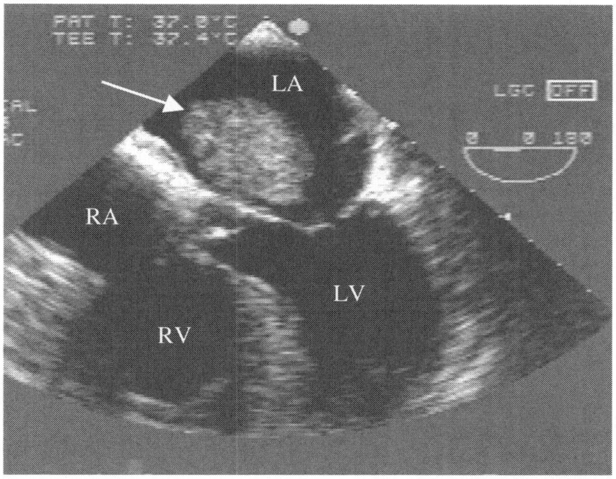

Figure 46–1 Transesophageal echocardiogram demonstrating a large (4.5 cm × 3.5 cm) atrial myxoma arising from the interatrial septum.

Physical Examination

The physical examination of patients with cardiac tumors is often unremarkable. However, several findings may be noted, including:

- **a tumor plop**, an early diastolic sound frequently confused with an opening snap or an S_3, may be heard in patients with large atrial tumors

- systolic or diastolic murmurs mimicking mitral regurgitation or stenosis may be present with left atrial tumors

- signs of heart failure may be present with large tumors of any cardiac chamber

With metastatic cardiac tumors, signs of the primary tumor may be identifiable on examination.

LABORATORY EVALUATION

Routine laboratory testing is not usually helpful in the diagnosis of cardiac tumors. Nonetheless, cardiac myxomas are often associated with anemia and an elevated erythrocyte sedimentation rate. These findings likely result from production of interleukin-6 by the myxoma.

DIAGNOSIS

The diagnosis of cardiac tumor is usually made by two-dimensional echocardiography. A **transthoracic echocardiogram** can provide information about tumor size, site of attachment, and mobility. When the transthoracic study is not definitive, **transesophageal echocardiography** (TEE) can provide improved resolution of the tumor and its attachment (see Figure 46–1). TEE can also detect smaller tumor masses not readily seen by transthoracic echocardiography. **Computed tomography** (CT) of the heart has also been used to evaluate cardiac tumors; it is most useful in determining the degree of myocardial invasion and the involvement of pericardial and extracardiac structures. In addition to visualization of the pericardium and extracardiac structures, **cardiac MRI** provides better definition of tumor prolapse and secondary valve obstruction, and can differentiate thrombi from tumors. **Cardiac catheterization and angiography** are not necessary in most cases of cardiac tumors, except to exclude coexisting coronary artery disease that may warrant revascularization at the time of tumor resection.

TREATMENT

For benign cardiac tumors, operative excision is the treatment of choice and, in most cases, is curative.

Peripheral embolization or dispersion of micrometastases remains the major surgical risk. Long term prognosis is good, although myxomas may recur after initial resection.

Operative resection is not an effective treatment for the majority of malignant primary or metastatic cardiac tumors owing to extensive tissue involvement or distal metastases. Prognosis is poor in general, with overall survival of 1–3 years following partial resection, chemotherapy, radiation, or combinations of these treatment modalities. Malignant pericardial effusions frequently recur after initial drainage and may require surgical pericardiotomy ("pericardial window").

◆ **KEY POINTS** ◆

1. Primary cardiac tumors are rare.
2. The most common primary cardiac tumor is an atrial myxoma.
3. The most common tumors to metastasize to the heart are lung, breast, and renal carcinomas; melanomas; and lymphomas.
4. Symptoms of cardiac tumors usually relate to their anatomic position rather than their histological type.

Questions

1. A 67-year-old veteran with a history of calf claudication and an abdominal aortic aneurysm repair presents to your office for a routine visit. He has no known coronary artery disease (CAD), diabetes, or family history of premature CAD. He stopped smoking 3 years ago. His blood pressure is 128/70 mmHg on an angiotensin-converting enzyme (ACE) inhibitor. His other medications include aspirin and multivitamins. His physical examination is notable for a well-healed abdominal surgical scar, and diminished bilateral dorsalis pedis and posterior tibial pulses. His wife mentions that his diet is "terrible," and she is concerned that his cholesterol level might be high. A fasting lipid profile is as follows:

Plasma total cholesterol	196 mg/dL
Plasma LDL cholesterol	140 mg/dL
Plasma HDL cholesterol	35 mg/dL
Serum triglycerides	105 mg/dL

   In addition to initiating therapeutic lifestyle changes, what is the most appropriate management?

   a. Repeat lipid profile in 3 months; target LDL < 130 mg/dL

   b. Repeat lipid profile in 3 months; target LDL < 100 mg/dL

   c. Initiate HMG-CoA reductase inhibitor; target LDL < 100 mg/dL

   d. Repeat lipid profile in 3–5 years

   e. Initiate a fibric-acid derivative agent

2. A 25-year-old woman presents to your clinic after "passing out" while standing in line at a bank. Immediately prior to the event, she recalls feeling nauseated and had a "warm sensation all over." She subsequently felt lightheaded and lost consciousness for approximately 30–40 seconds, following which she awoke and was aware of her surroundings. Witnesses told her that she attempted to hold onto a counter prior to collapsing. She denies previous syncopal episodes. Examination reveals normal BP and heart rate. Her pulmonary, cardiac, and neurological examination are all normal. Hematocrit, BUN, creatinine, and electrolytes are all normal. An echocardiogram and ECG performed in your office are unremarkable.

   What is the most appropriate next test to perform in this patient's evaluation.

   a. Holter monitoring

   b. electrophysiological study

   c. head CT scan

   d. tilt table testing

   e. carotid sinus massage

3. A 35-year-old nonsmoking male without significant past medical history presents with chest pain and

exertional dyspnea. Review of symptoms is notable for a one-week history of antecedent flu-like symptoms. Physical examination reveals a jugular venous pressure (JVP) of 15 cm H_2O, and rales halfway up the lung fields bilaterally. An S_3 and a III/VI holosystolic murmur at the apex are noted, as is pitting edema of bilateral lower extremities. Electrocardiogram reveals diffuse ST-T wave abnormalities. The initial creatine kinase (CK) is 586 with an index of 7%. The most likely diagnosis is:

a. pulmonary embolism

b. acute myocardial infarction

c. viral pericarditis

d. viral myocarditis

e. hypertrophic cardiomyopathy

4. You are asked to evaluate a 56-year-old man who has recently developed intermittent chest pain. He has a history of hypertension, smoking, and gastroesophageal reflux disease. Over the past three weeks he has noted several episodes of right-sided chest pain that occur at rest, are associated with mild diaphoresis, last 5–10 minutes, and spontaneously resolve. He has not noted exertional symptoms. His blood pressure is 140/80 mmHg, and his heart rate is 70 bpm. He has a prominent S_4 but an otherwise normal examination. An ECG reveals normal sinus rhythm and left ventricular hypertrophy with a "strain" pattern (anterolateral ST-T abnormalities). You make the diagnosis of atypical chest pain and schedule him for a stress test. Which of the following is the most appropriate type of stress test for this patient?

a. exercise ECG

b. dobutamine echocardiogram

c. adenosine stress with nuclear imaging

d. 24-hour ambulatory ECG monitoring

e. exercise stress with nuclear imaging

5. A 63-year-old male smoker presents to your clinic for a regularly scheduled appointment. On examination, his blood pressure is 140/90. His pulse is 70 and regular. His respiratory rate is 20. There is no jugular venous distension. His carotid pulses are 1+ bilaterally without bruits. Examination of his chest reveals diffusely decreased breath sounds with scattered rhonchi. Precordial examination is unremarkable. Abdominal examination reveals a pulsatile mass with an associated bruit. Peripheral pulses are diminished but symmetric. You obtain an abdominal ultrasound that reveals an abdominal aortic aneurysm. Which of the following factors would prompt you to recommend elective surgical repair?

a. coexistent coronary artery disease

b. family history of abdominal aneurysm

c. absence of symptoms

d. concomitant peripheral vascular disease

e. aneurysm diameter of 6 cm

The following options apply to questions 6–8:

a. acute myocardial infarction

b. unstable angina

c. stable angina

d. pulmonary embolism

e. spontaneous pneumothorax

f. pericarditis

g. costochondritis

h. aortic dissection

i. coronary artery spasm

6. A 60-year-old male with a history of hypercholesterolemia and smoking reports a 2-year history of substernal chest discomfort precipitated by exertion and relieved by rest. In the past several weeks, the pain has become more frequent and is precipitated by less exertion.

7. A 45-year-old man presents with sudden, severe, sharp chest pain that radiates to his back. On examination, his weight is 160 pounds; his height is 72 inches. His heart rate is 110 bpm. His blood pressure is 124/70 in the left arm and barely palpable in the right arm.

8. A 36-year-old man presents with intermittent, sharp, mid-sternal chest pain. The pain is somewhat worse with inspiration and is associated with mild dyspnea. Several weeks prior, he and his children had "cold" symptoms.

9. A 73-year-old man with a history of hypertension and peripheral vascular disease presents with acute onset of chest pain. The pain was initially epigastric, but then settled between his shoulder blades. On physical exam, he appears quite anxious. His blood pressure is 190/90 mmHg in both arms. Pulse is 98 bpm and regular. Respiratory rate is 20/min. His jugular veins are not distended, and his lungs are clear. Precordial exam reveals an S_4. No murmur is noted. Abdominal exam is notable for moderate tenderness with deep palpation and a peri-umbilical bruit. His right dorsalis pedis and posterior tibial pulses are 1+.

Laboratory studies include:

BUN: 40

Creatinine: 1.5

Hematocrit: 34%

ECG: Sinus tachycardia, left ventricular hypertrophy, no acute ischemic changes.

The most likely diagnosis is:

a. aortic dissection

b. acute myocardial infarction

c. acute arterial embolus

d. pulmonary embolism

e. pancreatitis

10. The patient in the preceding question undergoes a computed tomography (CT) scan that demonstrates a descending aortic dissection originating just distal to the aortic arch and extending to the aortic bifurcation. There is no significant vascular obstruction seen. The most appropriate initial therapy for this patient should include:

a. labetalol and nitroprusside

b. heparin

c. emergent surgical intervention

d. thrombolytic therapy

e. intravenous fluids and narcotic analgesics

11. A 41-year-old male smoker is referred to your clinic for the evaluation of claudication. This began several months ago and has steadily progressed since that time. Additional questioning reveals symptoms of cold-induced vasospasm. He has no history of diabetes or hypertension. On physical examination, the patient is a thin man in no acute distress. His blood pressure is 140/80 mmHg, and his pulse is 68 bpm. His chest is clear and cardiac examination is unremarkable. His abdomen is soft and nontender without masses or bruits. His extremities are warm but with diminished radial, dorsalis pedis, and posterior tibial pulses. Which of the following should you recommend?

a. atenolol 50 mg daily

b. diltiazem 30 mg four times daily

c. assessment of ankle-brachial indices

d. smoking cessation

e. surgical revascularization

12. A 70-year-old woman is admitted for progressive dyspnea. Physical examination reveals moderate respiratory distress. Her heart rate is 110 bpm and her blood pressure is 105/60 mmHg, but the systolic pressure falls to 90 mmHg with inspiration. Her radial pulse is 100 bpm, and the pulse volume varies significantly with the respiratory cycle. Her jugular venous pressure is elevated, and there is moderate lower extremity edema. Chest examination reveals distant heart sounds and faint crackles at the base of the left lung. This patient is most likely to benefit from:

a. intravenous diuretics and oral ACE inhibitors

b. nebulized albuterol and intravenous steroids

c. pericardiocentesis

d. aspirin, nitroglycerin, and beta-blockers

e. intravenous antibiotics

13. A 60-year-old male smoker presents with intermittent fevers over a several-week period. He has no significant past medical history, but was told that he had a murmur at some point in the past. His temperature is 100°F (37.7°C), heart rate 85 bpm, and blood pressure 135/70 mmHg. Physical examination reveals digital clubbing and splenomegaly. Small, erythematous, nontender spots are noted over the palmar aspect of his hands. His lungs are clear to auscultation. Cardiac examination reveals a mid-systolic click and a faint, apical, holosystolic murmur. What is the most likely diagnosis?

a.   pneumonia

b.   viral syndrome

c.   infectious endocarditis

d.   pericarditis

e.   congenital cardiac shunt

14.   A 44-year-old woman presents to the emergency room with complaint of increased pedal edema. She has a history of smoking, borderline hypertension, and class II heart failure resulting from a nonischemic cardiomyopathy. Her medications include a diuretic, a beta-blocker, and birth control pills. She lives in Mexico and recently came to the US to visit family. Shortly after her arrival she noted increased pedal edema. She denies any change in her baseline dyspnea, has been compliant with her medications, and denies any recent chest pain.

On examination, she is mildly uncomfortable but in no respiratory distress. Her blood pressure is 130/70 mmHg. Her pulse is 88 bpm and regular. Her JVP is elevated at 8 cm H_2O without hepatojugular reflux (HJR). Chest exam reveals moderate aeration but no evidence of consolidation. Precordial examination demonstrates distant heart sounds and a soft S_3. Her abdominal examination is benign. There is 1+ edema of the right lower extremity. The left lower extremity demonstrates 2–3+ edema with mild erythema and warmth. What is the most appropriate next step in her management?

a.   administer intravenous diuretics

b.   obtain blood cultures and start intravenous antibiotics

c.   obtain bilateral lower extremity ultrasound studies

d.   check 24-hour urine protein excretion

e.   start an ACE inhibitor and arrange follow-up with a local physician

15.   A 69-year-old man is referred to you for a recent episode of syncope. While walking on the beach in Florida, he had sudden loss of consciousness and awoke to find his family looking over him. He does not recall the event, but his daughter states that he "fell over" without warning. He has never had syncope in the past, but does admit to occasional

chest pain and exertional dyspnea. A physical examination reveals a blood pressure of 132/76 mmHg and a heart rate of 72 bpm. His lungs are clear. There are delayed and subdued carotid upstrokes with a loud, late-peaking, systolic crescendo-decrescendo murmur over the sternal border near the 2nd intercostal space. The second heart sound is faintly audible. Pulses are 1+ in all four extremities, there is no edema.

The most likely cause of this patient's syncope is:

a.   acute myocardial infarction

b.   vasovagal syncope

c.   orthostatic hypotension

d.   aortic stenosis

e.   mitral stenosis

16.   A 75-year-old woman with chronic atrial fibrillation presents to the ambulatory care clinic complaining of one week of fatigue and intermittent dizziness. She had previously been very active and normally walks around a small park every day. She denies any dyspnea or angina and reports no episodes of syncope. Her only other medical history is hypertension for which she takes hydrochlorothiazide. She also takes warfarin for her atrial fibrillation. An ECG in the clinic reveals atrial fibrillation with an average heart rate of 38–45 beats per minute.

The next appropriate step in the management of this patient would be:

a.   Holter monitoring

b.   echocardiogram

c.   implantation of a pacemaker

d.   implantation of an implantable cardioverter-fibrillator (ICD)

e.   no therapy other than reassurance

17.   You are asked to consult on a 70-year-old man who was recently admitted to the coronary care unit (CCU) following a cardiac arrest in a shopping mall. He was successfully resuscitated and brought to your hospital. He was initially unresponsive, but after 5 days, he has regained all neurological function. He has no known prior cardiac history, but admits to occasional dyspnea on exertion and pedal edema. Initial

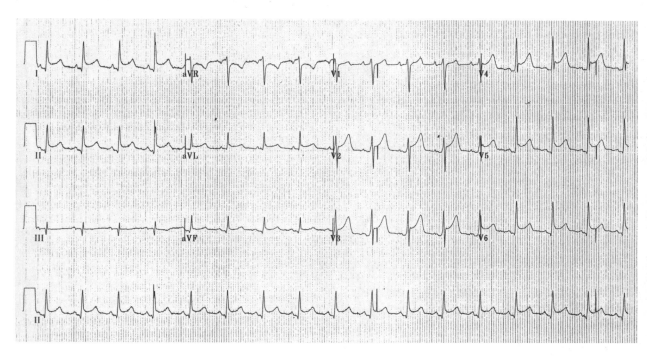

Figure Q–18

ECG revealed sinus rhythm with a left bundle branch block (LBBB). Laboratory evaluation in the CCU failed to demonstrate evidence of acute myocardial infarction. An echocardiogram was performed and demonstrated severely impaired left ventricular function (left ventricular ejection fraction [LVEF] 25%). Coronary angiography revealed only mild atherosclerotic disease of his coronary arteries.

In addition to optimizing medical therapy, you would recommend:

a. Holter monitoring

b. exercise stress test

c. implantation of an ICD

d. electrophysiological study

e. implantation of a pacemaker

18. A 35-year-old woman with systemic lupus erythematosus (SLE) complains of sharp left chest pain that is aggravated by breathing. She admits to having felt "under the weather" for the past week with a mild non-productive cough and rhinorrhea. She has also noted mild dyspnea with exertion. She denies

any recent injury, or other focal pains. Her lupus has been relatively quiescent and has not required treatment for several years. Physical examination demonstrates a temperature of 100.4°F (38.0°C), BP of 140/82 mmHg, and an HR of 80 bpm. Her JVP is normal, and her lungs are clear to auscultation. Cardiac examination reveals normal heart sounds and a faint, coarse murmur that is difficult to characterize. Her ECG is shown (see Figure Q–18).

The most likely diagnosis is:

a. acute myocardial infarction

b. acute pericarditis

c. mitral stenosis

d. pulmonary embolism

e. pneumonia

19. A 48-year-old obese man presents to the emergency room with dyspnea. He reports that the dyspnea began suddenly while he was sitting and watching television. He notes associated left lateral chest pain that is worse when he breaths deep. He denies fevers, chills, or cough. On examination, the

patient appears to be in moderate respiratory distress. Blood pressure is 110/70 mmHg, pulse is regular at 104 bpm, and respiratory rate is 28/min. His oxygen saturation is 93% on room air. Jugular venous pressure is 9 cm H_2O without HJR. His chest is clear, and his precordial exam is normal aside from tachycardia. His extremities are symmetric without edema or calf tenderness. Chest x-ray is normal, and ECG is without ST or T wave abnormalities. The most likely diagnosis is:

a. pneumonia
b. pneumothorax
c. pleurisy
d. pulmonary embolism
e. pericarditis

20. The most appropriate initial diagnostic study to confirm the diagnosis in question #19 is:

A. sputum culture
B. arterial blood gas
C. echocardiogram
D. lower extremity ultrasound
E. ventilation/perfusion (V/Q) scan

21. A 44-year-old man with alcoholic cardiomyopathy presents with dyspnea and increasing edema. Review of symptoms is notable for orthopnea and paroxysmal nocturnal dyspnea (PND). On exam he is in moderate respiratory distress. Blood pressure is 110/73 mmHg, pulse is 100 bpm and regular, respiratory rate is 24/min, and oxygen saturation is 93% on room air. JVP is markedly elevated and hepatojugular reflux is present. Examination of the chest reveals bibasilar rales. Precordial examination demonstrates tachycardia, a prominent S_3, and II/VI holosystolic murmur at the apex. His extremities are cool, and he has severe pedal edema. He is admitted to the coronary care unit, and right heart catheterization is performed. Initial pressures are:

right atrium: 20 mmHg
pulmonary artery: 72/36 mmHg
pulmonary capillary wedge: 33 mmHg
cardiac output: 2.2 L/min
systemic vascular resistance: 2218 dynes-sec-cm-5

In addition to oxygen and diuresis, the initial management of this patient should include:

a. enalapril and metoprolol
b. dopamine and dobutamine
c. dobutamine and sodium nitroprusside
d. digoxin and intravenous nitroglycerin
e. intra-aortic balloon pump

22. A 72-year-old man is referred for the evaluation of exertional dyspnea. History is notable for PND, orthopnea, lower extremity edema, and increasing abdominal girth. On examination, the patient appears comfortable, with blood pressure 130/80 mmHg, a heart rate of 90 bpm, a respiratory rate of 24/min, and an oxygen saturation of 94% on room air. His JVP is elevated and increases during inspiration. There are decreased breath sounds and dullness to percussion at the lung bases. Precordial examination is notable for a nondisplaced point of maximal impulse (PMI), normal S_1 and S_2 without additional heart sounds or murmurs. His abdomen is distended, and his liver is enlarged. There is severe bilateral lower extremity edema. Periorbital ecchymoses are also noted.

Laboratory studies are as follows:

K^+: 4.7; BUN: 48; creatinine: 2.6

Hematocrit 31; platelets 150,000

Chest x-ray: Normal cardiac silhouette. Bilateral pleural effusions.

ECG: Sinus rhythm at 90 bpm. Low limb lead voltage. Late transition and poor R wave progression.

Echocardiogram demonstrates thickened left and right ventricles with mildly reduced systolic function. There is no significant valvular disease. There is a small pericardial effusion noted.

The most likely diagnosis is:

a. idiopathic dilated cardiomyopathy
b. restrictive cardiomyopathy
d. constrictive pericarditis due to undiagnosed connective tissue disease
d. high output failure
e. pericardial tamponade

23. A 34-year-old woman is referred to your clinic for the evaluation of exertional dyspnea. She reports a two-month history of progressive dyspnea with an associated decline in exercise tolerance. She denies PND, orthopnea, or edema. She has no significant past medical history. She does not smoke, is unmarried, and has no children. She denies any history of recreational drug use.

On examination she appears comfortable at rest. Her weight is 190 pounds, her height is 5′3″. Her blood pressure is 130/90 mmHg, pulse is 90 bpm, respiratory rate is 20/min, and oxygen saturation is 94% on room air. JVP is 10 cm H_2O without HJR. Her lungs are clear. Precordial exam is notable for a right ventricular heave, a loud second heart sound, and a holosystolic murmur at the left lower sternal border that increases slightly with inspiration. Her extremities are without clubbing, cyanosis or edema.

Laboratory studies reveal normal electrolytes, renal function, coagulation profile, and urinalysis. She has a mild anemia. Chest x-ray reveals loss of the retrosternal air space, and prominent central vasculature with cropping of the peripheral pulmonary vessels. Her ECG demonstrates normal sinus rhythm at 90 bpm, right axis deviation and right atrial enlargement.

The most likely cause of this patient's dyspnea is:

a. coronary artery disease
b. asthma
c. pulmonary hypertension
d. anemia
e. acute pulmonary embolism

24. The patient in question #23 undergoes pulmonary artery catheterization that demonstrates a pulmonary arterial pressure of 76/45 mmHg. Echocardiogram demonstrates normal left ventricular function, but moderate right ventricular dysfunction and tricuspid regurgitation. An extensive evaluation does not reveal an obvious underlying cause, and she is diagnosed with primary pulmonary hypertension. The initial treatment of choice is:

a. angiotensin-converting enzyme inhibitor
b. vasodilating calcium channel blocker (i.e., nifedipine)
c. beta-blocker
d. epoprostenol
e. lung transplant

25. A 64-year-old man with hypertension and dyslipidemia presents to the emergency room with dyspnea. He has not had chest pain and denies abdominal pain, back pain, headache, visual changes, or paresthesias. His only medications are atenolol and simvastatin. He does not smoke and denies illicit drug use.

He appears in severe respiratory distress. His blood pressure is 230/120 mmHg in both arms; his pulse is 92 bpm and regular. Fundoscopic examination reveals changes consistent with hypertensive retinopathy. Jugular venous pressure is 12 cm H_2O. Lung examination reveals rales nearly to the apices bilaterally. Precordial examination demonstrates a prominent S_4 and a hyperdynamic apex without appreciable murmurs. Neurological examination is nonfocal.

Laboratory studies include:

BUN	25
Creatinine	1.5
Glucose	85
pH	7.44
pCO_2	35
pO_2	65

Urinalysis	
Specific gravity	1.011
pH	6.5
Protein	trace
RBC	0–2/hpf
WBC	0–2/hpf

Electrocardiogram reveals left ventricular hypertrophy with repolarization abnormalities.

The most appropriate initial management of this patient should include:

a.   oxygen, IV furosemide

b.   oxygen, IV furosemide, sublingual nitroglycerin

c.   oxygen, IV furosemide, intravenous sodium nitroprusside

d.   oxygen, IV furosemide, morphine

e.   oxygen, IV furosemide, oral metoprolol

The following options apply to questions 26–28:

a.   aortic stenosis

b.   aortic regurgitation

c.   mitral stenosis

d.   mitral regurgitation

e.   atrial septal defect

f.   patent ductus arteriosus

g.   hypertrophic obstructive cardiomyopathy

26. A 36-year-old woman from Trinidad presents with intermittent palpitations for several months. She also notes dyspnea on exertion and occasional orthopnea. Examination demonstrates a heart rate of 100 bpm and blood pressure of 110/60. Her lungs are clear but her jugular venous pressure is elevated at 8 mmHg. She has a loud second heart sound and a low-pitched diastolic murmur at the cardiac apex. An additional sound is heard shortly after S_2. What is the cause of her murmur?

27. A 75-year-old man presents for evaluation of dyspnea. He reports several years of occasional exertional chest pain and the recent onset of both exertional and rest dyspnea. He admits to a single episode of exertional syncope several weeks prior. Examination reveals a soft S_2, a III/VI, crescendo-decrescendo, systolic murmur at the upper sternal border that radiates to his carotids. What is the cause of his murmur?

28. A 40-year-old man presents for evaluation of a murmur. He has a history of hypertension for which he has been treated with diuretics. His brother died suddenly at the age of 38 years. On examination, his blood pressure is 148/90 mmHg. There is a III/VI mid-peaking systolic murmur along his left sternal border that does not radiate, but increases in inten-

sity during the strain phase of Valsalva. What is the cause of his murmur?

29. A 65-year-old man presents with fevers, chills, weight loss, and malaise. His examination demonstrates splinter hemorrhages in his nail beds and conjunctival petechiae. A III/VI HSM is heard at the cardiac apex. Echocardiography demonstrates a vegetation on his mitral valve and moderate mitral regurgitation. Blood cultures are obtained and grow *Streptococcus bovis*. He is placed on appropriate antibiotics and remains hemodynamically stable. Further evaluation at this stage should include:

a.   transesophageal echocardiogram

b.   thoracic CT scan

c.   CT scan of the head

d.   cardiac catheterization

e.   colonoscopy

30. A 35-year-old construction worker presents with several days of fevers and chills. Examination reveals a temperature of 102°F (38.8°C), heart rate of 110 bpm, and blood pressure of 120/85 mmHg. His teeth are in poor condition. His lungs are clear, and cardiac examination is unremarkable. Blood cultures are drawn and grow *Streptococcus viridans*. He is diagnosed with subacute bacterial endocarditis (SBE). Despite antibiotics, the patient continues to have persistent fever, and on the fifth hospital day he develops acute dyspnea. Physical examination is likely to reveal:

a.   a holosytolic murmur at the apex

b.   an early-peaking, crescendo-decrescendo murmur at the upper sternal border

c.   weak and delayed carotid upstrokes

d.   an apical mid-diastolic murmur with pre-systolic accentuation and opening snap

e.   a 3-component pericardial friction rub

31. A 62-year-old woman presents to the emergency room of a community hospital with 2 hours of dyspnea and diaphoresis. When specifically questioned, she also admits to mild chest heaviness and an uncomfortable feeling in her left shoulder. She has a history of hypertension, type 2 diabetes

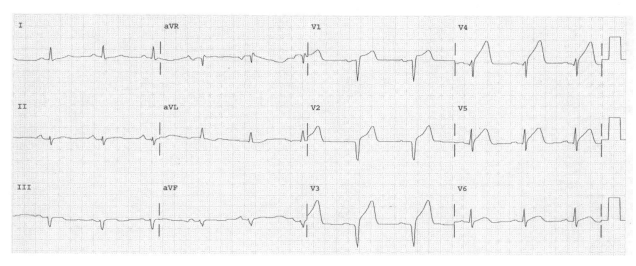

Figure Q–31

mellitus, and former tobacco use. Her medications include metformin, an ACE inhibitor, and hydrochlorothiazide.

On physical examination, her pulse rate is 96 bpm and regular, respiratory rate is 20/min, and blood pressure is 110/65 mmHg. Jugular venous pressure is not elevated. Lungs are clear to auscultation. There is an S_4, but no murmur is detected. Chest radiograph demonstrates normal cardiac and mediastinal silhouettes with clear lung fields. Her ECG is shown above (Figure Q–31). What is the most likely diagnosis?

a. pericarditis

b. acute myocardial infarction

c. unstable angina

d. left bundle branch block

e. pulmonary embolism

32. In addition to administering oxygen and chewable aspirin, initial therapy for the patient in question #31 should include:

a. beta-blockers and low-molecular-weight heparin

b. calcium-channel blockers and low-molecular-weight heparin

c. non-steroidal anti-inflammatory agents

d. nitrates and intravenous diuretics

e. dopamine and intravenous nitrates

33. After the above therapy is instituted, the patient continues to complain of chest discomfort, although the intensity is somewhat less. A repeat electrocardiogram is unchanged. Further history reveals that she suffered a mild stroke 6 months ago. What is the most appropriate next step in management?

a. Increase analgesics (morphine sulfate) until discomfort resolves.

b. Obtain a chest CT to rule out aortic dissection.

c. Administer intravenous thrombolytic therapy.

d. Arrange transfer to a tertiary care hospital for primary angioplasty.

e. Obtain ventilation-perfusion scan to rule out pulmonary embolism.

34. A 65-year-old woman is admitted to the hospital for progressive dyspnea and fatigue. She has a history of hypertension, smoking, and lung cancer and underwent a lobectomy 6 months previously. Initial evaluation demonstrated a blood pressure of 110/75 mmHg and a heart rate of 88 bpm. Her exam demonstrated decreased breath sounds at the left lower lung field and distant heart sounds. Initial laboratory evaluation was significant for:

White blood cell count:

$12.6 \times 10^3/mm^3$	(normal: 4–10)
Hematocrit: 27%	(normal: 42–52)

Initial chest x-ray demonstrated a left pleural effusion and a large cardiac silhouette.

She is treated with transfusion therapy. During her hospitalization, she develops acute hypotension with a BP of 80/50 mmHg and a heart rate of 115 bpm. She feel very light-headed but denies chest pain. Cardiac examination reveals faint heart sounds and elevated jugular venous pressure. Her lung examination is unchanged from previous.

The intervention likely to be of most benefit to this patient is:

a.   cardiac catheterization

b.   intravenous antibiotics

c.   pericardiocentesis

d.   intravenous heparin

e.   thoracentesis

35.   A 50-year-old man presents to the urgent care clinic for evaluation of substernal chest pain. Over the past 2 weeks, he has experienced similar chest discomfort that is brought on by light exertion, relieved with rest, and has increased in frequency and duration. He describes having had an episode of chest pain at rest, lasting for 40 minutes, which prompted him to seek medical care. He is currently pain free. He smokes 1 pack of cigarettes a day, and reports that his younger brother had suffered a "heart attack" at age 40. He does not know what his cholesterol status is. He is otherwise in good health but does not exercise regularly.

On examination, his pulse rate is 80/min and regular, respiratory rate is 20/min, and blood pressure is 150/95 mmHg. Pulse oximetry reveals an oxygen saturation of 98% on room air. An S_4 gallop is present, but the rest of his physical examination is unremarkable. Electrocardiogram reveals normal sinus rhythm with left ventricular hypertrophy, but without significant ST segment abnormalities.

You send him to the emergency department immediately for further evaluation. A chest radiograph shows mild cardiomegaly. His complete blood count is

normal, his creatinine is 0.9 mg/dL, his creatine kinase is 104 mg/dL with an MB index of 1.0, and his cardiac troponin is normal. What is the most likely diagnosis?

a.   acute myocardial infarction

b.   unstable angina

c.   stable angina

d.   acute pericarditis

e.   pulmonary embolism

36.   On arrival to the emergency room, he is given aspirin, low-molecular-weight heparin, and beta-blockers. Which of the following is the most appropriate next step in his management?

a.   emergent cardiac catheterization

b.   administration of thrombolytic therapy

c.   observe on telemetry and obtain further serum cardiac markers

d.   immediate exercise tolerance test with nuclear imaging for diagnosis

e.   transthoracic echocardiogram

37.   While waiting in the emergency department, he develops chest pressure radiating to his neck and associated with diaphoresis. A repeat electrocardiogram is obtained (Figure Q–37). His chest pain is relieved by two sublingual nitroglycerin tablets; however, a subsequent ECG is unchanged. Which of the following would you recommend?

a.   administration of thrombolytic therapy

b.   administration of glycoprotein IIB–IIIA inhibitor, then urgent cardiac catheterization

c.   administration of NSAIDs

d.   administration of intravenous nitroglycerin

e.   observation for 24 hours, followed by exercise tolerance test

38.   A 65-year-old man with type 2 diabetes mellitus presented with recurrent exertional chest discomfort that was felt to be consistent with angina pectoris. His medications included aspirin, atenolol, captopril, isosorbide mononitrate, glyburide, simvastatin, and an H-2 blocker. His pulse rate was 64/min and blood pressure 130/75 mmHg. A subsequent exercise tolerance test induced 3-mm of ST

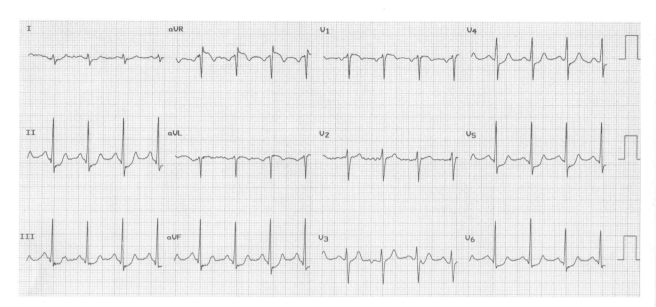

Figure Q–37

depression after 3 minutes of exercise. Cardiac catheterization is performed promptly and reveals high-grade obstruction (> 75%) of the proximal left anterior descending and right coronary arteries. Left ventricular function by echocardiography is mildly depressed with an ejection fraction of 45%. Which of the following should you recommend?

a. percutaneous transluminal coronary angioplasty (PTCA) +/– stent implantation

b. continuation of current medical therapy

c. transmyocardial laser revascularization

d. coronary artery bypass surgery (CABG)

e. intensification of current medical therapy

39. A 69-year-old woman presents to the emergency department with 3 hours of substernal chest tightness, associated with nausea and diaphoresis. Her history is significant for hypertension. Medications include diltiazem. On physical examination, her pulse rate is 100/min, and blood pressure is 120/75 mmHg. Jugular venous pressure is 10 cm H₂O. Lungs are clear to auscultation. Cardiac examination reveals a regular rhythm without murmurs or gallops. Electrocardiogram shows 2-mm ST-segment elevation in II, III, aVF with ST-segment depression in V₂. Chest radiograph is normal. Sublingual nitroglycerin is administered.

She becomes pale, clammy, and lightheaded. Repeat blood pressure is 80/60 mmHg. She is placed in the Trendelenberg position and an intravenous fluid bolus is given. Her blood pressure increases to 90/62 mmHg. What is the most likely diagnosis?

a. acute inferior myocardial infarction with RV infarct

b. aortic dissection

c. pulmonary embolism

d. cardiac tamponade

e. papillary muscle rupture with mitral regurgitation

40. How can you confirm the above diagnosis (question #39) promptly?

a. ultra-fast CT scan

b. transesophageal echocardiogram

c. transthoracic echocardiogram

d. 12-lead ECG with right-sided precordial leads

e. MRI of the chest

41. A 45-year-old woman from Haiti arrives at your clinic complaining of dyspnea and a dry cough for 2–3 months. She has been unable to walk more than

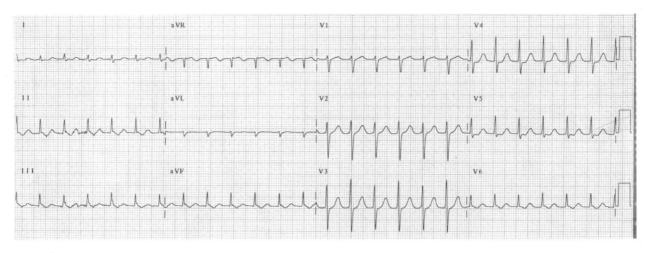

Figure Q–43

about 200 feet before developing severe shortness of breath. She denies any fevers, but has episodic night sweats. She tells you she has been in this country for about 6 weeks. Physical examination demonstrates elevated jugular venous pressure with prominent waveforms. Notably, there is an increase in the venous distention with inspiration. Her heart sounds are faint with an early diastolic third sound present. No murmur is heard. The right upper quadrant is tender, and the liver is pulsatile. ECG reveals sinus tachycardia, but is otherwise normal. Chest x-ray reveals mild scarring of the right upper lobe of the lungs and calcification of the periphery of the cardiac silhouette. PPD is positive.

The most likely cause of her dyspnea is:

a.   pericardial tamponade

b.   pulmonary tuberculosis

c.   constrictive pericarditis

d.   acute pericarditis

e.   severe mitral stenosis

42.   The best manner in which to confirm the diagnosis in the patient in question #41 would be:

a.   chest CT scan

b.   ECG

c.   echocardiogram

d.   bronchoscopy

e.   cardiac catheterization

43.   A 60-year-old woman is seen in the emergency department (ED) for acute onset of palpitations without dyspnea or chest discomfort. She has no known cardiac history. She states the palpitations began one hour prior to her arrival to the ED and recalls no inciting factor. She ad-mits to mild associated lightheadedness. Her BP is 140/80 mmHg. There is no increase in her JVP, and her lungs are clear. Cardiac examination reveals no abnormal sounds. ECG in the ED is shown in Figure Q–43.

Carotid sinus massage is attempted and has no effect. Which of the following is the next best treatment option:

a.   oral nifedipine

b.   electrical cardioversion

c.   intravenous lidocaine

d.   intravenous diltiazem

e.   intravenous enalaprilat

44.   A 37-year-old woman arrives at your clinic with a 6 month history of progressive dyspnea on exertion and fatigue. She also notes occasional irregular palpitations and recent onset of pedal edema. Her past medical history is significant for asthma and a childhood murmur. She has not seen a physician in many years. On examination, her HR is 75 bpm and irregularly irregular. BP is 135/60 mmHg. Her JVP is 10 cm H_2O. Palpation of her precordium reveals a prominent left parasternal impulse. She has a normal

S_1 and a prominent S_2. The second heart sound is persistently split, without respiratory variation. There is a 2/6 systolic ejection murmur localized to the base of her heart. Her PMI is normal. The liver is enlarged to 3 cm below her costal margin and is pulsatile. ECG reveals atrial fibrillation and an incomplete right bundle branch block.

The most likely cause of her right heart failure is:

a. primary pulmonary hypertension

b. atrial septal defect

c. ventricular septal defect

d. aortic stenosis

e. aortic coarctation

45. The most appropriate initial method to confirm your suspected diagnosis in question #44 is:

a. echocardiogram

b. exercise stress test

c. cardiac catheterization

d. chest x-ray

e. cardiac MRI

46. A 15-year-old girl is evaluated for a fever and joint pains. Three weeks ago, she had a sore throat that resolved without treatment. Four days ago, she developed pain and swelling of the right ankle and the right elbow. Two days ago, she developed pain and swelling of the left ankle. Today, the affected joints have improved, but she developed pain and swelling of the left knee. Physical examination reveals a temperature of 101°F (38.3°C) and a heart rate of 110. A soft holosystolic murmur and an S_3 are audible at the cardiac apex. The left knee is erythematous, tender, and has an effusion. Laboratory evaluation demonstrates a mildly elevated white blood cell count, an erythrocyte sedimentation rate of 60 (normal <20), and an elevated anti-streptococcal antibody. You make the clinical diagnosis of acute rheumatic fever.

In regard to this patient, which of the following statements is true?

a. Blood cultures are likely to be positive for group A streptococci.

b. Cardiac examination is also likely to disclose an opening snap and a low pitched mid-diastolic murmur at the cardiac apex.

c. Acute antibiotic treatment is not required, as the patient's sore throat has resolved.

d. She should receive benzathine penicillin every three weeks until she is 25 years old.

e. She may have residual deformity of her left knee.

47. A 58-year-old postmenopausal woman comes to your office for a routine physical examination. She does not have a history of CAD or diabetes mellitus. She smokes one pack of cigarettes per day. Family history is negative for premature CAD. Her physical examination is unremarkable. Blood pressure is 130/85 mmHg.

Laboratory data shows:

Plasma glucose (fasting)	100 mg/dL
Plasma total cholesterol	238 mg/dL
Plasma HDL cholesterol	45 mg/dL
Plasma LDL cholesterol	166 mg/dL
Serum triglycerides	135 mg/dL
Liver function tests	normal

Which of the following is most appropriate?

a. no specific therapy

b. smoking cessation and repeat lipid profile in 3 months

c. smoking cessation and therapeutic lifestyle changes (TLC) with goal LDL of <160 mg/dL

d. smoking cessation, TLC, and repeat lipid profile in 3 months, with goal LDL of <130 mg/dL

e. initiation of pharmacological therapy with goal LDL of <100 mg/dL

48. A 55-year-old man is admitted to the coronary care unit with an inferior wall myocardial infarction. He receives intravenous tissue plasminogen activator (tPA) with successful reperfusion and resolution of ST-segment elevation. On his 3rd hospital day, he develops sudden-onset shortness of breath without any chest discomfort. His current medications are

aspirin, metoprolol, captopril, and simvastatin. His pulse rate is 110/min and regular, respiratory rate is 32/min, and his blood pressure is 100/70 mmHg. Oxygen saturation is 90% on room air. Rales are present bilaterally. Cardiac examination reveals a III–IV/VI holosystolic murmur heard best at the apex with radiation to the axilla and back. An S_3 gallop is present. Electrocardiogram shows sinus tachycardia, with inferior Q waves and T wave inversions, but unchanged when compared with an earlier ECG. What is the most likely diagnosis?

a. ventricular septal rupture

b. left ventricular free wall rupture

c. papillary muscle rupture with acute mitral regurgitation

d. recurrent myocardial infarction

e. pulmonary embolism

49. Which of the following is the most appropriate course of action for the patient in question #48?

a. digoxin

b. furosemide

c. heparin

d. pericardiocentesis

e. intra-aortic balloon pump placement and emergent surgery

50. A 58-year-old post-menopausal woman with a history of chronic stable angina, hypertension, and type 2 diabetes mellitus, presents to your office for a routine visit. Her anginal symptoms have remained stable since her last visit 3 months ago. She brisk-walks for 45 minutes 3–5 times per week. She does not smoke and is compliant with her medications, which include aspirin, atenolol, lisinopril, and insulin. On examination, her pulse rate is 60/min and blood pressure is 118/75 mmHg. Fasting laboratory data is notable for an Hb_{A1C} of 7.2%, blood glucose of 150 mg/dL, total cholesterol of 200 mg/dL, HDL of 35 mg/dL, and LDL of 140 mg/dL. Which of the following would be most appropriate?

a. addition of clopidogrel

b. initiation of HMG-CoA reductase inhibitor ("statin")

c. increase atenolol

d. increase lisinopril

e. increase insulin

51. A 26-year-old woman who is in the 2nd trimester of her 1st pregnancy is referred to you because of a cardiac murmur. She is asymptomatic aside from exertional fatigue. On physical examination, her pulse rate is 85 bpm, and blood pressure is 116/64 mmHg. Jugular venous pressure is 6–7 cm H_2O. Lungs are clear. Cardiac examination reveals a hyperdynamic apex and a grade II/VI early-peaking, systolic ejection murmur heard best at the upper left sternal border. S_1 and S_2 are normal. Additional heart sounds are not heard. Mild bilateral lower extremity edema is present. ECG is essentially normal. Which of the following is most appropriate?

a. obtain a chest x-ray to evaluate the cardiac silhouette

b. start diuretic therapy

c. obtain an echocardiogram to evaluate for structural cardiac abnormalities

d. antibiotic prophylaxis for endocarditis

e. no specific cardiac therapy

f. obtain lower extremity vascular ultrasound to rule out deep vein thrombosis

52. You are seeing a 38-year-old woman who is in the 3rd trimester of her 3rd pregnancy. She has a history of mild hypertension that is treated with hydrochlorothiazide, although this has been discontinued by her obstetrician. She is currently asymptomatic. On physical examination, her pulse rate is 84/min, and her blood pressure is 140/96 mmHg on multiple readings. The rest of her examination is unremarkable other than a gravid uterus. Her serum creatinine is normal. No proteinuria is present.

In addition to recommending sodium restriction and rest, which of the following anti-hypertensive medications would you prescribe at this time?

a. atenolol

b. captopril

c. hydrochlorothiazide

d. methyldopa

e. labetalol

Answers

1. c

Recognize CAD risk equivalents according to current guidelines. Peripheral arterial disease, abdominal aortic aneurysm, symptomatic carotid artery disease, and diabetes mellitus are considered CAD risk equivalents. The goal LDL level should be <100 mg/dL in these patients. In addition to therapeutic lifestyle changes (TLC), drug therapy should be considered simultaneously in such patients. In order to achieve the LDL goal, a 30% reduction in LDL level is necessary; TLC alone is unlikely to achieve this level. HMG-CoA reductase inhibitors lower LDL levels effectively (18–55%). Fibric-acid derivatives (fibrates) lower triglycerides effectively, although LDL reduction is relatively small (5–20%).

2. d

Recognize the presentation of vasovagal syncope and know the appropriate diagnostic test. This type of syncope is common in younger patients and is frequently associated with a stressful event or prolonged standing. It is often preceded by lightheadedness, dizziness, and vasodilatation ("warm feeling"). Other causes to be considered in this patient include hypertrophic cardiomyopathy, congenital long-QT syndrome, and seizure, although the normal ECG and echo exclude the first two options and the history does not suggest seizure activity. The best test to confirm the diagnosis of vasovagal syncope is a tilt table test. In this setting it is 70–75% sensitive. Electrophysiological study (EPS) is not indicated in syncope patients without structural heart disease, because the test is neither sensitive nor specific. Head CT is usually unhelpful in the evaluation of syncope unless the patient has neurological signs or symptoms. Holter monitor is useful if bradyarrhythmias and tachyarrhythmias are suspected. This patient's history is not suggestive of carotid sinus hypersensitivity syndrome, and, thus, carotid sinus massage is not indicated.

3. d

Recognize the presentation of viral myocarditis. The typical patient with acute myocarditis is an otherwise healthy, young adult. Although the clinical presentation varies widely, symptomatic patients usually present with heart failure of recent onset. Other presenting symptoms include palpitations, chest pain, syncope, and sudden cardiac death. Patients may recall a preceding viral syndrome. Echocardiography typically demonstrates ventricular systolic dysfunction that may be either global or regional. Acute myocarditis can mimic acute myocardial infarction (chest pain, ST-T wave changes, myocardial enzyme elevation, and regional wall motion abnormalities on echocardiogram). A careful history must be obtained to distinguish between the two entities. Pericarditis usually presents with chest pain and diffuse

ST segment elevation, but does not cause heart failure. Neither pericarditis nor hypertrophic cardio-myopathy are associated with an elevation in crea-tine kinase-MB fraction (CK-MB). Pulmonary emboli rarely result in left heart failure or significant CK-MB elevation.

---

4. e

Determine the appropriate stress test modality, and rec-ognize the indications for adding an imaging modality to a stress test. In general, if a patient can exercise, an ex-ercise test should be performed. If the patient can't exercise, pharmacological stress testing is required (adenosine, dipyridamole, dobutamine). If an exercise test is performed and there are no significant ST abnormali-ties on the resting ECG, then ECG monitoring alone is usually adequate for the detection of ischemia. However, if there are abnormal ST segments on the resting ECG (e.g., left bundle branch block, left ventricular hypertro-phy with a "strain" pattern, digoxin effect, persistent ST depression, paced rhythm), the ECG is not adequate to identify ischemia and an imaging modality is necessary. The use of echocardiographic or nuclear imaging im-proves the sensitivity and specificity of the test in this setting. If pharmacological stress is performed an imaging modality is always required.

---

5. e

Recognize indications for surgical repair of abdominal aneurysms. The indications for surgical repair of abdom-inal aneurysms include: diameter >5.5 cm; rate of growth >0.5 cm in 6 months; symptoms; and thrombotic or embolic complications. Randomized trials have compared surgery to watchful waiting in patients with asympto-matic aneurysms of <5.5 cm and have not found a sur-vival benefit with early surgery. Small, asymptomatic aneurysms may be managed medically with aggressive blood pressure control and beta-blocker therapy. Beta-blockers decrease shear stress in the aorta and may decrease the rate of aneurysm expansion and risk of rupture. In patients managed medically, serial imaging is required to assess for aneurysm expansion. Patients with coexisting CAD may need to undergo coronary revas-cularization prior to aneurysm repair.

6. b

7. h

8. f

Anginal chest pain is usually a mid-sternal or left-sided discomfort that comes on with exertion and is relieved with rest. Stable angina occurs at a reproducible level of exertion. Unstable angina is that which occurs at rest, with increased frequency, or with less exertion. The pain of myocardial infarction is similar to angina but is more severe and prolonged. An aortic dissection usually causes severe, sharp, sometimes tearing pain that radiates to the back. It may be associated with pulse discrepancies owing to impairment of blood flow in branch vessels. Peri-cardial pain is usually pleuritic, positional, and may be associated with a friction rub. Pericarditis is often pre-ceded by a viral illness. Pain from a pulmonary embol-ism or pneumothorax may mimic angina but is usually pleuritic and associated with dyspnea. Chest pain from coronary spasm tends to occur at rest, with variable relationship to exertion.

---

9. a

Recognize the presentation of an acute aortic dissection. Most patients with acute aortic dissection present with the abrupt onset of severe pain that is localized to the chest or back and described as sharp, ripping, or tearing. The pain often radiates to the neck, jaw, flanks, or legs. Hypertension is the most common finding in patients with descending aortic dissections, whereas those with ascending aortic dissections frequently present with hypotension. Other physical findings may include: pulse deficits; asymmetric extremity blood pressures (>30 mm Hg); short decrescendo diastolic murmur (due to acute aortic insufficiency); left pleural effusion (hemo-thorax); paraparesis or paraplegia; neurologic deficits consistent with cerebrovascular accident; abdominal pain (mesenteric ischemia); flank pain (renal infarction); acute lower extremity ischemia; cardiac tamponade (rupture into pericardial space); and Horner's syndrome (compression of superior cervical sympathetic ganglion).

---

10. a

Know the initial medical management of a descending aortic dissection. In general, descending aortic dissections can be managed conservatively unless they are complicated by acute end-organ ischemia or aneurysm rupture, whereas ascending aortic dissections require emergent surgical therapy. Initial medical management is aimed at promptly lowering blood pressure and decreasing left ventricular contractility (dP/dT). Intravenous beta-blockers are the treatment of choice; nitroprusside may also be required. Heparin and thrombolytic therapy are absolutely contraindicated in this setting. Intravenous fluids and analgesia may be required but do not treat the underlying problem.

11. d

Diagnose and manage thromboangiitis obliterans. Thromboangiitis obliterans (TAO), also known as **Buerger's disease**, is a vasculitis of the small and medium-sized arteries and veins of the upper and lower extremities. Cerebral, visceral and coronary vessels may also be involved. Young, male smokers (<45 years of age) are most commonly affected. Patients with TAO frequently present with the triad of claudication, Raynaud's phenomenon, and migratory superficial thrombophlebitis. Physical examination typically reveals reduced or absent distal pulses, trophic nail changes, digital ulcerations, and digital gangrene. The etiology of TAO is unknown but there appears to be a definite relationship to cigarette smoking and an increased incidence of HLA-B5 and HLA-A9 antigens in patients with the disease. No specific therapy exists for TAO. Smoking cessation appears moderately effective at halting disease progression. Surgical reconstruction is of limited applicability due to the distal nature of the disease. In severe cases, amputation may be required.

12. c

Recognize the presentation and treatment of pericardial tamponade. This patient has mild hypotension, muffled heart sounds, and elevated JVP (Beck's triad). Additionally, there is marked respiratory variation in her pulse volume and systolic blood pressure (pulsus paradoxus), and findings consistent with right heart failure. These features are all characteristic of pericardial tamponade, a diagnosis that can be confirmed with an echocardiogram. Emergent pericardiocentesis is the treatment of choice.

The systolic pressure normally may fall by as much as 10 mmHg during inspiration. An exaggerated pulsus paradoxus may also be seen in constrictive pericarditis, or severe airway obstruction. Choices a, b, c, and e are the treatments for heart failure, chronic obstructive pulmonary disease (COPD) exacerbation, acute cardiac ischemia, and pneumonia, respectively.

13. c

Recognize the features of subacute bacterial endocarditis. This patient's physical examination demonstrates peripheral manifestations of endocarditis, including digital clubbing and Janeway lesions. Other lesions that may be seen include splinter hemorrhages, Roth spots, and Osler's nodes. The most common predisposing factors for SBE are structural heart diseases, including mitral valve prolapse. His mid-systolic click and apical murmur are indicative of this disorder. Although pneumonia, pericarditis, and viral syndromes may cause febrile illnesses, they are not associated with the peripheral findings noted here. Although a ventricular septal defect or patent ductus arteriosus may predispose to SBE, they are not associated with the murmur of mitral valve prolapse. SBE should always be considered in patients presenting with a fever of unknown origin.

14. c

Recognize the clinical features and risk factors for venous thromboembolic disease. The increase in this patient's edema likely results from a deep venous thrombosis. Although worsening of her heart failure must also be considered, the asymmetric nature of the edema and the clinical scenario are much more consistent with a DVT. The diagnosis can be confirmed with a bedside lower extremity ultrasound. A number of acquired conditions are associated with venous thromboembolic disease. These conditions result in stasis of blood, vascular injury, and/or hypercoagulability, and include immobilization (stroke, spinal cord injury, prolonged travel); obesity; pregnancy; advanced age; heart failure; trauma; surgery; indwelling vascular catheters; prior deep venous thrombosis; malignancy; oral contraceptives; smoking; and, nephrotic syndrome. Additionally, hereditary hypercoagulable states may contribute (e.g., Factor V Leiden mutation, activated protein C resistance, protein C deficiency, protein S deficiency, antithrombin III deficiency, hyperhomocyst(e)inemia, antiphospholipid antibody syndrome).

15. d

Recognize the signs and symptoms of severe aortic stenosis (AS). This patient experienced the common symptoms of significant aortic stenosis including syncope, angina, and dyspnea on exertion (possible congestive heart failure [CHF]). In addition, his examination is consistent with severe to critical AS with a late peaking systolic ejection murmur and **pulsus parvus et tardus**. As AS becomes more severe, the second heart sound becomes faint, and may altogether disappear. Although the other choices are possible causes of syncope in this man, this clinical presentation is classic for syncope resulting from significant AS.

16. c

Recognize the indications for permanent pacemaker implantation. This patient has symptomatic bradycardia, likely a result of a tachy-brady syndrome. She is on no medications that could induce the bradycardia, and her conduction system disease is irreversible; thus, she has a clear indication for pacemaker implantation. Holter monitoring is not indicated, as the resting ECG is diagnostic. ICDs are reserved for those with life-threatening ventricular tachyarrhythmias. Simple reassurance without further therapy is inappropriate, as the patient is at risk for progressive bradycardia and syncope without pacemaker therapy.

17. c

Understand the treatment of patients who have survived a cardiac arrest. One of the approved indications for ICDs is for the treatment of survivors of sudden cardiac death. Other indications include for the management of patients with a history of myocardial infarction, depressed LV function, and non-sustained VT, who are inducible to sustained VT during EP study. Holter monitoring and EP study in sudden cardiac death survivors is unnecessary, as the possibility of recurrent cardiac arrest

is sufficiently high to warrant empiric implantation of an ICD. Exercise stress testing will likely be unhelpful, because angiography did not reveal significant coronary artery stenoses. The patient has no conduction disease described that would necessitate implantation of a pacemaker.

18. b

Recognize the symptoms and signs of pericarditis. Pericarditis classically causes sharp, **pleuritic** chest pain, and may be associated with a sensation of dyspnea. The presence of a pericardial friction rub is pathognomonic for pericarditis. This rub is often confused with a murmur, but is difficult to characterize because it occurs in both systole and diastole and may have one to three components. The ECG demonstrates the classic findings of PR segment depression and diffuse ST segment elevation. In this particular case, the pericarditis may be related to her SLE, or may be post-viral in etiology. Although an acute myocardial infarction may be associated with pericardial irritation, the clinical history and ECG are much more consistent with pericarditis. Mitral stenosis frequently causes exertional chest pain and dyspnea, but it is not pleuritic. Pneumonia can cause pleuritic chest pain, but is not associated with a pericardial friction rub or ECG changes. A pulmonary embolism is a distinct possibility; however, the ECG abnormality is essentially diagnostic of pericarditis.

19. d

Diagnose pulmonary embolism (PE). The most common presenting symptom of PE is sudden dyspnea, which occurs in approximately 80% of patients. Additional symptoms include pleuritic chest pain, cough, hemoptysis, and syncope. Physical examination of patients with PE may be normal but often demonstrates signs of pulmonary hypertension or right heart failure including tachypnea, tachycardia, elevated JVP, tricuspid regurgitation murmur, accentuated pulmonic component of S_2 (P_2), and a right ventricular heave. A pulmonary rub may be heard over the involved area of lung when pulmonary infarction has occurred. The normal chest x-ray essentially excludes pneumonia or pneumothorax as the cause, and the absence of ECG changes makes pericarditis very unlikely. Pleurisy is a frequent cause of pleuritic chest pain but is not associated with acute short-ness of breath or signs of right heart failure.

20. e

Recognize the appropriate test to confirm the diagnosis of PE. Ventilation/perfusion (V/Q) lung scan remains the most frequently employed diagnostic test for PE. Although V/Q scans may yield inconclusive results, normal and near-normal tests virtually exclude the diagnosis of PE, while a high-probability test confirms the diagnosis. Arterial blood gas analysis in a patient with a PE typically demonstrates respiratory alkalosis, hypocapnea, and hypoxemia, but is of low specificity. Echocardiography is an insensitive means of diagnosing PE; however, it provides a rapid assessment of right ventricular function in patients with an established diagnosis of PE. Venous ultrasonography for the detection of deep venous thrombosis (DVT) may be helpful in patients with intermediate clinical probability and indeterminant V/Q scan results, or clinical signs suggestive of DVT. Although venous ultrasonography has high sensitivity (90–100%) and specificity (90–100%) for the detection of DVT, a negative result does not exclude the diagnosis of PE; up to 50% of patients with PE may have no sonographic evidence of DVT.

21. c

Understand the management of decompensated heart failure based on hemodynamic measurements. This patient is volume-overloaded with high left and right heart filling pressure, low cardiac output, and high systemic vascular resistance (SVR), but has an adequate systemic blood pressure. He clearly requires diuresis; however, his markedly reduced cardiac output and elevated SVR are the predominant hemodynamic abnormalities. He requires inotropic support (dobutamine) as well as afterload reduction (nitroprusside). Although beta-blockers have favorable effects on chronic heart failure, they are contraindicated in decompensated heart failure. This patient's blood pressure is adequate, and, therefore, he does not need a vasopressor (dopamine). Digoxin is a very weak inotrope and is unlikely to be of any value in acute heart failure. An intra-aortic balloon pump would likely improve this patient significantly; however, it should be considered only after aggressive medical therapy has failed.

22. b

Recognize restrictive cardiomyopathy. The clinical presentation of restrictive cardiomyopathy is similar to that of severe constrictive pericarditis with exertional dyspnea and signs of biventricular heart failure. Additional symptoms may include orthopnea, paroxysmal nocturnal dyspnea, anorexia, and fatigue. Physical examination frequently reveals signs of right and left venous congestion. Kussmaul's sign (a paradoxical rise in JVP with inspiration) may be present. Echocardiography typically reveals thickened ventricles with relatively preserved systolic function. With idiopathic dilated cardiomyopathy, the heart is dilated and the systolic function is usually moderately to severely depressed. With constrictive pericarditis, the left ventricle is usually small, non-thickened, and hyperdynamic. Pericardial tamponade is rarely the result of a small pericardial effusion and is not associated with Kussmaul's sign. High-output failure is usually associated with hyperdynamic ventricular function and is not associated with biventricular thickening.

23. c

Recognize the features of pulmonary hypertension. This patient's physical findings of an RV heave, loud second heart sound, tricuspid regurgitant murmur, and elevated JVP, all suggest elevated pulmonary arterial and right heart pressures. The chest x-ray demonstrates right ventricular enlargement and pulmonary vascular changes consistent with pulmonary hypertension. Coronary artery disease would be distinctly unusual in a 34-year-old woman, especially in the absence of risk factors, chest pain, or ECG abnormalities. Right heart failure from asthma would be unlikely in the absence of a long history of severe bronchospastic disease. Anemia may cause dyspnea but does not produce the physical findings of pulmonary hypertension and right heart failure. Chronic pulmonary emboli may result in pulmonary hypertension and the findings noted in this patient. An acute pulmonary embolism would be unlikely given the several month history of dyspnea.

24. b

Understand the treatment of primary pulmonary hypertension (PPH). PPH is an incurable disease with a relatively poor prognosis. Vasodilators are the mainstay of treatment, although not all patients exhibit a significant treatment response. The oral vasodilators of choice include nifedipine and diltiazem in doses of 120–240 mg/day and 540–900 mg/day, respectively. In patients who have an inadequate response to these agents, a continuous infusion of epoprostenol, a vasodilating prostaglandin, may be beneficial. Epoprostanol acts by increasing intracellular levels of cyclic AMP, and produces both acute and sustained hemodynamic improvement, symptomatic improvement, and prolonged survival in patients with PPH. It may be used either as primary treatment or as a bridge to lung transplant. Single lung and combined heart-lung transplantation remains the only definitive therapy for PPH, and is used for patients who fail vasodilator therapy. One-year survival following lung transplantation approaches 65–70%. Beta-blockers and angiotensin-converting enzyme inhibitors do not have a role in the treatment of PPH.

25. c

Recognize and manage hypertensive emergency. This patient has marked hypertension with concomitant symptoms/target organ damage (acute pulmonary edema) and requires immediate blood pressure reduction. Although oxygen and diuresis are clearly necessary, they are not adequate, and intravenous antihypertensive agents such as sodium nitroprusside, nitroglycerin, or enalaprilat, should be administered expeditiously. The initial goal should be a 25% reduction in mean arterial pressure within the first two hours. Further reduction in blood pressure should proceed more slowly as rapid reductions in blood pressure can lead to end organ hypoperfusion. Sublingual nitroglycerin is not an effective method of controlling blood pressure and most oral agents are not absorbed fast enough to produce the desired effect in a short period of time. Beta-blockers should be used with caution in patients with decompensated heart failure.

26. c

27. a

28. g

The 36-year-old woman has the classic findings of mitral

stenosis with a loud P_2 (from pulmonary hypertension), an opening snap in early diastole, and a diastolic rumble. Tachycardia and dyspnea are commonly seen with MS and her palpitations likely reflect paroxysmal atrial fibrillation. The 75-year-old man has severe aortic stenosis as evidenced by the late-peaking systolic murmur that radiates to the carotids, and the soft S_2. Diminished carotid upstrokes might also have been present. His symptoms of chest pain, dyspnea, and syncope are the cardinal symptoms of AS. The 40-year-old man has hypertrophic cardiomyopathy. This murmur may mimic AS but does not radiate to the carotids and/or result in diminished carotid upstrokes. Additionally, the murmur of hypertrophic cardiomyopathy (HCM) is the only murmur that increases with Valsalva. The murmur of aortic insufficiency (AI) is a decrescendo diastolic murmur at the left sternal border. Mitral regurgitation produces a holosystolic murmur at the cardiac apex that radiates to the axilla. An ASD results in a systolic flow murmur at the upper sternal border (owing to increased flow across the pulmonary valve) and a fixed split S_2. A patent ductus arteriosus produces a continuous (systolic and diastolic) "machine-like" murmur at the left upper sternal border that radiates to the back.

29. e

Know the appropriate tests for the evaluation of endocarditis and recognize the significance of specific causative organisms. Patients with S. bovis endocarditis frequently have colonic neoplasms and should be screened with colonoscopy. CT of the chest may be useful to evaluate for lung abscess in a patient with right-sided SBE and abnormal chest x-ray, but is unlikely to be of value in this patient. Although SBE may be associated with cerebral abscesses and intracranial aneurysms, routine scans are not indicated in the absence of CNS symptoms. Cardiac catheterization would be indicated only in the event of a complication requiring cardiac surgery (i.e., progressive valvular disease).

30. a

The course of events suggests that antibiotics have failed to eradicate the infection and progressive valvular dysfunction has occurred that resulted in heart failure. Acute valvular dysfunction is almost always regurgitant.

The only answer that is consistent with a regurgitant lesion is the apical holosystolic murmur of MR. The crescendo-decrescendo murmur is indicative of a flow murmur. The weak and delayed carotids are indicative of aortic stenosis. A mid-diastolic murmur and an opening snap are features of mitral stenosis, while the 3-component rub indicates pericarditis.

---

31. b

Recognize the ECG of a patient with an acute ST elevation MI. This ECG demonstrates 2–3 mm of ST segment elevation in leads V_1–V_5. This is consistent with an acute infarction of the anterior wall of the left ventricle. This most likely resulted from an acute thrombotic occlusion of the left anterior descending coronary artery. The presence of Q waves in V_1–V_3 suggests that the infarct has been evolving for more than a few hours. Although pericarditis is also associated with chest pain and ST elevation on ECG, the ST elevation is usually diffuse and is concave upward in morphology. Additionally, PR segment depression is frequently seen with pericarditis but is not present on this ECG. Unstable angina is associated with ST segment depression on ECG, not ST segment elevation. A left bundle branch block can produce ST segment elevation in the anterior precordial leads; however, it is always associated with a wide QRS complex (not present here). Pulmonary emboli can be associated with a variety of ECG changes, most commonly tachycardia and signs of right heart strain (right bundle branch block, T wave inversions in the inferior and anterior leads, S1Q3T3 pattern), but rarely cause regional ST elevation.

---

32. a

Know the acute pharmacological management of an acute myocardial infarction. Immediate therapy should include aspirin and supplemental oxygen. Morphine sulfate can help reduce the sympathetic outflow during an acute MI and is the analgesic of choice. Beta-blockers should be given to reduce the heart rate, providing the BP is >90 mmHg and the patient is not in heart failure. The reduction in HR reduces myocardial oxygen demand, and may limit ischemia/infarction. Anticoagulation with either unfractionated heparin or low-molecular-weight heparin should be initiated as soon as possible if there are no contraindications. Calcium channel blockers are not routinely indicated in the setting of an AMI although they may be useful for heart rate control for patients who have contraindications to beta-blockers (e.g., severe bronchospasm or beta-blocker allergy). Nitrates would be reasonable for symptom control in this patient; however, diuretics are not indicated given the lack of congestion and the relatively low blood pressure. NSAIDs are the treatment of choice for pericarditis but are contraindicated in an AMI.

---

33. d

Recognize the different reperfusion strategies for acute MI. Reperfusion therapy is indicated for acute ST-elevation MI (STEMI) presenting within 6 hours of onset of symptoms. Thrombolytic therapy and primary angioplasty are considered equivalent strategies in STEMI, provided that angioplasty can be done in a timely manner (<90 minutes after presentation). Primary angioplasty is associated with a lower incidence of intracranial hemorrhage as well as a trend toward a lower mortality. Unfortunately, it is not readily available in many community hospitals. Thrombolytic therapy would usually be the preferred strategy in this setting; however, it is contraindicated in this patient because of her recent CVA. Thus, immediate transfer to a facility that has angioplasty capability is indicated. Although aortic dissections and pulmonary emboli may result in chest pain, the history is more consistent with myocardial ischemia and the ECG findings are diagnostic of an acute STEMI. Further diagnostic testing to exclude aortic dissection or pulmonary embolism would only delay the time to myocardial reperfusion. Liberal use of analgesia is an important adjunctive therapy for acute MI; however, the primary goal is to salvage the ischemic myocardium by reestablishing blood flow to the occluded coronary artery.

---

34. c

Recognize the features and treatment of cardiac tamponade. This patient exhibits the classic signs of cardiac tamponade including hypotension, elevated JVP, and faint heart sounds (Beck's triad). She would also likely have exaggerated respiratory variation of her systolic blood pressure (**pulsus paradoxus**). Patients with tamponade may rapidly deteriorate unless an emergent pericardiocentesis is performed. Cardiac tamponade may be confirmed with echocardiography; however, it is a clinical diagnosis that requires emergent therapy. Although she has a small pleural effusion, it is not the cause of her deterioration, and, thus, thoracentesis would not be helpful. Cardiac catheterization is not indicated in this setting. It is noteworthy that the cause of tamponade in this woman is likely recurrent lung cancer. The most common tumors that metastasize to the pericardium are lung, breast, lymphoma, and melanoma.

35. b

Recognize the difference between an acute coronary syndrome and chronic stable angina. This patient presents with classic crescendo exertional angina of recent onset, followed by a prolonged episode of rest angina (>20 minutes). The accelerating nature of his anginal pattern as well as rest angina are characteristic of **unstable angina**. His electrocardiogram does not demonstrate ST segment abnormalities, and, therefore, is not consistent with an ST-elevation MI or pericarditis. Although he had a relatively prolonged episode of rest angina, and may subsequently "rule-in" for a non-ST-elevation MI by serial assessment of cardiac markers (CK-MB or troponin), the ECG itself does not suggest an acute MI. The presentation of an acute pulmonary embolism is usually that of sudden, sharp, pleuritic, chest pain that is associated with dyspnea.

36. c

Know the appropriate management of unstable angina. Aspirin, beta-blockers, and anticoagulation with heparin or low-molecular-weight heparin are all indicated and recommended in the initial management of unstable angina. Patients with unstable angina, especially those having had a prolonged episode, require admission to the hospital for telemetry monitoring and for serial measurement of CK-MB and troponin levels. Patients who subsequently develop elevated cardiac enzymes are at a higher risk of recurrent events and have a worse long-term prognosis. Non-emergent cardiac catheterization is often performed in this setting. Emergent cardiac catheterization in unstable angina is only indicated when angina is refractory to medical therapy or when hemo-dynamic instability is present. Thrombolysis is not indicated for the treatment of unstable angina or non-ST

elevation MI; in this setting, it is associated with an increased mortality. Exercise stress testing is contraindicated in patients with **active** unstable angina, but may be performed once the patient is stabilized. Transthoracic echocardiogram can identify regional wall motion abnormalities if active ischemia or prior MI is present, but does not add significant diagnostic information in this case as the patient is currently pain-free.

37. b

Recognize the high-risk features of unstable angina, and how the presence of these features alters the management. The ECG demonstrates 1–2 mm of ST segment depression in leads V_4–V_6, II, III, and aVF. This patient's prolonged rest angina, and persistent ST-segment depression after resolution of his chest pain place him in a higher risk category. Other high-risk features include congestive heart failure, hemodynamic instability, and positive CK-MB or troponin. Patients with high-risk features should receive GpIIB-IIIA inhibitors and proceed to urgent cardiac catheterization, while intermediate- to low-risk patients may undergo further risk stratification with stress testing to determine their need for catheterization and revascularization. Intravenous nitroglycerin may be effective in preventing further ischemic episodes, but it is not a definitive treatment. NSAIDs or thrombolytic therapy are not indicated for the treatment of unstable angina.

38. d

Recognize the indications for coronary artery bypass grafting (CABG) in patients with coronary artery disease. This patient's angina was easily provoked on stress testing despite multiple anti-ischemic medications, suggesting that his current medical regimen is inadequate for the control of his ischemia. Additionally, his heart rate and blood pressure at rest are well controlled and unlikely to allow further up-titration of his medications without inducing bradycardia or hypotension. He has, thus, failed medical management and will require revascularization. Both percutaneous and surgical revascularization are effective in the treatment of CAD. However, patients with left main CAD, triple-vessel CAD, and double-vessel CAD with high grade stenosis of the left anterior descending coronary artery stenosis experience long-term mortality benefit from CABG when compared with multivessel PTCA or medical therapy. This is especially true for diabetic patients and patients who have depressed left ventricular systolic function. Transmyocardial laser revascularization (TMR) is only reserved for patients with refractory angina who are not CABG candidates (usually due to poor target vessels).

39. a

40. d

Know the presentation of RV infarction. RV infarction is most commonly associated with inferior wall MI. This patient presents with an acute inferior wall MI and signs of RV infarction, including hypotension (commonly after nitroglycerin administration owing to RV preload reduction), and elevated JVP with clear lungs. RV infarction should be suspected and excluded in all patients with acute inferior wall MI. A 12-lead ECG with right-sided precordial leads should be performed. ST-elevation of >0.5 mm in V_{4R} is diagnostic of RV infarction. Pulmonary embolism can present similarly with chest pain, hypotension, and elevated JVP; however, ECG would not demonstrate ST-elevation characteristic of acute MI. Aortic dissection characteristically presents with sharp chest pain radiating to the back. Cardiac tamponade may complicate the course of an acute MI when free wall rupture is present, although its presentation tends to be more dramatic. If an ECG with right-sided precordial leads is not diagnostic and tamponade remains high on the differential diagnosis, a quick bedside echocardiogram can be performed. Papillary muscle rupture complicating acute MI usually presents with dyspnea, pulmonary edema, and a loud holosystolic mitral regurgitation murmur.

41. c

Recognize the symptoms and signs of constrictive pericarditis. Constrictive pericarditis results from thickening of the pericardium and inability of the ventricles to completely expand in diastole. Thus, cardiac output is reduced and right heart pressures are significantly elevated. The paradoxical rise in JVP with inspiration is known as **Kussmaul's sign** and is commonly seen in patients with constrictive pericarditis. The "prominent" venous

pulsations are to the result of rapid x- and y-descents that are characteristic of this disease. Right heart failure and hepatic congestion are common findings in these patients. Tuberculosis is a common cause of this syndrome and is the likely cause in this patient. The clinical presentation is not that of acute pericarditis, and, although some of the features could also be seen with pericardial tamponade, the pericardial calcification makes constrictive disease much more likely. Although a pericardial knock may be confused with an opening snap, the absence of a diastolic rumble makes MS unlikely.

42. e

Identify the test of choice by which to diagnose constrictive pericarditis. Cardiac catheterization allows for direct measurement of the ventricular pressures, and, in the presence of constrictive pericarditis, will demonstrate **equalization** of the LV and RV diastolic pressures with a dip-and-plateau pattern. Chest CT scan may be the best study by which to visualize the thickened pericardium, but this finding alone is not diagnostic of constrictive pericarditis without the hemodynamic confirmation. Echocardiography may demonstrate some typical findings associated with constriction, but it is also not diagnostic. Bronchoscopy may reveal tuberculosis but it does not prove the patient has constrictive physiology.

43. d

Identify AVNRT on ECG and recognize the treatment options. Her ECG demonstrates AVNRT. This is an SVT (narrow complex tachycardia) caused by a microreentrant circuit within the AV node. The atria and ventricles are often simultaneously activated and P-waves are not usually obvious on the ECG (retrograde P waves are seen after the QRS complex in lead II and aVF on this patient's ECG). However, a "pseudo-R" may be noted in lead V1 that is actually a P-wave superimposed on the terminal portion of the QRS complex. The tachycardia is dependent on the AV node for its perpetuation; therefore, any therapy that slows or blocks AV nodal conduction (e.g., calcium channel blockers, beta-blockers, adenosine, carotid sinus massage) may terminate or reduce the rate of this tachycardia. Of the listed medications, only diltiazem has effects on the AV node.

Although synchronized electrical cardioversion is very effective at terminating this arrhythmia, it is generally reserved for hemodynamically unstable patients or patients that fail pharmacological therapy.

44. b

Recognize the signs and symptoms of an ASD. Atrial septal defects are common congenital abnormalities in adults. In childhood, the only manifestation may be a murmur. If the ASD is large and left uncorrected, it can result in progressive right heart enlargement, pulmonary hypertension, and eventually right heart failure. As the right heart pressures rise, right-to-left shunting of deoxygenated blood may occur and cyanosis may develop (Eisenmenger's syndrome). The physical findings of a systolic ejection murmur and fixed split S_2 are characteristic of an ASD, especially in the presence of an incomplete right bundle branch block on ECG. The right ventricular heave (prominent left parasternal impulse) and loud P_2 suggest associated pulmonary hypertension, and the elevated JVP and hepatomegaly suggest that this patient also has right heart failure. Although a VSD may produce a fixed split S_2, the associated murmur is usually louder, holosystolic, and may have an associated thrill, whereas the murmur of an aortic coarctation is usually localized to the interscapular region, may be both systolic and diastolic, and is not associated with a split S_2 or right heart failure. Primary pulmonary hypertension may result in right heart failure, but is not associated with a fixed split S_2.

45. a

Identify the most appropriate initial test to confirm the presence of an ASD. Echocardiogram is an excellent method to detect an ASD. It is easily performed and non-invasive, and can quantify the severity of the interatrial shunt. Cardiac MRI can also identify an ASD, but is costly and less easily accessible. Chest x-ray and ECG may be suggestive, but are not diagnostic. Cardiac catheterization is useful to assess the severity of the shunt after initial diagnosis, and to assess concomitant CAD if surgical correction is anticipated. Exercise stress testing is not helpful for the diagnosis of an ASD.

46. d

The patient has two of the major criteria for rheumatic fever—migratory polyarthritis and evidence of carditis—and has evidence of a recent streptococcal infection. Other major criteria include chorea, erythema marginatum, and subcutaneous nodules. Rheumatic fever follows streptococcal pharyngitis by several weeks, so blood cultures are unlikely to be positive. However, a course of penicillin should be administered to all patients with rheumatic fever to eradicate all residual infection. The risk of recurrent rheumatic fever is high in these patients and they should receive prophylaxis against streptococcal pharyngitis for at least 15 years. A mitral mid-diastolic murmur and an opening snap are features of mitral stenosis, which develops years to decades after rheumatic fever. The polyarthritis of rheumatic fever is non-erosive, and is not associated with long-term deformity.

47. d

Recognize the major risk factors for CAD, goal LDL levels, and need for therapeutic lifestyles changes (TLC) as well as drug therapy. According to the Adult Treatment Panel (ATP) III guidelines for cholesterol management, this patient has 2 major risk factors, namely cigarette smoking and age ≥55 years. The LDL goal for this patient is <130 mg/dL. Initial recommendations should include smoking cessation and TLC (including the TLC diet, weight management, and increased physical activity). If the goal LDL can not be achieved with these interventions after 3 months, drug therapy should then be considered.

48. c

49. e

Recognize the presentation and management of papillary muscle rupture complicating an acute MI. Papillary muscle rupture in acute MI is rare, but classically occurs 3–5 days after the initial infarction (earlier following thrombolysis). Its presentation is usually very dramatic, with the development of acute pulmonary edema resulting from acute severe mitral regurgitation. The holosystolic murmur at the LV apex is characteristic of MR. It

but can sometimes be difficult to distinguish this murmur from that of a ventricular septal defect, although the latter is usually more central and not associated with pulmonary edema. Ventricular free wall rupture is usually heralded by cardiac tamponade or sudden cardiac death, and is not associated with a new murmur or pulmonary edema. The diagnosis can easily be confirmed by echocardiography. Treatment of papillary muscle rupture is surgical; IABP placement preceding surgery is usually necessary to maintain hemodynamic stability.

50. b

Know the importance of risk factor modification in secondary prevention of CAD. This is a patient with multiple cardiac risk factors including diabetes mellitus (DM), hypertension, and hypercholesterolemia, all of which are modifiable. Patients with known CAD or DM should have a target LDL of <100 mg/dL. HMG-CoA reductase inhibitors are considered 1st line therapy for LDL reduction in these patients. Tighter blood glucose control can also be achieved in this patient, although its cardiovascular benefit is not as well established as that of statins. Her blood pressure is well controlled and there is no need for any adjustment of her anti-hypertensive regimen at this point. Clopidogrel is a platelet inhibitor similar to aspirin, but with a different mechanism of action. It is equivalent to aspirin in reducing mortality in CAD. However, it is unclear if it offers any additional benefit when it is added to aspirin in patients with **stable** CAD (recent data suggests that addition of clopidogrel to aspirin in unstable angina and NSTEMI reduces reinfarction rate and mortality).

51. e

Recognize the cardiovascular findings of normal pregnancy. Normal pregnancy leads to an increase in plasma volume and cardiac output, and may result in elevated JVP, a hyperdynamic apical impulse, and systolic murmurs. These benign murmurs are early peaking and non-radiating, and are associated with normal heart sounds. A cervical venous hum and a continuous murmur over the breasts (mammary souffle) may also be present. The expanded blood volume is normal and does not require diuretic therapy. Chest x-ray is relatively contraindicated in pregnancy. Echocardiography is safe, but not necessary in this setting. Because these murmurs are related to increased flow and not due to abnormal valves, there is no need for antibiotic prophylaxis.

52. d

Know the indications for pharmacological therapy and its safety in pregnant hypertensive patients. This patient meets the indication for anti-hypertensive drug therapy with repeatedly elevated BP measurements. She is not pre-eclamptic or eclamptic. Methyldopa has the best-established safety record in pregnancy, and is recommended as 1st-line therapy. Hydralazine may also be used. Beta-blockers may lead to fetal growth retardation. ACE-inhibitors are associated with fetal death and renal failure in newborns and are contraindicated in pregnancy. There have also been reports of neonatal bradycardia, hyponatremia, and thrombocytopenia associated with maternal hydrochlorothiazide use.

Index

Left ventricular end diastolic volume, 84
Left ventricular failure, 200
Left ventricular hypertrophy, 28, 29
Left ventricular systolic dysfunction, 7
Left ventricular tumors, 224
Leriche's syndrome, 180
Leukocytosis, 152
Levine's sign, 3
LHC. *See* Left heart catheterization, 37–39
Lidocaine, 116
Lifestyle modification, hypertension and, 177
Lightheadedness, 117
Limb ischemia, 151
Lipid-laden plaque, 55, 56
Lipid-lowering agents, 61
Lipid metabolism, 57
Lipid profile, 59, 61, 177
Lipomas, 224, 225
Lipoprotein (a), 57, 58
Lipoprotein metabolism, 57, 58
Lipoproteins, 58
Lisinopril, 178
Liver disease, 118
Liver function tests, 61, 201
LMWH. *See* Low-molecular weight heparin
Lone atrial fibrillation, 114
Long QT syndrome, 128, 129
Loop monitors, 41
Losartan, 178
Low-density lipoproteins, 55, 57, 58, 64
Low-molecular weight heparin, 70, 72, 198
Low-output heart failure, 88
Lung cancer, 164, 224
Lung disease, 201
Lungs, 17
Lung transplant, 202, 211
LVEDP. *See* Left ventricular end-diastolic pressure
Lyme disease, 97, 98
Lymphadenopathy, 98, 138
Lymphedema, 197
Lymphoma, 164, 224, 225

Macrophages, 55
Magnesium, 79, 116
Magnetic resonance angiography, 181, 186, 189, 193, 198

Magnetic resonance imaging, 5, 6, 48–49, 144, 189
Malaise, 151
Male gender
    aortic aneurysms and, 184
    coronary artery disease and, 64
    hypertension and, 175
    peripheral arterial disease and, 180
Mammary souffle, 217
Marfan's syndrome, 4, 143, 148, 186, 188
MAT. *See* Multifocal atrial tachycardia
Mechanical prosthetic valves, 157
Media, 54
Medications, as cause of palpitations, 10, 11
Medtronic-Hall valve, 157
Melanoma, 164, 224
Mesotheliomas, 224, 225
Metabolic abnormalities, 11, 91, 111
Metabolic equivalents, 29
Metabolic stress test, 8
Metastatic tumors, 224
Methacholine challenge, 8
Methyldopa, 219
Metoprolol, 94, 178, 191, 219
METs. *See* Metabolic equivalents
MI. *See* Myocardial infarction
Migratory superficial thrombophlebitis, 183
Milrinone, 94
Minoxidil, 178
Mitral annular calcification, 148
Mitral regurgitation, 147–149
    as cause of heart failure, 88
    hypertrophic cardiomyopathy and, 101
    murmurs and, 16
    pulmonary hypertension and, 200
    rheumatic fever and, 138
Mitral stenosis, 15, 16, 122, 145–147, 200
Mitral valve, 150
Mitral valve disease, 138, 200
Mitral valve disorders, 145–149
Mitral valve prolapse, 15, 16, 147, 148, 150
Mitral valvotomy, 147
Mobitz I (Wenckebach) heart block, 119
Mobitz II heart block, 119
Modified Duckett Jones criteria, 139

Morphine, 69–70
MPVs. *See* Mechanical prosthetic valves
MRA. *See* Magnetic resonance angiography
MRI. *See* Magnetic resonance imaging
MUGA. *See* Multiple gated blood pool imaging
Muller's sign, 144
Multifocal atrial tachycardia, 13, 112, 113
Multiple gated blood pool imaging, 44–46
Mural thrombi, 77
Murmurs, 14–17
    aortic insufficiency and, 143
    aortic stenosis and, 142
    Austin-Flint, 144
    cardiac tumors and, 225
    Carey-Coombs, 138
    classification of, 16
    holosystolic, 148
    infective endocarditis and, 151–152
    intensity of, 14–15
    palpitations and, 10
    pregnancy and, 217–218
    systolic, 17
Musculoskeletal pain, 4, 5
MVO. *See* Myocardial oxygen demand
MVP. *See* Mitral valve prolapse
Myalgias, 151
Myocardial contusion, 221, 222
Myocardial infarction
    angina and, 63
    aortic dissection and, 188
    cardiac tamponade and, 166
    chest pain and, 3–4, 5
    coronary artery disease and, 53
    infective endocarditis and, 151
    non-ST elevation myocardial infarction, 67–70
    pulmonary embolism and, 197
    ST-elevation myocardial infarction, 71–74
    ST segment in, 25
    stress testing and risk of, 26
    tachyarrhythmias and, 111
    unstable angina and, 69
    ventricular tachycardia and, 115
Myocardial infarction complications, 75–80